THEORY, PRACTICE,

and

TRENDS

in

HUMAN SERVICES: AN INTRODUCTION

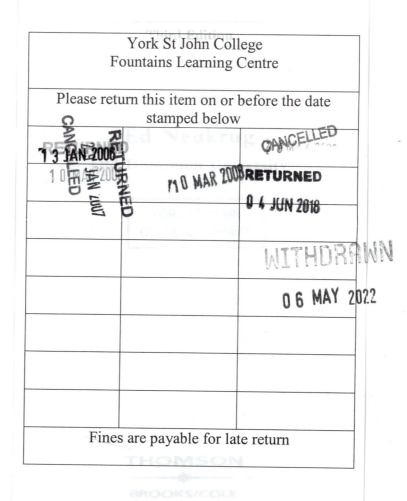
Australia • Canada • Mexico • Singapore • Spain

THOMSON

BROOKS/COLE

THOMSON

™

BROOKS/COLE

Executive Editor: *Lisa Gebo*
Acquisitions Editor: *Julie Martinez*
Assistant Editor: *Shelley Gesicki*
Editorial Assistant: *Amy Lam*
Technology Project Manager: *Barry Connolly*
Marketing Manager: *Caroline Concilla*
Marketing Assistant: *Mary Ho*
Advertising Project Manager: *Tami Strang*
Project Manager, Editorial Production:
  Stephanie Zunich

Print/Media Buyer: *Jessica Reed*
Permissions Editor: *Bob Kauser*
Production Service: *Buuji, Inc.*
Photo Researcher: *Terry Wright*
Copy Editor: *Robin Gold*
Cover Designer: *Lisa Henry*
Cover Image: *José Ortega*
Compositor: *Buuji, Inc.*
Printer: *Webcom, Limited*

For more information about our products,
contact us at:
Thomson Learning Academic Resource Center
1-800-423-0563

For permission to use material from this text,
contact us by:
Phone: 1-800-730-2214 **Fax:** 1-800-730-2215
Web: http://www.thomsonrights.com

Library of Congress Control Number:
2002117212

ISBN 0-534-53384-1

Brooks/Cole—Thomson Learning
511 Forest Lodge Road
Pacific Grove, CA 93950
USA

Asia
Thomson Learning
5 Shenton Way #01-01
UIC Building
Singapore 068808

Australia/New Zealand
Thomson Learning
102 Dodds Street
Southbank, Victoria 3006
Australia

Canada
Nelson
1120 Birchmount Road
Toronto, Ontario M1K 5G4
Canada

Europe/Middle East/Africa
Thomson Learning
High Holborn House
50/51 Bedford Row
London WC1R 4LR
United Kingdom

Latin America
Thomson Learning
Seneca, 53
Colonia Polanco
11560 Mexico D.F.
Mexico

Spain
Paraninfo
Calle/Magallanes, 25
28015 Madrid, Spain

Dedicated to all of the hard-working
human service professionals of the world

Contents

Preface

Welcome to the third edition of *Theory, Practice, and Trends in Human Services: An Introduction*. Although I maintained the core subject matter and the general theme of the text, I made a number of changes in this edition that I believe make it stronger. For example, in this edition, I replaced the term *human service worker* with *human service professional*, which better reflects the professional knowledge and training of this mental health professional. In addition, I updated the text by revising and expanding the ethical vignettes at the end of each chapter, updating information when appropriate, and updating references throughout the text. I also made a number of specific changes in each chapter, to the appendixes, and to the glossary.

In Chapter 1, "Defining the Human Service Professional," I updated information on the various mental health professionals and on the roles and functions of the human service professional. In addition, after reviewing the research on the characteristics of the effective human service professional, I revised some of the qualities and now include the following: being empathic, open-minded, accepting, cognitively complex, psychologically adjusted, genuine, a relationship builder, and competent. I believe these characteristics better match the current information that can be found in the literature.

Chapter 2, "The Human Service Profession: History and Standards" continues to offer a brief history of the fields of psychology, counseling, and social work and how their respective histories affected the creation of the human services field.

The discussion of history leads into an examination of the current status of the human service field followed by an updated discussion concerning four important standards in the field today: skills standards, credentialing, ethics, and accreditation.

Chapter 3, "Theoretical Approaches to Human Service Work," has maintained much of what was in the previous editions, including a discussion of the differences between counseling and psychotherapy, the individual versus systemic approach to treating clients, and the meaning of theory in counseling. A number of major theoretical approaches are examined, including the psychodynamic approach, behavioral approach, humanistic approach, and cognitive approach. This is followed by a review of some major cross-theoretical approaches including integrative approaches (eclecticism), brief and solution-focused approaches, and gender-aware counseling

Chapter 4, "The Helping Interview: Skills, Process, and Case Management" starts with a discussion of the helping environment, including office environment, personal characteristics of the helper, and the importance of nonverbal behaviors. This is followed by a review of major counseling techniques including listening skills; empathy; encouragement and affirmation; self-disclosure; the use of questions; giving information, advice, and offering alternatives; and confrontation. The chapter then examines the stages of the helping relationship and offers an updated examination of case management techniques when working with clients.

In Chapter 5, "The Development of the Person, "I have revised the section on defining development, and I now refer to *DSM-IV-TR* instead of *DSM-IV*. However, the body of this chapter remains largely intact and includes an examination of child development, cognitive development, moral development, personality development, life-span development, and a comparison of normal and abnormal development.

Chapter 6, "Systems: What Are They, and How Do We Work with Them?" continues to examine family systems, group counseling, and community systems. In this chapter I discuss how general systems theory can be applied to all kinds of systems and distinguish some of the varying kinds of family counseling and group counseling approaches that exist today. The major change in this chapter has to do with how I approach community systems in that I note that clients can be affected by communities in two major ways: by creating change in clients via community agencies or by working with communities to create wider systemic change that will positively affect clients.

In Chapter 7, "Human Service Professionals in a Pluralistic Society," I've updated the information on diversity in the United States and globally, and I offer an argument for helpers to be multiculturally aware. In this chapter I again discuss some models that can be useful when working with diverse clients, and I have added some practical suggestions for working with a number of diverse client groups including ethnic and racial groups, individuals from diverse religious backgrounds, women, men, gays and lesbians, individuals who are HIV positive, the homeless and poor, older persons, the mentally ill, and individuals who are disabled.

Chapter 8, "Research, Program Evaluation, and Testing," has been streamlined. The chapter starts with a description of the research process and goes on to contrast quantitative and qualitative research. The quantitative research section examines true experimental research, causal-comparative (ex post facto) research, correlational research, and survey research. The qualitative section examines ethnographic and historical research. The next section of the chapter offers an overview of process evaluation and outcome evaluation, two types of program evaluation. Finally, the chapter concludes with an overview of testing, including ability and personality, and the four qualities essential for any test: validity, reliability, cross-cultural fairness, and practicality.

In Chapter 9, "The Human Service Professional and the World of Work," I have updated and simplified the definitions related to career development; however, the body of the chapter remains the same. Thus, we continue to examine the importance of work and of career development; the history of career development and the career counseling theories that have been generated over the years; the tremendous expansion in the use of all types of career-related information, especially computer generated information; and ways to optimize helping clients, and ourselves, find a career.

Chapter 10, "A Look to the Future: Trends in the Function and Roles of the Human Service Professional" has been greatly revised. For instance, I have updated or added information on trends in working with a number of increasingly important client populations, including the incarcerated, their families, and victims of crime; individuals who are HIV positive; the homeless and the poor, older persons; the chronically mentally ill; people with disabilities and individuals at risk for chemical dependence. The section on standards in the profession now discusses program accreditation instead of program approval, credentialing, ethics, and skills standards. The chapter also examines the developmental emphasis in human services and its relationship to primary prevention as well changes in managed health care and its effect on the human services profession. In this chapter there is a new section on how medical breakthrough will affect the work of the human service professional as well as a continued focus on multicultural issues and its effect on human services. The chapter again examines the issues of stress, cynicism, and burnout and we offer a new model, "The Wheel of Wellness," to help professionals examine their well-being. Near the end of the chapter we present the job outlook in the human services and offer some suggestions on how to apply for a job or for a graduate program. The chapter concludes with a discussion of the importance of continuing education.

Finally, some additions and changes have been made to the appendices. Appendix A is new and offers the Web sites for a number of important mental health related professional organizations. Appendix B provides the reader with the Ethical Standards for Human Service Professionals. All students are encouraged to read them and discuss these guidelines in class. Appendix C offers an overview of the Council for Standards in Human Service Education (CSHSE), and Appendix D is an overview of accreditation standards of CSHSE. Appendix E is a copy of the Global Assessment of Functioning Scale (GAF) from *DSM-IV-TR*. Finally Appendix F offers "Understanding Your Holland Code," to better facilitate the Holland code analysis suggested in Chapter 9. Following Appendix F is a detailed glossary that should be helpful in understanding and studying many of the concepts introduced in the text.

As with the first and second editions, a unique aspect of this text is that near the end of each chapter you will have an opportunity to reflect on your level of "developmental maturity." You will be able to compare yourself to what might be considered to be the "ideal" human service professional; the professional who embodies the best characteristics of the professional in the field. As life is a continual growth process, I hope that instructors will encourage students to view this section as offering a "model" toward which all of us can strive and will discourage students from feeling that they are inadequate if they currently do not embody some of these traits. If you are an instructor, prior to having your students read Chapter 1, you might encourage them to complete the questionnaire entitled "Assessing Your Adult Developmental Level," which can be found in the experiential section of the chapter.

Near the end of each chapter is a section on professional and ethical issues. This section provides ethical and professional concerns that are relevant to the chapter topic.

Each chapter ends with "Experiential Exercises" designed to aid the reader's understanding of the material presented. This section presents ethical and professional dilemmas, vignettes, and/or questions to contemplate that allow students to continue to reflect upon these important issues. If you are an instructor, you might want your students to complete some of these exercises prior to their reading of the chapter. As I have found that there is simply not enough time to do all of the exercises, you might want to assign those activities that will best augment your teaching style. As a student, I would encourage you to read each exercise and complete as many as you have time for.

ACKNOWLEDGMENTS

I am grateful for the helpful comments of the many reviewers of this third edition. Their critical read of the second edition and the manuscript for the third edition was quite helpful in lending me direction in this new edition. Thus, I thank Deborah Altus, Washburn University; Rebecca Angle; Juanita Gomez, South Texas Community College; Sandra Haynes, Metropolitan School of Denver; Melvin T. Henderson, Metropolitan State University; Susan Kinsella, Georgia Southern University; Nan Littleton, Northern Kentucky University; Polly McMahon, Spokane Falls Community College; Barbara Peterson, Tacoma Community College; Roberta Petrie, St. John's University; Audrey Ringer, Berkshire Community College; Bonnie Smith, Greenville Technical College; Harry Smith, Baltimore City Community College; April West-Baker, Highline Community College.

To all the individuals associated with Brooks/Cole and Wadsworth Publishing, my considerable thanks for the support you have given to me. I would especially like to give thanks to Scott Rohr, Buuji, Inc., who helped to improve the text in immeasurable ways. Thank you, Scott, for your hard work! In addition, I would like to thank a number of individuals from Brooks/Cole, including Stephanie Zunich. And a very special thanks to Julie Martinez, whose support, friendship, and hard work helped to make this third edition come to life.

As always, a number of individuals have helped me in my research, writing, and editing. Hunter Bolling, my graduate assistant, was truly remarkable in her perseverance as she sought to obtain copyright permissions, assisted in the editing, updated and expanded the glossary, and worked tirelessly on the index. Hunter, you were truly remarkable! Thanks to Dawn, Sandi, and Bunny, who assisted me in numerous day-to-day issues. And thanks to all of my colleagues and friends who have supported me in the revision of this third edition.

ABOUT THE AUTHOR

Born and raised in New York City, Dr. Ed Neukrug obtained his B.A. in psychology in 1973 from SUNY Binghamton, his M.S. in counseling from Miami University of Ohio, and his doctorate in counselor education from the University of Cincinnati.

After teaching and directing a graduate program in counseling at Notre Dame College in New Hampshire, he accepted a position at Old Dominion University in Norfolk, Virginia, where he currently chairs the Department of Educational Leadership and Counseling. In addition to teaching, Dr. Neukrug has worked as a counselor at a street-front, walk-in crisis center; an outpatient therapist at a mental health center; an associate school psychologist; a school counselor; and a private practice psychologist and licensed professional counselor.

Dr. Neukrug has held a variety of positions in local, regional, and national professional associations in counseling and human services. He has published numerous articles in state and national journals. In addition to *Theory, Practice, and Trends in the Human Services: An Introduction,* Dr. Neukrug has written *The World of the Counselor* (2003), *Experiencing the World of the Counselor: A Workbook for Counselor Educators and Students* (2003), and *Skills and Techniques for Human Service Professionals: Counseling Environment, Helping Skills, Treatment Issues* (2002). Dr. Neukrug has also received a number of human service related grants and contracts.

Dr. Neukrug is married to Kristina Williams-Neukrug and has two children, Hannah who is eight and Emma who is three. He has an older sister, Carole, and a younger brother, Howard. His father, Joseph, died in 1976, and his mother, Eleanor, currently resides in Florida.

1

Defining the Human Service Professional

High school was a rough time in my life. Although I did well in school, my personal life was less than satisfactory. I was overweight, was afraid of dating, was particularly concerned with how I appeared to my friends, and had low self-esteem. I spent little time thinking about what major I would choose when I went to college. Although my mom would period- ically threaten to take me to a psychologist (a threat that today I wish she had carried out), I mostly kept my fears to myself. My school counselor, although nice, did not seem tuned into my problems and instead appeared more concerned with my schedule. In fact, one time when facing a problem, I found I had no one to whom I could turn. I considered going to my phys- ical education teacher because he seemed like a nice guy, but instead I went to my father. Thankfully, he came through for me. I hoped things would change in college.

Having done well in the sciences in high school, I decided to start college as a biology major. With little personal reflection and a lack of adequate career services at my college, I decided dentistry was the way to go. At least I would make some money. It was 1969, the end of the '60s. Turmoil abounded around college campuses; drugs for "consciousness rais- ing" were everywhere. Hare Krishnas and Zen Buddhists enticed you to follow them to "the answer." (If you did let them lead you down the path, you soon found out that the answer was that there was no answer.) "The times, they were a changin'." It was a time to confront the traditional values of society, and soon I found myself confronting my own choices in life—my own traditional values. Did I really want to be a dentist or was there another path for me? Suddenly, studying psychology seemed to be my natural path. Why, of course, didn't I want to help people, help mankind (later to be called humankind), help the evolution of the planet? I quickly changed my major. Was I disappointed—I wasn't learning how to help others; I was memorizing the anatomy of the brain and the eye, learning how rats find their way through mazes, and exploring theories on why people do the things they do. Although I was promised that this knowledge was the basis of the helping professions, I wasn't con- vinced. Indeed, even today I'm not convinced.

During those times, I was never taught how to respond to someone in a "counseling" way. I felt displaced and disappointed. Unfortunately, during the 1960s, there were few human service programs. What led me on my search for a field that hardly even existed at that time? What intuitive sense did I have that there was another career path for me, in which I would be teaching 20 years later? What characteristics did I possess at the time that made me an effective human service professional, and what skills would I need to develop? In this chapter, we will explore many of these questions as we discuss the skills, characteris- tics, and values of the human service professional, as well as the broad field of human service work.

This chapter will explore the identity of the human service professional. Specifically, we will examine the beginning of the profession, contrast it with other mental health professions, and discuss professional associations that serve the various mental health professionals. Next, we will examine those characteristics that have been shown to be important in being an effective helper and discuss ways of acquiring such qualities. The chapter will conclude with a discussion of our professional relationships to related professions and the importance of being willing to continually examine ourselves as professionals.

IDENTIFYING THE HUMAN SERVICE PROFESSIONAL

The Beginning:
The Human Service Professional Degree Emerges

Although human services have been around for hundreds of years (see Chapter 2), a professional degree in human services didn't evolve until the mid-1960s. During the 1960s, there was an increased sense of social responsibility toward the poor, minorities and women, and the mentally ill. This social awareness was one factor that led to President Johnson's **Great Society**[1] initiatives and resulted in the establishment of federal grants for a variety of social welfare programs (Fullerton, 1990a, b; Osher, 1990). With the social welfare system greatly expanding, it soon became apparent that the established graduate programs in counseling, psychology, and social work would not be able to handle the increasing need for trained mental health professionals. Thus, we saw the beginnings of the human service degree. Although both associate's and bachelor's programs arose at this time, their orientations were somewhat different (McClam, 1997a). The associate's degree was geared toward training the mental health aide, or paraprofessional, whereas the bachelor's degree was seen as more broadly based and considered a professional degree (Fullerton, 1990a, 1990b).

As the need for human service professionals expanded, so did educational programs that would train such professionals. From these programs a "human service curriculum" that borrows from other related fields, yet trains human service professionals in a unique way, evolved. Today, there are approximately 380 certificate and associate degree programs in human services fields, and 400 programs offer a bachelor's degree in human services (U.S. Department of Labor, Bureau of Labor Statistics 1998–1999a). A small number of graduate programs in human services are also available. In this chapter, and in Chapter 2, we will have the opportunity to take a closer look at the history, roles and functions, and overall standards of the human services profession.

Who Is the Human Service Professional Today?

Generally, the human service professional is a person who has an associate's or bachelor's degree in human services or a closely related field. Although specific course work varies from program to program, most human service degree programs offer an introductory course in human services as well as course work in interviewing, family counseling, group counseling, crisis intervention, counseling skills, and some type of supervised field placement. Other major areas that are sometimes covered include social welfare history and policy, human development, career development, research, testing, counseling theories, ethics, and multicultural issues (Clubok, 1997; McGrath, 1991–92).

---

[1]Boldface terms are defined in the glossary at the end of the book.

The human service professional of today is seen as a generalist who can work side by side with a number of other professionals and take on a wide range of roles in the helping professions (Diambra, 2000; Greene, 1995; Woodside & McClam, 1998a). Although the human service professional generally does not do in-depth counseling and psychotherapy, he or she is well equipped to facilitate client change and growth. One might find human service professionals in dozens of places, although some of the more prominent fields include mental health, mental retardation, substance abuse, aging/gerontology, domestic violence, youth service, child care, correction/criminal justice, education/schools, health care, recreation/ fitness, and vocational rehabilitation (McClam & Woodside, 2001; McGrath, 1991–92).

Usually, human service professionals help clients problem solve and do not facilitate personality reconstruction. Table 1.1 shows a visual representation of some differences in how human service professionals, counselors, social workers, and psychologists might approach working with a client.

Roles, Functions, Competencies, and Skills of the Human Service Professional

Thirteen Roles and Functions   Usually, the work of the human service professional is focused around one or more of 13 roles and functions as identified by the **Southern Region Education Board (SREB)** (SREB, 1969). These include the following:

1. **Outreach worker** who might go into communities to work with clients
2. **Broker** who helps clients find and use services
3. **Advocate** who champions and defends clients' causes and rights
4. **Evaluator** who assesses client programs and shows that agencies are accountable for services provided
5. **Teacher/educator** who tutors, mentors, and models new behaviors for clients
6. **Behavior changer** who uses intervention strategies and counseling skills to facilitate client change
7. **Mobilizer** who organizes client and community support to provide needed services
8. **Consultant** who seeks and offers knowledge and support to other professionals and meets with clients and community groups to discuss and solve problems
9. **Community planner** who designs, implements, and organizes new programs to service client needs
10. **Caregiver** who offers direct support, encouragement, and hope to clients
11. **Data manager** who develops systems to gather facts and statistics as a means of evaluating programs

Table 1.1 Comparison of Select Professionals' Orientations to Working with Clients*

	Human Service Worker	Counselor/ Social Worker	Psychologist
Supportive	High	Moderate	Low
Problem-focused	High	Moderate	Low/Moderate
Works with conscious	High	Moderate	Low/Moderate
Focused on present	High	Moderate	Low/Moderate
Directive	Moderate	Moderate/Low	Low
Facilitative	Moderate	Moderate/High	High
Nondirective	Moderate/Low	Moderate/High	High
Insight-oriented	Moderate/Low	Moderate/High	High
Works with unconscious	Low	Moderate/High	High
Focused on past	Low	Moderate	High

*Note: These are generalizations. The focus of any particular professional may vary as a function of the individual's personality and theoretical orientation. For instance, it is not unusual to find some psychologists being very directive and problem-focused. And, one can readily find a human service professional who is highly nondirective.

12. **Administrator** who supervises community service programs

13. **Assistant to specialist** who works closely with the highly trained professional as an aide and helper in servicing clients (Mandel & Schram, 1985; Schram & Mandel, 1996; Diambra, 2001)

Skills Standards and Competencies In addition to these roles and functions, in a recent national project to develop **skills standards**, 12 competencies have been identified as important to the work of the human service professional (Diambra, 2001; Taylor, Bradley, & Warren, 1996). The competencies include (1) participant empowerment; (2) communication; (3) assessment; (4) community and service networking; (5) facilitation of services; (6) community and living skills and supports; (7) education, training, and self-development; (8) advocacy; (9) vocational, educational, and career support; (10) crisis intervention; (11) organization participation; and (12) documentation. These 12 competencies and the skills needed to accomplish them will be discussed in more detail in Chapter 2.

Clearly, there is much overlap between the roles and functions as identified by the SREB and the more recent competencies. However, there are also some significant differences, and perhaps what is more important, because the competencies are broken down into a large number of skills needed to accomplish them, the competence can greatly assist the human service professional in understanding his or her role and can be a guide for training programs.

OTHER MENTAL HEALTH PROFESSIONALS

Although there is some overlap in the training of the many different professionals in the social service field, great differences also exist. Let's briefly review some of these different kinds of mental health professionals.

Psychiatrist

Psychiatrists are physicians who generally have completed a residency in psychiatry. This means that they have completed extensive training in some kind of mental health setting. As physicians, psychiatrists have expertise in prescribing medication for emotional problems. Their affiliated professional association is the **American Psychiatric Association (APA).**

Psychologist

Psychologists generally have doctoral degrees in psychology, have completed internships at a mental health facility, and have passed specific state requirements to obtain licensure as psychologists. Their professional association is the **American Psychological Association (APA).**

Social Worker

Although the term **social worker** can apply to a person holding either an undergraduate or graduate degree in social work or a related field (for example, human services), more generally social workers have master's degrees in social work **(MSW).** With additional training and supervision, social workers can become members of the **Academy of Certified Social Workers (ACSW),** which means they have obtained national certification. In addition, most states have specific requirements for becoming a **licensed clinical social worker (LCSW),** which is usually a separate process from that of becoming an ACSW. Their professional association is the **National Association of Social Workers (NASW).**

Counselor

Although many individuals may call themselves counselors, generally a **counselor** is an individual who has a master's degree in counseling. Many subspecialties exist in the counseling field. A few of the more common ones are **school counseling** (formerly called guidance counseling), **mental health counseling, college counseling,** and **rehabilitation counseling.** Counselors can become certified as a **National Certified Counselor (NCC),** and can also become **licensed professional counselors (LPCs)** in most states. Certification and licensure usually require additional training and supervision to practice, although one credential is generally not a prerequisite for the other. The professional association of counselors is the **American Counseling Association (ACA).**

Couple and Family Counselors

Couple and family counselors are specifically trained to work with systems and can be found in a vast array of agency settings and in private practice. These professionals tend to have specialty course work in systems dynamics, family therapy, family life stages, and human sexuality, along with the more traditional course work in the helping professions. Many couple and family therapists are members of the **American Association for Marriage and Family Therapy (AAMFT).** Others often join a couple and family division of the professional association to which their degrees are associated (e.g., psychologist—APA, counselors—ACA, social workers—NASW).

Psychiatric Nurse

Trained primarily as medical professionals, psychiatric nurses are also prepared to provide education, prevention, and treatment for mental health services (APNA, 2002; Davidson, 1992). Psychiatric nurses can be found in a number of roles including nurse practitioner, clinical nurse specialist, head nurse, educator, administrator, director of nursing, researcher, staff nurse, therapist, and consultant. Although some psychiatric nurses have an associate or bachelor's degree in nursing, most hold an advanced degree in nursing. Certification of psychiatric nurses can be held in a number of mental health areas. The professional association of psychiatric nurses is the **American Psychiatric Nurses Association (APNA).**

Psychotherapist

Because most states do not have laws that regulate the term **psychotherapist,** individuals with no training, experience, or even a degree can call themselves psychotherapists. On a practical level, psychotherapists usually have advanced degrees in psychology, social work, or counseling and work in mental health settings or in private practice, providing individual, group, or marital counseling. However, if someone tells you he or she is a psychotherapist, it would be wise to inquire what his or her degree is in.

PROFESSIONAL ASSOCIATIONS
IN HUMAN SERVICES AND RELATED FIELDS[2]

Purpose of Associations

There are a number of professional associations in the social services, many of which the human service professional can join. Professional associations serve a number of purposes, including the following:

---

[2]See Appendix A for the URLs of important organizations in the field of human services.

- To provide a political base (for example, lobbying efforts) that helps secure jobs for human service professionals and to advocate for political agendas important to the profession (for example, client rights issues)
- To offer conferences and workshops to foster innovative ideas in the areas of client services, teaching, and advocacy
- To publish newsletters and journals to keep members abreast of the latest innovations in the field
- To provide a process that encourages networking and mentoring
- To offer grants for special projects related to the field

The Associations

The **National Organization for Human Service Education (NOHSE)** (see www.nohse.org). Founded in 1975, NOHSE is a relatively new association whose main purposes are

- To provide a medium for cooperation among Human Service organizations and individual faculty, practitioners, and students
- To foster excellence in teaching, research, and curriculum development for improving the education of human service delivery personnel.
- To encourage, support and assist the development of local, state and national organizations of Human Services.
- To sponsor forums through conferences, institutes, publications and symposia that foster creative approaches to human service education and delivery (NOHSE, 2002, Purpose section)

Although NOHSE is geared mostly toward faculty in human service programs, undergraduates are encouraged to join, and those who are pursuing a graduate degree in human services might also find this association interesting.

NOHSE has six regional associations (Mid-Atlantic, Midwest, Northeast, Northwest, South, and West). Each of these regions has its own professional meetings, and they operate somewhat independently in offering workshops, conferences, and other professional activities. Membership in NOHSE entitles you to a number of benefits including

- Subscription to *Human Service Education*, NOHSE's journal
- Subscription to *The Link*, NOHSE's newsletter
- Professional development workshops and conferences
- Scholarships and grants for professional development
- *Resource Directory of Consultants in Human Services*
- Information and referral services
- Networking
- Recognition awards

If you are interested in becoming more involved professionally as a human service professional, you should join NOHSE and the regional chapter.

The American Counseling Association (ACA) (see www.counseling.org) Today, with 52,000 members, ACA is the world's largest counseling association. This not-for-profit association is an umbrella organization that serves the needs of all types of counselors in an effort to "enhance the quality of life in society by promoting the development of professional counselors, advancing the counseling profession, and using the profession and practice of counseling to promote respect for human dignity and diversity" (ACA, 2002, Mission and Vision Statement, ¶2).

ACA publishes one journal, *The Journal of Counseling and Development*. In addition, ACA currently sponsors 17 divisions, all of which maintain newsletters, and most publish a journal. The association has numerous conferences and workshops at the state, regional, and national level. Although the association is geared toward master's- and doctoral-level counselors, counselor trainees, and counselor educators, undergraduates who are interested in the counseling field are welcomed.

The National Association of Social Workers (NASW) (see www.naswdc .org) The NASW was founded in 1955 as the result of the merger of seven membership associations in the field of social work. Servicing both undergraduate- and graduate-level social workers, NASW has nearly 155,000 members, and its purpose is "to create professional standards for social work practice; advocate sound public social policies through political and legislative action; provide a wide range of membership services, including continuing education opportunities and an extensive professional program" (Associations Unlimited, 2002a). The association publishes four journals and other professional publications. Only professionals with an undergraduate or graduate degree in social work or social work students are allowed to join this association.

The American Psychological Association (APA) (see www.apa.org) Founded in 1892 by G. Stanley Hall, APA started with 31 members and now maintains a membership of 83,000. Undergraduate and graduate students can join as affiliate members. The main purpose of this association is "to advance psychology as a science, a profession, and as a means of promoting human welfare" (Associations Unlimited, 2002b). The association has 46 divisions in various specialty areas and publishes numerous psychological journals.

The American Psychiatric Association (APA) (see www.psych.org) Founded in 1844, today the APA has almost 40,000 members. The association's main purpose is to "further the study of the nature, treatment, and prevention of mental disorders." (Associations Unlimited, 2002c). The association accomplishes this by offering programs and workshops on psychiatric disorders, evaluating and publishing statistical data related to psychiatric disorders, and supporting educational and research activities in the field of psychiatry. The association is active in advocacy work for mental health issues and has a number of councils and committees to focus on mental health concerns. The APA publishes journals in the field of psychiatry and is responsible for the development and publication of the **Diagnostic and Statistical Manual–IV–Text Revision (DSM–IV–TR),** a major publication for mental health diagnosis.

The American Association of Marriage and Family Therapists (AAMF) (see www.aamft.org) In recent years, the American Association of Marriage and Family Therapy (AAMFT) has become the prominent professional association in the field of marriage and family counseling. AAMFT was established in 1945 by family therapy and communication theorists to develop standards for their field and to offer an association that could bring together people with varying professional backgrounds who had an interest in marriage and family therapy (Associations Unlimited, 2001e). Today, AAMFT has 23,000 members, publishes the Journal of Marital and Family Therapy, sponsors a yearly conference, and offers many other professional activities. Although geared toward licensed marriage and family therapists, AAMFT also allows others to join.

The American Psychiatric Nurses Association (APNA) (see www.apna.org) A relatively young association, the American Psychiatric Nurses Association was founded in 1987 with 600 members. Today, APNA comprises almost 4000 members. The main purpose of APNA is to provide "leadership to advance psychiatric mental health nursing practice, improve mental health care for culturally diverse families, individuals, groups and communities, and shape health policy for the delivery of mental health services" (Associations Unlimited, 2002e). APNA offers a number of continuing education and professional development activities and publishes the *Journal of the American Psychiatric Nurses Association.* The association provides advocacy for psychiatric nurses to improve the quality of mental health delivery.

CHARACTERISTICS OF THE EFFECTIVE HUMAN SERVICE PROFESSIONAL

Whether you are thinking about entering, or have already decided to enter the human service field, as I did 25 years ago, you probably have some intuition that this field somehow fits your sense of who you are. You may have some image of the human service professional. Perhaps you think he or she is a person who wants to help others; who cares about people and the state of the world; who is introspective, intuitive, and social; or who has other similar qualities. On the other hand, you probably also think that the human service professional is not a cold person, does not hold rigidly sterile views, and is not concerned only with himself or herself. In fact, the qualities of the helping professional have been researched over the years (Gladstein, 1983; Goldstein & Higginbotham, 1991; Highlen & Hill, 1984; Lambert & Bergin, 1983; Neukrug & McAuliffe, 1993; Rowe, Murphy, & De Csipkes, 1975; Sexton, 1993; Sexton & Whiston, 1991, 1994). Although the reviews are exhaustive, unfortunately, too often the results seem inconclusive and the number and type of factors that might have some effect on client outcomes almost seem too numerous to draw any firm conclusions. However, given these inherent difficulties, and based on the current state of research on what makes an effective helper, I have generated eight characteristics that may be empirically or theoretically related to effectiveness as a helper. The characteristics I have picked include (1) **empathy,** (2) **open mindedness,** (3) **acceptance,** (4) **cognitive complexity,** (5) **psychological adjustment,** (6) **genuineness,** (7) **relationship building,** and (8) **competence.** As research in these areas becomes more refined, some of these characteristics might change, but let's take a close look at these.

Empathy

Empathic persons have a deep understanding of another person's point of view. These people can "get into the shoes" of another. For those of you who have watched *Star Trek: The Next Generation,* you may know the "counselor," the epitome of the empathic person, with her ability to understand another's perspective on the world. **Carl Rogers** (1957) liked to say that the empathic person could sense the private world of clients as if it were his or her own, without losing the "as if" feeling. Empathic individuals can accept people in their differences and can communicate this sense of acceptance. For the helping relationship, empathy is seen as a skill that can build rapport, elicit information, and help the client feel accepted (Carkhuff, 2000; Egan, 2002).

Open-Mindedness

Individuals who are **open minded,** or **nondogmatic,** allow others to express their points of view. Although these individuals may have strong opinions of their own, they do not feel as if they need to change others to their viewpoints. Such people are open to criticism, to change, and to hearing the views of others in a way that will allow them to adapt their own values and beliefs. Certainly, one readily thinks of people like Hitler or Stalin as examples of close-minded, dogmatic individuals, but these people are the extreme. Most of us have a kind of tempered **dogmatism**—there are areas in which we have extremely strong convictions, yet we aren't constantly trying to convince people to change to our points of view. It is important to look at our dogmatic areas and ask ourselves, "Why do I have so much energy in this area?" Individuals who are close-minded cannot effectively listen to another. If I am trying to convince you of something, how can I hear your point of view? Some research shows an inverse relationship between dogmatism and empathy; that is, dogmatic people tend not to be empathic (McAuliffe & Eriksen, 2000; Neukrug & McAuliffe, 1993).

Acceptance

People who have high regard for others can accept people in their differentness regardless of dissimilar cultural heritage, values, or belief systems. When in a helping relationship, individuals with a high regard for others are able to accept the helpee (the person needing help) unconditionally, without having "strings attached" to the relationship. Rogers (1957) calls this **unconditional positive regard.** Leo Buscaglia (1972) calls this responsible love: "Responsible love is accepting and understanding. . . . [L]ove helps us to accept the fact that the other individual is behaving only as he [or she] is able to behave at the moment" (p. 119).

Having high regard for others does not mean that one necessarily likes everything a person has done. For instance, one would most certainly not like the actions of the convicted murderer or rapist; however, the person with high regard can come to understand how the felon came to commit those actions. This deep understanding comes from being empathic and is like having a window that leads deep inside the soul of the other individual—a window that allows the helper to see the hurts and pains of the other. This window into the other's being assists the helper to accept the helpee unconditionally and with high regard.

Cognitive Complexity

Individuals who have complex cognitive skills have the ability to understand the world, and ultimately their clients, in complex and abstract ways (Kegan, 1982, 1994; King, 1978). Such individuals view learning as a mutual and reciprocal process whereby experts can share knowledge with others and learn from others. In addition, those who are cognitively complex have a strong sense of self, can hear feedback from others, and are willing to learn, teach, share, and be open with others.

Research on the development of **cognitive complexity** also shows that individuals who are complex cognitively tend to embrace many of the personal characteristics already highlighted as important, such as empathy and openness (Lovell, 1999; McAuliffe & Erikson, 2000; Neukrug & McAuliffe, 1993). The research also suggests that cognitively complex individuals are able to view a client from multiple perspectives. For instance, such a person can understand an individual from his or her point of view, from the point of view of others, and see how the system (e.g., family and community) might affect the person. Clearly, a person who is cognitively complex also has the tools to positively affect his or her clients' courses of treatment.

One of the most exciting aspects of cognitive complexity is the notion that all individuals can grow and change and become more complex thinkers over time. This has fantastic implications for training programs because such programs can help students gain in cognitive complexity and ultimately become better helping professionals (McAuliffe & Erikson, 2000)!

Psychological Adjustment

Helpers who have a high level of **psychological adjustment** are willing to look deeply within themselves. This means that they have the courage to receive feedback from others and are willing to be self-critical. **Introspective** individuals are open to their deeper feelings and are willing to examine their own hurts and pains. In researching the ability of helpers to be self-examining, investigators have examined helpers' rates of attendance in therapy. Generally, the results have been positive, with a number of studies showing that between 64 and 83% of counselors, social workers, psychologists, and psychiatrists had been in therapy (Deutsch, 1984; Neukrug & Williams, 1993; Norcross, Strausser, & Faltus, 1988; Prochaska & Norcross, 1983). And, in a study of human service students, educators, and professionals, 75% reported having been in counseling, with women seeking counseling at higher rates than men (Neukrug, Milliken, & Shoemaker, 2001)

Participation in one's own therapy has a number of benefits for the helper. First, it can assist the helper in dealing with his or her own personal difficulties. "For a counselor to set themselves up as a helper to others, without having resolved major difficulties of their own, would appear to be farcical" (Wheeler, 1991, p. 199). Second, the helper can gain a first-hand sense of whether what he or she does will work. Third, it enables the helper to identify and empathize with the experience of sitting in the client's seat. Fourth, personal therapy yields great insight of self, which is likely to have a positive effect on the helping relationship. Finally, it helps to prevent **countertransference,** or the process whereby the helper's own issues interfere with effectively helping his or her clients.

Studies have shown that a fairly large percentage of helping professionals had been in therapy before entering training programs (Guy & Liaboe, 1986; Neukrug & Williams, 1993). This likely indicates that many helpers have wounds from childhood that they have been willing to examine, thus lessening the likelihood of countertransference.

Is therapy the only road to psychological adjustment? Probably not; however, it is a very special relationship not achievable through friendships or other significant relationships. Other activities, such as support groups, meditation, exercise, and journaling, have all been shown to have positive effects on our psychological adjustment. Therapy is not the only way, but it is one of a few activities that can lead to good mental health and more effective counseling relationships.

Genuineness

At times, I am caught in the dilemma of saying and acting in the way that I feel versus saying and acting in the way that I think another person wants me to be. Do I express my true feelings, or do I hide them to protect another person—or perhaps, more accurately, to protect myself? Do I tell my boss that I am angry at her and take the chance that I might get fired? Do I tell my client that what he shares with me makes me feel sad and take the chance that such a revelation might make him feel uneasy? Do I risk a friendship by telling my friend that I feel manipulated by him? Rogers (1961, 1980) felt that being in sync with your feelings and behaviors, being **genuine** or **congruent,** was crucial to healthy relationships. Individuals who embody such characteristics are **transparent;** that is, they readily show their feelings to others (Greenberg, 1994; Jourard, 1971; Rogers, 1957). Although it may be prudent at times not to share certain feelings with your boss, friend, or client, a relationship that emphasizes nongenuineness can have little substance and, in the case of the helping relationship, will be less likely to promote growth in clients.

Compared with the individual who is congruent and real, nongenuine people do not have their feelings, thoughts, and actions in sync. How they feel is not represented by what they say or how they act. These individuals are fake—living life with subtle deceptions, often deceiving themselves. Afternoon soap operas, for example, represent the exaggeration of nongenuineness. Here we see individuals "acting" at life—being terribly dishonest in their relationships—not for fear of hurting the other but for fear that their lives would be ruined if they were truthful. These "lies" are often not conscious. They have become part of the individual's way of living in the world.

Unless people are horribly caught up in a nongenuine way of living, they usually have a sense that they are living incongruently. There is a slight (sometimes more than slight) internal tug saying "Something's not right inside" or "I know I'm trying to put something over on this person." Clients often come for help to have the human service professional assist them in becoming more in sync. Therefore, if the helper is nongenuine, assisting the client along his or her path would be difficult.

In the book *People of the Lie,* Peck (1998) felt that what can begin as "small white lies" could snowball over time, become a nongenuine lifestyle, and eventually represent evil. Although rare, he even felt that this nongenuine lifestyle could take over one's life and lead to possession by Satan. He sees therapy as "mini-confessionals" where people can cleanse themselves of their incongruities. Although you may not believe that lying can lead to possession by the devil, most people would agree that living a nongenuine lifestyle is not healthy.

Relationship Building

The relationship between the helper and client may be the most significant factor in creating client change (Safran & Muran, 2000; Sexton & Whiston, 1991; Whiston & Coker, 2000). Such a relationship is closely related to the ability of the client and helper to build an emotional bond and to work on setting attainable goals. The impact of the helper's ability to build an emotional bond is felt throughout the helping relationship, regardless of whether it is acknowledged by the counselor and the client.

The well-known family therapist **Salvadore Minuchin** (1974) has always stressed the importance of building an alliance with clients. Using the term "joining" to describe the building of the client-helper relationship, he says that the helper must join with the family if therapeutic goals are to be reached. Although Minuchin has his own characteristic manner of joining with a family, all helpers build an alliance based on their unique ways of helping. The challenge for all helpers is to have the emotional fortitude to build strong relationships, to know how to build such bonds within the context of their theoretical framework, and to be able to understand how these bonds dramatically affect work with clients.

Competence

Helper expertise has been shown to be a crucial element for client success in counseling (Whiston & Coker, 2000), and perceived competence has been consistently chosen by helpers as the most important factor in picking a helper

(Grunebaum, 1983; Neukrug, Milliken, & Shoemaker, 2001; Neukrug & Williams, 1993; Norcross et al., 1988). Thus, it should not be surprising that **competence** is the final characteristic I have chosen as crucial for helpers to embrace.

Competent helpers have a thirst for knowledge. They desire to examine the newest trends, the newest approaches, to be on the cutting edge of the field. Such helpers exhibit this thirst through their study habits, their desire to join professional associations, their reading of professional journals, their view that education is a lifelong process, and their ability to view their own approach to working with clients as something that is always broadening and deepening.

Competence is consistently acknowledged as a crucial ethical concern by most professional associations (Corey, Corey, & Callanan, 2003). (See also Appendix B, Statements 26, 27, 30, and 31.) Therefore, having the desire to learn skills as well as the specific techniques needed to work with certain problems is essential for the effective human service professional.

During my years of teaching counseling and helping skills, I have found that some students seem reluctant to learn these necessary skills. They seem to think that their personality characteristics are enough to "get them by." However, truly effective human service professionals are not willing to just "get by." These professionals have a thirst for knowledge. They exhibit this through their studies, their desire to join professional associations and read professional journals, and their ability to broaden and deepen their own approach to clients.

These eight characteristics of empathy, open mindedness, acceptance, mindfulness, psychological adjustment, genuineness, relationship building, and competence are qualities to which human service professionals should aspire. Few if any of us are already there. More likely, these qualities can be nurtured and developed as we travel our own unique paths through life. But how do we begin to acquire some of these qualities? Let's examine some possible ways.

PERSONALITY DEVELOPMENT
OF THE EFFECTIVE HELPER

Are some of us born with the previously described characteristics that lead us toward the human service field, or can they be learned, or are these qualities the combination of genetic and acquired traits? When I became a psychology major and still felt something was amiss, was I searching for this elusive human service field because I already possessed some of these characteristics and it was a natural place for me to be? Or, perhaps because of my own emotional wounds, I unconsciously sought a field that dealt with emotional pain. In the latter case, it might mean that I didn't already possess these characteristics and needed to cultivate them.

Many theorists and philosophers have struggled with trying to understand this nature of the person. **Carl Rogers** and **Abraham Maslow** (1954), two of the founders of the field of **humanistic counseling and education,** thought we were born with a natural actualizing tendency and that if we were reared in a nurturing environment, many of the described characteristics would naturally

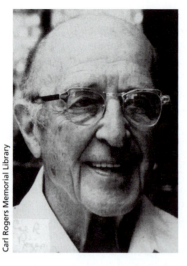

Carl Rogers Memorial Library

Carl Rogers, one of the founders of the field of humanistic counseling and education

develop. They also thought that even if the nurturing environment was not present in early childhood, the qualities could still develop if such an environment was available later in life. On the other hand, **Sigmund Freud,** the founder of psychoanalysis, thought that people constantly struggled with instinctual aggressive and sexual drives and that these drives, in combination with early childhood experiences, determined our temperament. Therefore, he would have believed that a human service professional's personality is formed in early childhood. Others, such as **B. F. Skinner** (1953), the famous behaviorist, and **Albert Ellis** (1996), the well-known cognitive therapist, believed that, although we might not be born with these qualities, they could be developed through certain learned experiences. These differing views of human nature and how they relate to the helping professions will be discussed in more detail later in Chapters 3 and 5. However, regardless of how you believe personality is formed, the eight qualities noted earlier are clearly important if one is to be an effective helper.

An Adult Development Approach

Adult developmental theorists such as **William Perry** (King, 1978), **Robert Kegan** (1982, 1994), and **Gail Sheehy** (1976) have proposed that the way individuals view the world can change throughout the life span if the individual is afforded opportunities for personal growth. These theorists would state that many of the characteristics listed earlier are the outgrowth of a natural developmental process. They assert that if given an environment that supports and yet challenges the individual's way of constructing reality, he or she would naturally develop many of these characteristics. Borrowing from some of the other developmental theorists such as **Jean Piaget** (1954), who examined child development, and **Lawrence Kohlberg** (1969), who examined moral development, these adult developmental theorists state that adult cognitive abilities are sequential and build on themselves. In other words, current ways of viewing the world are based on completion of past stages, and as we evolve we can broaden and expand our ways of viewing the world.

Adult cognitive theorists such as Perry and Kegan hypothesize that the way we think moves in stages from a concrete, rigid type of thinking toward an abstract, more flexible, "relativistic" type of thinking. Research on adult cognitive development seems to support some of Perry's and Kegan's hypotheses because it shows that individuals who are at higher stages of adult cognitive development tend to embrace many of the characteristics of the effective helper (Lovell, 1999; McAuliffe & Eriksen, 2000; Neukrug & McAuliffe, 1993). Therefore, it would seem imperative for human service programs to afford students opportunities to move forward on these cognitive schemes.

Perry's Scheme of Adult Cognitive Development

Perry's theory of intellectual and ethical development (King, 1978) has particularly emphasized the learning process of college students. His theory has three stages encompassing nine positions. In **dualism,** the first stage, students view the world as black or white, or right or wrong, and have little tolerance for ambiguity. Students in this stage might believe the professor has "the answer" and would expect learning to come mostly from the professor teaching it to the students.

The second stage is **relativism.** Here students move away from viewing the world in an absolutist, right or wrong fashion. The relativist thinks abstractly, allows for differing opinions, and understands that there may be many ways of viewing the world. Students in this stage expect learning to be more of a sharing process and would explore the opinions of others to formulate their own outlooks on life.

The final stage is **commitment in relativism.** Although relatively few individuals are in this stage, those who are maintain their relativistic outlook and can commit to specific values and behaviors in which they live their lives. In other words, they may take specific religious stances, job orientations, or personality characteristics while maintaining an accepting attitude toward others' lifestyles (Widick, 1975). Students in this stage, who are committed in relativism, may have strong opinions, yet they are still open to learning from others.

Research on the Perry scheme seems to indicate that the higher the stage one is in, the more likely it is that he or she embodies many of the characteristics important in the human service professional (Benack, 1988; Lovell, 1999; Neukrug & McAuliffe, 1993). Also, it has become clear that as students go through college and graduate school, they advance on the Perry scheme (Magolda & Porterfield, 1988).

Kegan's Constructivist View
of Adult Cognitive Development

Similar to Perry but using a more interpersonal model, Kegan (1982, 1994) suggests there are six stages of cognitive development (Stages 0 through 5), with Stages 3, 4, and 5 representing ways in which most adults view the world. Kegan's **incorporative, impulsive,** and **imperial stages** (Stages 0, 1, and 2) deal mostly with child development and focus on how the individual moves from total self-involvement toward the beginning awareness of a shared world with other people (although some adults can still be seen acting out these earlier states). These stages will be dealt with in more detail in Chapter 5.

Kegan's third stage is the **interpersonal stage,** which represents the individual who is embedded in his or her relationships. Individuals in this stage cannot truly separate their sense of who they are from their families, friends, or community groups. Kegan's fourth stage, the **institutional stage,** represents the person who has separated his or her values and sense of self from parents, peers, or community groups. These individuals have a strong sense of personal autonomy and self-reliance. Kegan's final stage is the **interindividual stage.** Here, individuals are able to maintain a separate sense of self and have the capability of incorporating feedback from others, feedback that allows for growth and change. They are not embedded in their autonomous self-reliant way of living as are Stage 4 institutional persons.

The Woody Allen movie *Zelig* clearly shows an individual in transition from Stage 3 to Stage 4. Zelig is the epitome of Stage 3, the interpersonal person. He takes on the persona of whomever he is around. He is afraid to be himself. If he's around an African-American, he becomes African-American; if he's around a Chinese person, he speaks fluent Chinese. He becomes obese when around someone who is obese, and he becomes a psychiatrist attempting to treat the psychiatrist who is treating him. What seems to be a lighthearted movie soon becomes serious when we see the reasons why Zelig becomes whomever he is around. Under hypnosis, Zelig reveals the reasons he becomes the person he is with—he is afraid to be himself. A lifelong history of ridicule every time he expressed his own opinion made him too scared to be himself. After intensive therapy, Zelig becomes "cured." Finally, the big day arrives when Zelig is to meet a number of renowned psychiatrists who will examine him to see if he is actually cured. At first, things seem successful because Zelig does not take on the persona of the psychiatrists. But as the meeting continues, one of the psychiatrists remarks on what a beautiful day it is. Zelig, who has become his "own person" and is now very assertive, states, "It is not a nice day." Indeed, Zelig has become too much of his own person because he soon starts a fight with the psychiatrist to prove his point. Although Zelig has changed and grown, he is now embedded in another developmental level—Kegan's Stage 4, the institutional stage.

If this film were to show Zelig moving into Kegan's final stage, the interindividual stage, we would see him being able to hear other points of view and incor-

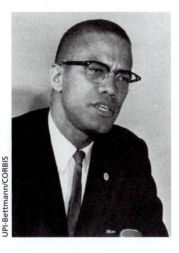

UPI-Bettmann/CORBIS

The life of Malcolm X reflects movement through Kegan's stages of development

porate them into his view of the world, if he so chooses. In Maslow's terms, he would then be the self-actualized person—a person who is in touch with himself, can hear feedback from others, is nondogmatic, has an internal locus of control, is empathic and introspective—in other words, an individual who embodies many of the characteristics of the effective human service professional.

Although Zelig represents a comedic example of movement through the Kegan stages, finding a real-life illustration is not difficult. Consider, for example, the life of **Malcolm X** (X & Haley, 2001). As a young adult, Malcolm X found himself involved in a life of crime and drug addiction. While serving a 10-year prison sentence for robbery, he was introduced to the Nation of Islam, the Black Muslim religion headed by Elija Muhammad. Malcolm readily gave up his former lifestyle and became embedded in the values of the Nation of Islam. He lived, slept, and breathed their values, and his identity became the values held by the Nation of Islam (Kegan's interpersonal stage). However, as he developed, he realized that he did not agree with some of their ideas, and he moved from embeddedness in their values to a strong sense of his own religious, cultural, and moral values. Still somewhat closed to other points of view, Malcolm X had matured to the point where he could now embrace his own set of values (Kegan's institutional stage).

Following a pilgrimage to Mecca, he changed his name to **Al Hajj Malik al-Shabazz** and again modified his views "to encompass the possibility that all white people were not evil and that progress in the black struggle could be made with the help of world organizations, other black groups, and even progressive white groups" (*Encyclopedia of Black America,* 1981, p. 544). Clearly, Al Hajj Malik al-Shabazz had evolved to Kegan's interindividual stage (and Perry's commitment to relativism stage). He now could hear other points of view, be open to feedback, and yet have a clear sense of his own uniqueness in the world.

ACQUIRING THE CHARACTERISTICS
OF THE EFFECTIVE HELPER

A Values Clarification Approach

Helping students develop the characteristics of the effective human service professional is crucial if they are going to graduate as skilled professionals with social consciousness. Embodying the characteristics of empathy, open mindedness, acceptance, cognitive complexity, and genuineness and being able to build relationships, be psychologically adjusted, and competent is no easy task. To develop these characteristics, you usually have to obtain some feedback concerning how others view you. These characteristics need to be slowly nurtured and developed within a supportive yet somewhat challenging environment. For instance, Zelig needed to discover the therapeutic setting to feel the support and challenge that allowed him to transcend his previous way of living.

Although personal counseling is one avenue people can use to facilitate personal growth, change can also occur through other experiences. For instance, college can offer the environment conducive for growth, with the classroom as the necessary supportive environment that is also challenging to the student. **Values clarification,** one approach easily used in the classroom, challenges students to understand and embrace their unique perspectives while offering potential new lenses through which to view the world. The classroom environment can assist students in their development as successful human service professionals who embody the eight characteristics listed earlier. At the same time, this environment can assist the development of the emerging adult personality as represented by Perry and Kegan. The values clarification process is seen as a three-step process whereby individuals are challenged to (1) choose their values, (2) prize their choices, and (3) act on the choices they make (Raths, Harmin, & Simon, 1966; Simon, Howe, & Kirschenbaum, 1995).

Understanding the valuing process was brought home to me when I participated in a five-day workshop sponsored by **Sid Simon,** one of the founding figures of the values clarification movement. During that time, we were asked not to reveal some essential components of what made us who we were. Therefore, it was suggested that we not reveal to other workshop participants basic facts such as our level of education, the type of work we did, and other major identifying features. Because I was a doctoral student at the time, I soon realized how much of my ego was wrapped up in being in a doctoral program. I began to ask myself some basic questions: "Would people still like me if they didn't know I was highly educated?" More important, "Would I like myself without the persona of the doctoral degree?" As the workshop continued, certain exercises were designed to bring us increased awareness. For instance, we all participated in a two-hour blind walk in which we had an assistant who aided us. During those two hours, we ate lunch (my aide fed me) and walked around the grounds with the help of our assistants. This exercise showed me how I take my able body for granted, how I don't use my senses to the fullest, and how I limit my capabilities in general.

ACTIVITY 1.1   Values Clarification

First, find a partner—someone you don't know well. Tell him or her a little about your life. You might want to talk about such things as how you perceive your future career path, what is important to you in life, how you find meaning in your life, people who have influenced you the most, and events that have had a great impact on you. Try to listen carefully to each other, and when you are finished, do the following activity.*

1. Of the eight human service professional characteristics, rate how important you think each characteristic is for the effective functioning of the human service professional. (Although I believe these qualities are all essential, you may have a different opinion.)
2. Rate yourself next on how well you think you embody these characteristics.
3. Now, here comes the hard part. Have your partner rate you on how well he or she thinks you embodied the characteristics during the role play. (Remember, a person who is Stage 3 on the Kegan scale will want to be liked and will be reticent to rate low, even if he or she really feels that the student should be rated low.)
4. Next, rate yourself based on whether you think you exhibited those qualities as you went through your life today.

5. When you have completed your ratings, examine the scores. Are there areas that you state you value but do not exhibit through your behavior? In other words, have you prized and cherished the things you state you value or are there areas you can improve?
6. Because we all can improve parts of our lives, what ideas do you have to work on those areas? Write them in the last column of the chart. In other words, what action can you take to enhance the values that you state you prize?

When rating, use the scale below. A high rating indicates that you embody the characteristic, believe it is important, or exhibited the particular characteristic today.

1. An extremely high rating
2. A very high rating
3. A moderately high rating
4. A somewhat high rating
5. Neither high nor low
6. A somewhat low rating
7. A moderately low rating
8. A very low rating
9. An extremely low rating

	Importance	Self-Rating	Other's Rating	Exhibit Today?	What You Can Do to Improve Scores
Empathy					
Open-Mindedness					
Acceptance					
Cognitive Complexity					
Psychological Adjustment					
Genuineness					
Relationship Building					
Competence					

*Note: This exercise can also be done by asking someone you know well to complete the ratings.

Workshops like these help us understand what we value and how we define ourselves. They help us focus on those things in our lives that are important to us. For instance, through this workshop, I began to ask myself the following questions: "How important is my doctoral degree in defining me as a person?" "How important is a healthy and able body?" "If it is important, do I tend to treat my body in healthy ways?" Values clarification exercises like these help us identify those parts of ourselves that we treasure and can challenge us to prize, cherish, and treat sacredly those parts of ourselves that we have identified as important. In addition, these exercises teach us to examine why we may not be prizing certain identified values and help us make decisions either to change our values or to find ways in which we can act to embrace those identified values.

Activity 1.1 is an example of a values clarification exercise that pulls together many of the major themes of this chapter. To determine how you value the eight characteristics of the human service professional, whether you embrace the characteristics you value, and what action you can take to enhance the values you identify as important, take a moment to complete this activity.

Because these exercises are important to help you stretch developmentally and, concurrently, to cultivate the human service professional's characteristics, there will be experiential exercises at the end of each chapter to facilitate your own personal growth while you learn some basic facts and principles of the human service field.

ETHICAL, PROFESSIONAL, AND LEGAL ISSUES

Knowing Who We Are and Our Relationship to Other Professional Groups

Human service professionals have a unique identity that is reflected through the field's body of knowledge. By knowing who we are, we also have a clear sense of who we are not. When we identify ourselves as human service professionals, we are able to clearly define our professional limits, know when it is appropriate to consult with colleagues, and recognize when we should refer to other professionals.

> Human service professionals know the limit and scope of their professional knowledge and offer services only within their knowledge and skill base. (See Appendix B, Statement 26).

THE DEVELOPMENTALLY MATURE HUMAN SERVICE PROFESSIONAL

Willing to Meet the Challenge

The developmentally mature (Kegan's Stage 5) human service professional looks at his or her own behavior, risks obtaining feedback from others, and is open to change. This person views life as affording opportunities for growth and transformation. Although this individual's goal may be to embody the characteristics of the effective human service professional, he or she realizes that the "healthy" individual is always "in-process"—that is, he or she realizes that life is a continual, never-ending growth process.

As Perry notes, the developmentally mature individual has commitment in relativism. This person has a clear sense of his or her values relative to the human service profession and knows himself or herself. However, despite this firm sense of self, this person is willing to change if offered other ideas or concepts that make sense. "Firm yet flexible" is this person's credo.

Finally, developmentally mature human service professionals are committed to excellence in themselves and in the profession. Therefore, they look for avenues of personal and professional growth and are willing to give of themselves to promote the profession.

SUMMARY

We began this chapter by defining the human service professional. We briefly discussed the early development of human service education and how it was a response to the need for more helping professionals during the 1960s. We highlighted some of the typical kinds of jobs performed by the human service professional and also delineated some of the differences in focus between the human service professional and other social service professionals. In defining the work of the human service professional, we delineated the 13 roles as identified by SREB as well as the 12 recently identified skills standards.

Comparing and contrasting the human service professional with related mental health professionals was another focus of this chapter. We thus briefly examined some of the roles and functions of psychiatrists, psychologists, social workers, counselors, psychiatric nurses, and psychotherapists. We also highlighted their respective professional associations including the American Psychiatric Association (APA), the American Psychological Association (APA), NASW, the ACA, and APNA. In addition, we paid particular attention to NOHSE, the association of human service educators, practitioners, and students.

The last half of this chapter emphasized the importance of the human service professional embodying the eight characteristics of the effective helper. These include empathy, open mindedness, acceptance, cognitive complexity, psychological adjustment, genuineness, relationship building, and competence. We then discussed how those qualities could be explained through the cognitive development theories of Perry and Kegan. We considered ways of enhancing our personality characteristics while increasing our developmental level. Avenues such as therapy and values clarification exercises were seen as potential vehicles for change because they support and challenge our perceptions of the world. A values clarification exercise was offered to assist students in increasing self-knowledge.

As we neared the conclusion of the chapter, we stressed the importance of knowing our professional identity, for it assists us in defining who we are and in setting professional limits on ourselves. We noted that this ethical and professional issue is highlighted in the Ethical Standards of Human Service Professionals (see Appendix B). Finally, we concluded this chapter by examining what it means to be a developmentally mature human service professional, noting that such an individual is open to change and views life as a continual transformational process. Mature human service professionals are personally and professionally committed to excellence and willing to expend the energy needed to improve both themselves and the profession.

EXPERIENTIAL EXERCISES

1. Comparisons of Social Service Professionals

1. We often have varying perceptions of the training, education, and salary of the different social service professions. To see whether your perceptions are correct, fill in the items requested for the social service professionals listed in the following chart.
2. Obtain a Sunday newspaper and circle all the want ads that are social service oriented. In class, make a list of the types of jobs being advertised; the education, training, and experience needed for the job; and the salary being offered.

	Education	Types of Courses	Additional Training?	Licensed/Certified (Yes/No)	Salary
Human Service Worker					
Psychologist					
Psychiatrist					
Mental Health Counselor					
School Counselor					
College Counselor					
Social Worker					
Psychotherapist					

2. Interviewing Professionals in the Field

Using the following questions as a guideline, have one-fourth of the class interview a human service professional, one-fourth a social worker, one-fourth a psychologist, and the remainder, a counselor. Then, with one student representing each of the disciplines, divide into groups of four. In your small groups, discuss the similarities and differences you find in the professions.

1. Why did he or she decide to enter the chosen profession?
2. What degree(s) was (were) obtained?
3. What is the theoretical orientation of the professional?
4. What are the job roles and functions as defined by the professional?
5. What was his or her entry-level salary?
6. What is his or her current salary?
7. What is his or her view on the differences among the four professions?

3. SREB's 13 Roles and Functions

Using the 13 roles and functions of human service professionals as identified by SREB, describe an activity that might correspond to each role and function. Use the interview completed in Exercise 2 if you need some assistance in identifying specific activities.

1. Outreach worker
2. Broker
3. Advocate
4. Evaluator
5. Teacher/educator
6. Behavior changer
7. Mobilizer
8. Consultant
9. Community planner
10. Caregiver
11. Data manager
12. Administrator
13. Assistant to specialist

4. Discussing the Difference Between Counseling and Psychotherapy

In class, the instructor will put the words *counseling* and *psychotherapy* on the board. Free-associate to these words and the instructor will write these associations on the board. Then, as a class, discuss the differences between the two terms. What do you think the counseling limitations are of the human service professional? Do you think the human service professional does counseling? Refer to Table 1.1 when discussing this question.

5. Joining Professional Associations

What professional association(s) do you want to join? Why might you join one association rather than another?

6. The Characteristics of the Effective Human Service Professional

The following sets of activities have to do with the characteristics you think make an effective human service professional, as well as the qualities you possess that will make you an effective human service professional. To each question, write responses that you can bring to class. In class, you will be given the opportunity to discuss your responses in small groups.

1. Make a list of the personality characteristics you believe the effective human service professional should embody.

2. Make a list of the skills and techniques you think the effective human service professional should have.

3. What personality characteristics do you currently possess that will make you a successful human service professional?

4. What skills do you currently possess that will make you a successful human service professional?

5. Choosing one of the quotes from the chapter, (a) analyze its meaning and (b) discuss, in class, its meaning relative to the eight characteristics of the effective human service professional.

7. Acquiring the Characteristics of the Effective Human Service Professionals

The following sets of questions concern the acquisition of the qualities of the effective human service professional. Write responses for each question that you can bring to class. In class, you will be given the opportunity to discuss your responses in small groups.

1. How have the influences listed below affected your desire to enter the human service field? (If you are not entering the field, base your response on the field you think you will eventually enter.)

   a. Parents' education

   b. Parents' occupations

   c. Placement in family (for example, middle child, youngest child)

   d. Educational experiences

   e. Work experiences

   f. Volunteer experiences

   g. Your values and beliefs

   h. Your gender and ethnic background

2. Often, individuals enter the helping professions because they have gone through their own painful experiences and want to assist others with theirs. What personal experiences have made you sensitive to other individuals' difficult life situations?

3. Many of the eight characteristics of the effective human service professional are developed through modeling the behavior of people who have significantly affected our lives. In the following chart, write the names of four people in your life that have most affected you in a positive way. These individuals can be friends, parents, religious leaders, politicians, movie figures, literary figures, and so on. Then, fill in the chart, noting how the individuals modeled one or more of the characteristics. Finally, in class, share with another student how you have taken on some of the behavior modeled by each person.

SIGNIFICANT PERSON

Characteristic	1.	2.	3.	4.
Empathy				
Open-mindedness				
Acceptance				
Cognitive complexity				
Psychological Adjustment				
Genuineness				
Relationship Building				
Competence				

8. Assessing Your Adult Developmental Level

Directions. The following inventory is designed to give you a self-assessment of your degree of dogmatism, empathy, internality, and openness to feedback. These qualities have been shown to be important in building an effective helping relationship and tend to increase as a function of age, education, and experience. It is extremely important to answer honestly on the instrument. After you have taken the instrument, have your instructor review the importance of these qualities in the helping relationship. The instrument has not been researched to show its validity and should only be used to give you a rough sense of a conglomerate score on these qualities. Use the following scale when responding to each item.

1. Strongly agree   4. Slightly disagree
2. Slightly agree   5. Strongly disagree
3. Neither agree nor disagree

_____ 1. I believe that my opinions are almost always right.

_____ 2. It is not unusual for people to seek me out to talk about their problems.

_____ 3. When I receive feedback from a professor, I almost always learn from it.

_____ 4. The professor almost always has the answer.

_____ 5. In making major life decisions, I usually trust my own "inner sense."

_____ 6. In life, others are usually better at decision making than I am.

_____ 7. Usually, when I try to listen to someone, I make it a point to ask a lot of questions.

_____ 8. The best type of learning takes place when the professor gives us the facts.

_____ 9. The church, synagogue, or mosque I most identify with always espouses the right views.

_____10. When I am listening to someone, I usually know from the opening statement what that person is going to say.

_____11. I can almost always determine the value of a person's belief system based on his or her appearance.

_____12. Usually, my friends' opinions are more important than my own.

_____13. In coming to my views on life, I have spent much time gathering information from others, reflecting, and being introspective.

_____14. Usually, when I am listening to someone who is struggling with an issue, I try to tell him or her what would be the best solution to the problem.

_____15. My views are solid and no one can change them!

_____16. Things that happen in my life are out of my control.

_____17. I have chosen my values following deep reflection; however, I am still open to examining them further.

_____18. Life is what I make it to be.

_____19. When listening to someone, I usually disregard the person's feelings and listen more to "the facts" of the situation.

_____20. Generally, I think students can offer much to the knowledge base of a class.

_____21. I have rarely questioned the views of my parents.

_____22. When in a work group, in an effort to complete tasks efficiently, it is often necessary to make decisions with little or no collaboration.

_____23. Most clients need to be given strong advice and firm direction from the beginning of the helping relationship.

_____24. The most important quality of the helping relationship is understanding the inner world of the client.

Scoring the inventory. For items 2, 3, 5, 13, 17, 18, 20, and 24 give yourself *1* point if your response was a "5," *2* points if your response was a "4," *3* points if your response was a "3," *4* points if your response was a "2," and *5* points if your response was a "1." For all other items, give yourself the number of points that you rated the item. The highest score on this inventory is a 120. The closer you are to this score, the more you are empathic, internally oriented, nondogmatic, open to feedback, and able to view learning as a reciprocal process. Undergraduate students in human services usually average between 75 and 85 on this instrument. In class, your instructor might want you to anonymously hand in your score so you can compare it with the rest of the class. This will give you a sense of your score as it compares with your peers'.

9. Assessing Our Values

In class, divide into triads. In your triad, you will be given the number *1, 2,* or *3.* Those who have been given the number *1* will be "pro," and those who have been given the number *2* will be "con." Number *3*s are to help numbers *1* and *2* if they have trouble doing the task. Your task is to take one of the following situations (or come up with one of your own) and role-play your feelings about the situation. If you are pro, role-play the situation as if you are for it, even if you actually are against it. If you are con, role-play the situation as if you are against it, even if you are for it. It is important not to tell the members of your triad how you actually feel about the situation. Role-play for about 5 minutes.

Then do the same thing, but this time take a new situation; number *2* will be pro, and number *3* will be con. Number *1* will be the helper. Finally, take a third situation and this time, number *3* will be pro, number *1* con, and number *2* will be the helper.

Situations:

1. Abortion
2. Capital punishment
3. Opening an X-rated bookstore in your neighborhood
4. The war on terrorism
5. National health insurance
6. Affirmative action
7. Increased tuition

Processing the exercise. In class, generate a list of reasons why you couldn't effectively listen to the other person at times. For instance, someone might say, "I was so upset that I just wanted to tell the other person how I felt." The instructor can put a list of "hindrances" to effective listening on the board. In class, discuss the following:

1. Why is it difficult to hear someone who holds differing values from your own?
2. How can you learn to accept differing values?

3. What techniques can you use to listen more effectively to an individual who holds values that vary from your own?

4. Why is acceptance of diversity important when you are in the role of helper?

10. Ethical and Professional Vignettes

Read the ethical dilemmas below. Using the *Ethical Standards of Human Service Professionals* in Appendix B, write a response to the dilemma.

1. A human service professional is making disparaging remarks about social workers, saying things like "They don't know what they're doing" and "Their training is inferior." Is this ethical? Professional? Legal? What should you do?

2. You are working with a client who is also seeing another human service professional at a different agency for the same problem. Is this ethical? Is this professional? What should you do?

3. You have heard one of your colleagues make racist remarks. What should you do? What can you do?

4. A colleague of yours seems to have rigid views about his clients and refuses to participate in continuing education activities. He says, "I've been in this field a long time, I know what I'm doing." Is he acting ethically? Professionally? What, if anything, should you do?

5. A client of yours is asking you to advocate for her child who she suspects is learning disabled. Your client asks you to call the school and request testing for the child. The school has thus far refused such testing. Should you do this? Is this ethical? Is this professional?

6. You decide to go to a pro-choice (or pro-life) rally despite the fact that you know some of your clients may see you and be turned off by your political affiliation. Is what you're doing ethical? Professional? Legal?

7. Your agency has implemented a new policy that states that all clients who are using illegal drugs will be reported to the police. You vigorously oppose such a policy and decide to ignore it. Are you acting ethically? Professionally? Legally?

8. A colleague of yours states that she is a credentialed human service professional. Actually, the state in which you work has no credentialing process. Is she acting ethically? Professionally? Legally? What, if anything, should you do?

2

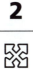

The Human Service Profession: History and Standards

There I was, finishing college as an idealistic, energetic young man trying to decide what to do next. Rather than work, I decided to go to graduate school (although a few years of work experience probably would have been good for me). I knew I wanted to work in the helping professions, so I asked my psychology professors for advice. They suggested I pursue a doctoral degree in psychology. They offered no alternatives—there were no alternatives as far as they were concerned. I thought there must be some other options, so I went to the career center where I was given the same advice. In the early 1970s, these advisers felt there was only one choice for men going into the helping professions—psychology. Now I realize that these good-intentioned advisers were likely sexist, uninformed, and perhaps a little elitist in their views about the helping professions. For them, men became psychologists and women went into social work. For those who couldn't make it into the few doctoral programs in psychology—well, they could become counselors. And at that time, few ever heard of this relatively new profession called human services.

Fortunately, today options are many in the mental health professions; thus, in this chapter, we will explore the history of the fields of psychology, social work, and counseling; examine some of the stereotypes that have emerged based on their histories; and look at how these three fields have greatly affected the emergence of the recent field of human services. We will then examine the relatively short history of the human service profession and see what trends have taken place in this developing field. Finally, we will examine the emergence of standards in the profession and reveal how such standards are a mark of the maturity of a profession.

HISTORY

Why Look at History?

Can you imagine a woman burned as a witch because she was mentally ill, or placed in a straitjacket and thrown into a filthy, rat-infested cell for the remainder of her life? Can you envision a man placed in a bathtub filled with iron filings to cure him of mental illness; or bled to rid him of demons and spirits that caused him to think in "demonic ways"? What about having a piece of your brain scraped out to change the way you feel? These examples are a part of the history of our profession.

Unfortunately, I've taught long enough to know that when history is approached, it often is not as interesting as what you just read. In fact, my experience has been that half the class mentally steps out. Why is this? Learning names, dates, and a few facts is just plain boring for many people. If you're a student who is dreading this chapter, you may be asking yourself, "Why learn it?"

In 1962, **T. S. Kuhn** wrote a book called *The Structure of Scientific Revolutions.* This book had a profound effect on me because it helped put my ideas about knowledge and change in perspective. In particular, Kuhn's concept of the **paradigm shift** intrigued me. He said that knowledge builds upon itself and that new discoveries are based on the evolution of past knowledge. However, Kuhn went

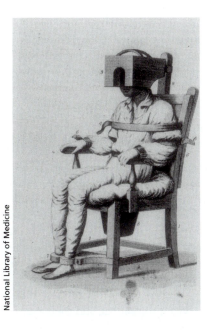

Early treatment of the mentally ill

on to note that sometimes current knowledge does not adequately explain the way things work. At this time, circumstances are ripe for a change in our understanding of the world—ripe for a paradigm shift. For instance, for hundreds of years individuals were at ease with the concept that the earth is flat. However, the advent of new scientific equipment seemed to contradict this model of viewing the world. A new explanation was needed. Thus, it was explained that the earth must be round. Similarly, in the social sciences, past theories adequately worked for a while. For instance, for many years psychoanalysis was the treatment of choice for mental illness. However, research on the effectiveness of treatments and the advent of new theories and new treatment procedures revealed that psychoanalysis often should not be the treatment of choice. In other words, a paradigm shift took place in the mental health field.

The human service field has had and will have paradigm shifts. By studying the history of the field and by gaining knowledge about its roots, perhaps you will be the person to develop the next paradigm shift!

Antecedents to the Human Services Profession

Since the dawn of time, people have attempted to understand the human condition. Before the advent of religion, people used myths, magic, beliefs in spirits, ritualism, and sacred art as implements for thought and introspection and to make sense out of this complex world—"tools with which to think, talk, and know about self and world" (Ellwood, 1993, p. 20). Over the centuries, **shamans,** or individuals who had special status because of their mystical powers, were considered to be caretakers of the soul and were thought to have knowledge of the future. Later in history, the concept of soul gave way to the concept of psyche.

The modern day understanding of the psyche began to emerge in the last 200 years and has been applied by a number of professions related to human services, including counseling, social work, and psychology. The human service profession emerged much more recently and has drawn heavily from the fields of counseling, social work, and psychology:

> The human service knowledge base is derived as much from psychology, guidance and counseling, nursing, etc., as it is from social work. (Clubok, 1984, p. 3)

Today, we can see that the human service profession has borrowed an understanding of the counseling process and a rich appreciation for testing and research from the field of psychology; a deep caring for the underprivileged and an awareness of the power of social and family systems from the social work profession; and a holistic and wellness approach that attempts to understand the individual within the context of his or her career, love relationships, and group interactions from the counseling profession. Although, today, these fields share much in common, their somewhat divergent histories have strongly affected the human service professional. In the following sections, we will briefly examine the history of these three fields, discuss how they affect today's human service professional, and then examine the recent history of the human services.

A Brief History of the Psychology Profession   The field of psychology has a rich history founded in religion, philosophy, and science, and the concepts that have evolved from psychology are often seen as representing the underpinnings of many, if not all, of the social service fields today. As you review the following condensed history of the field of psychology, consider how much of what you read may have affected the work of today's human service professional.

Hippocrates (B.C.E. 460–377) was one of the first individuals in recorded history to reflect on the human condition. Whereas many of his contemporaries believed that possession by evil spirits was responsible for emotional ills, Hippocrates thought differently, and some of his suggestions for the treatment of the human condition might even be considered modern by today's standards. For instance, for melancholia he recommended sobriety, a regular and tranquil life, exercise short of fatigue, and bleeding, if necessary. For hysteria, he recommended marriage—an idea with which many in today's world would certainly argue.

As with Hippocrates, one might think that some of Plato's (B.C.E. 427–347) ideas came right out of a text on modern psychoanalysis. He believed that introspection and reflection were the keys to understanding knowledge and reality and that dreams and fantasies were substitutes for desires not satisfied. In addition, he considered problems of the human condition to have physical, moral, and spiritual origins. Although Plato's views were enlightening, some consider his student Aristotle (B.C.E. 384–322) to be the first psychologist because he attempted to objectively study knowledge and his writings were psychological in nature (Wertheimer, 1978). In fact, he wrote essays on how people learn through association and the role that the senses play in learning.

Although individuals such as **Augustine** (354–430 C.E.) and **Thomas Aquinas** (1225–1274 C.E.) highlighted consciousness, self-examination, and inquiry as philosophies that dealt with the human condition, there were actually very few records of innovative thinking regarding the psychology of the mind during the 800 years between them. This was partly the result of the rise of Christianity, which renewed the focus on the supernatural and advanced a movement away from any attempts to view the person objectively, as Aristotle had proposed. Following this quiet period in the history of science, the Renaissance and the era of modern philosophy arose in Europe. Here was a rediscovery of the Greek philosophies and a renewed interest in questions regarding the nature of the human condition.

Soon after the Renaissance, we saw the beginnings of modern psychology. In the early to mid-1800s individuals like **Wilhelm Wundt** (1832–1920) and **Sir Francis Galton** (1822–1911), two of the first experimental psychologists, developed laboratories to examine physical differences among people for such things as height, head size, and reaction time. The natural outgrowth of this movement was the testing era, where individuals' traits and abilities were compared with each other using tests. The rise of the testing movement saw individuals like **Alfred Binet** (1857–1911) develop the first individual intelligence test, which was used to help the French Department of Education separate those children who were "normal" from those who were "abnormal" (Hothersall, 1995). Later, ability tests such as school achievement tests and personality tests were developed. Today, tests are found everywhere and are often an important component to a deeper understanding of our clients.

The beginnings of the testing movement paralleled the rise of psychoanalysis, the first comprehensive approach to doing therapy. Developed by Sigmund Freud (1856–1939), psychoanalysis held the new view that an individual's problems may in part have psychological origins. Freud was greatly influenced by people like **Franz Mesmer** (1734–1815) (from whom the word mesmerize was derived), who were practicing a new phenomenon called hypnosis. Until this time, mental illness was generally thought to be of a physical nature, and the treatment of mental illness often was quite odd (see Box 2.1). However, when some individuals with certain kinds of physical illnesses were placed under a hypnotic trance, their ailments would disappear, suggesting the illness had psychological origins. Freud later gave up the use of hypnosis and developed psychoanalysis, which attempted to explain the origins of human behavior. His new view on mental health and mental illness was revolutionary and continues to profoundly affect the ways in which we conceptualize client problems (Appignanesi & Oscar, 1999).

Freud's theory, which tended to be somewhat pessimistic concerning the nature of the individual and the ability of people to change, emphasized instincts and early child-rearing patterns in understanding personality development. Partly in response to Freud's bleak views concerning the individual's development, contemporaries and students of his such as **Alfred Adler** (1870–1937) and **Erik Erikson** (1902–1994) developed theories that were more humanistically based and stressed the influences of social forces on the development of the individual.

BOX 2.1   The Beginnings of the Modern Mental Hospital

In 1773, the "Publik Hospital for Persons of Insane and Disordered Minds" admitted its first patient in Williamsburg, Virginia. The hospital, which had 24 cells, took a rather bleak approach to working with the mentally ill. Although many of the staff of these first hospitals had good intentions, their diagnostic and treatment procedures left much to be desired. For instance, some of the leading reasons that patients were admitted included masturbation, womb disease, religious fervor, intemperance, and domestic trouble—hardly reasons we'd use today for admission to a mental institution. Normal treatment procedures were to administer heavy dosages of drugs, to bleed or blister individuals, to immerse individuals in freezing water for long periods, and to confine people with straitjackets or manacles. Bleeding and blistering were thought to remove harmful fluids from the individual's system (Zwelling, 1990). It was believed important to cause fear in a person, and even individuals like **Dr. Benjamin Rush,** known for his innovative and relatively benign treatment of the mentally ill, spoke of the importance of staring a person down:

The first object of a physician, when he enters the cell or chamber of his deranged patient, should be, to catch his EYE . . . The dread of the eye was early imposed upon every beast of the field. . . . Now a man deprived of his reason partakes so much of the nature of those animals, that he is for the most part terrified, or composed, by the eye of a man who possesses his reason. (cited in Zwelling, 1990, p. 17)

Although many believed in these rather extreme procedures with the mentally ill, some tried tirelessly to employ more humane methods. **John Minson Galt II,** the hospital's administrator from 1841 to 1862, believed that comfortable surroundings, social interaction, and job-related activities could help the mentally ill get better. **Dorothea Dix** also fought for humane treatment of the mentally ill and helped to establish 41 "modern" mental institutions.

Today, there are many approaches to psychotherapy, a good number of which are an outgrowth of or a reaction to Freud's psychoanalytic approach. (See Chapters 3 and 5 for a further discussion of Freud and psychoanalysis.)

The 20th century has seen a great expansion in the field of psychology. Today, we still find experimental psychologists working in laboratories trying to understand the psychophysiological causes of behavior and clinical psychologists working directly with clients doing therapy. In addition, we find other highly trained psychologists doing testing in schools, working for business and industry on organizational concerns, and working in many other areas.

The American Psychological Association (APA), which was founded by G. Stanley Hall more than 100 years ago, has expanded dramatically and today is a major force in the social service field (Sokal, 1992). For instance, APA offers divisions for individuals who have an interest in just about any aspect of psychology, lobbies for a wide array of mental health concerns, and publishes numerous research journals through which an attempt is made to understand human behavior. Along with the American Psychiatric Association, APA has supported the development and continued refinement of the *Diagnostic and Statistical Manual of Mental Disorders–Text Revision (DSM-IV-TR)* (APA, 2000). This manual is instrumental in helping the clinician understand the individual, and insurance companies use it for diagnosis when processing mental health claims.

Although in the beginning the field of psychology was dominated by white men, recently we have seen the emergence of women and minorities as prominent psychologists. Along with the field of psychiatry, psychology has been one of the most important fields that has attempted to unravel some of the mysteries toward the understanding of mental health and mental illness. Today, the field of psychology continues to lead the way in the development of new theories of working with the individual and of attempting to explain normal and abnormal behavior.

Psychology's Impact on the Human Service Field For the human service professional, the field of psychology has had many practical implications. From providing the theoretical underpinnings that help us understand the nature of the person, to assisting us to understand human behavior, to helping us find better ways of working with our clients, the field of psychology has been a major force in the social sciences. Psychologists often may be our employers, our supervisors, our colleagues, or individuals with whom we consult. Acknowledging their relationship to our beginnings is important.

A Brief History of the Social Work Profession The emergence of the social work field grew out of concern for the underprivileged and deprived in society. In contrast with the psychology field, which focused more on understanding the nature of the person, the field of social work originated in the desire to help the destitute.

In England, until the 16th century, providing relief to the poor was voluntary and usually overseen by the church. However, given the dismal social conditions, the English government, under Henry VIII, established one of the first systems of social welfare (Burger & Youkeles, 2000). The **Poor Laws** of 1601 established local "overseers of the poor" within each parish. These individuals were responsible for finding work for the poor, aiding those who could not work, and providing shelter or **almshouses** for those who were incapable of taking care of themselves. Although crude in its initial establishment, this law later became a model for social welfare programs. As a carryover from the English system, during the colonial period, local governments in the United States enacted laws to help the poor. During this same time, organized charities, usually affiliated with a religious group, arose in the United States.

During the 1800s, as populations in cities grew, an increasingly large underclass developed in the United States. Because the traditional charitable organizations could not meet the needs of these individuals, politicians applied mounting pressure to create specialized institutions. Thus, reform schools, lunatic asylums, and other specialized institutions were established.

Two major approaches arose to help the underprivileged who were not institutionalized. **Charity organization societies (COSs)** maintained a list of volunteers who would enter the poorer districts of cities, become acquainted with the people, aid in educating the children, give economic advice, and generally assist in alleviating the conditions of poverty. Usually, the poor were not given money but were given advice, support, and, at times, a few "necessities." The volunteers, who were often called **friendly visitors,** also stressed moral judgment and religious values. Sometimes these friendly visitors would spend years assisting one family. The COSs are seen as the beginning of social casework, which is the process by which the needs of a client are examined and a treatment plan is designed.

In contrast to the COSs, the **settlement movement** had staff members who actually lived in the communities in which they sought to help the poor and immigrants:

> The settlements claimed to deal in brotherhood, not philanthropy; their spirit was fraternalistic, not paternalistic. . . . The settlement worker, [stated Jane Addams] . . . learned not alone from firsthand observation and the compiling of evidence but from sharing the common lot of the disinherited; the resident must "have genuine sympathy and continued relations with those who work day after day, year after year." Through a shared life, the settlement workers would come in time, not to speak for the slum dwellers, but to help them "express themselves and make articulate their desires." (quotes from Addams, 1911, p. 310) (Chambers, 1963, p. 15)

These idealistic young staff members believed in community action and tried to persuade politicians to provide better services for the poor. One of the best-known settlement houses was **Hull House,** established by **Jane Addams** in 1899 in Chicago (Addams, 1911; Macht, 1990). Addams was a social activist known for her liberal views and progressive ideas.

Out of this involvement with the underprivileged came articles and books concerned with methods of adequately meeting the needs of the underclass. Following the development of these "casebooks," and spearheaded by **Mary Richmond** at the turn of the century, the first social work training program was established at Columbia University. By 1919, there were 17 such programs in the country. During the next 30 years, the social work field grew in many different directions, with some of its main areas focusing on social casework, social group work, and community work.

Starting in the 1940s and continuing to the present, an increased emphasis on understanding social and family systems has emerged in this country. Because social workers had already been intimately working with social systems and with families, this increased emphasis on the functioning and dynamics of these systems became a natural focus for many social work programs. Such programs were the first to view the individual in a contextual or systems framework, rather than seeing the individual in isolation as did many of the early philosophers and psychologists. One social worker in particular, **Virginia Satir** (1967), was instrumental in reshaping some of the practices of the mental health profession by including a greater systems focus.

In 1955, a number of social work organizations combined to form the National Association of Social Workers (NASW). In 1960, NASW established the Academy of Certified Social Workers (ACSW), which set standards of practice in the field for master's-level social workers. Today, NASW has 155,000 members, of which approximately 61,000 are certified social workers. Social workers can be

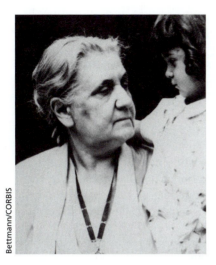

Bettmann/CORBIS

Jane Addams, one of the first "modern day" social workers, was a social activist known for her humane and liberal ways.

found in a variety of social service settings from hospitals, to mental health centers, to homeless shelters—the roots of the social work profession. In addition, although many social workers today do individual psychotherapy and family therapy, some work in community settings doing advocacy work and others administer social service organizations.

Because the social work field grew out of charity organizations and volunteerism and because women in the 1800s did not work outside the home, many women found their sense of meaning through these charitable efforts. Thus, for many years the field had the reputation of being a "woman's occupation." Recently, this has drastically changed as the field and American values have transformed.

Social Work's Impact on the Human Service Field The field of social work brings much to the human service profession. The beginnings of the social work field in many ways echo the essence of much of what today's human service professional does. Like the early social worker, today's human service professional helps the poor, the deprived, the underprivileged, and the mentally ill. And, like the early social worker, much of the human service professional's major emphasis is on support, advocacy, and caretaking. On a more practical level, the social work field has taught us casework approaches, how to work with systems, how to advocate for our clients, and the importance of respect and caring for our clients. One might say that the human service professional of today has taken on many of the functions and roles that the social worker used to embrace. Today, like psychologists, social workers are often our supervisors, administrators, colleagues, or consultants. The human service field is clearly a cousin to the social work profession.

A Brief History of the Counseling Profession The Industrial Revolution, which began in the United States after the Civil War, changed the social and economic structure of the country. Many rural Americans, as well as immigrants—most of whom came from Europe to escape oppression—were drawn to urban factory centers in search of a better life. By the turn of the 20th century, we saw the spread of the use of tests. These events set the stage for the very beginning of the counseling profession, which at that time was focused on vocational guidance. Teachers and administrators were soon using tests in the schools to help individuals understand their skills and abilities and to "guide" them to appropriate professions. One of the leaders of this guidance movement was **Frank Parsons**, often said to be the founder of vocational guidance (Jones, 1994; McDaniels & Watts, 1994; Parsons, 1989). These events led to the founding in 1913 of the **National Vocational Guidance Association** (NVGA), considered the forerunner of the American Counseling Association (ACA). As early as 1911, Harvard offered the first graduate courses for guidance specialists, and soon after, in Boston and New York, counselors were certified (Gladding, 2000).

Until the 1940s, most "counselors" were still doing vocational guidance. But during this decade, Carl Rogers (1942, 1951) and his nondirective, humanistic approach greatly affected the field of counseling. This client-centered revolution dramatically changed the way counselors were working, and they soon were giving less advice, focusing more on the "here and now," doing less testing and evaluation, and doing more facilitating. This **humanistic** approach to counseling starkly contrasted with the psychoanalytic approach of Freud. With the advent of World War II came an increased need for counselors and psychologists to work with war veterans. Thus, we soon saw counselors working outside the schools, practicing this new humanistic approach to counseling.

Probably the decade that most affected the counseling field was the 1950s. The **National Defense Education Act (NDEA)** of 1958 was a direct response to the Soviet Union's launching of humankind's first satellite, *Sputnik,* and funded the expansion of school counseling programs to identify gifted students. As a result, school counselors at the middle and secondary levels proliferated. The **American Personnel and Guidance Association (APGA)** was also founded during this decade. APGA was formed out of NVGA and other related counseling associations that were prevalent at the time.

In the 1960s, President Johnson's **Great Society** initiatives funded many social service programs. Partly in response to the greater need for counselors, the field diversified and counselors were increasingly found working in mental health, rehabilitation, higher education, and other related disciplines. In this decade, the **Association for Counselor Education and Supervision (ACES),** a division of APGA, delineated standards for a master's-level counseling program (Sweeney, 1992). Also in this decade, differing types of group counseling expanded.

The end of the 1960s decade and the beginning of the 1970s saw a new approach to training counselors, known as "microcounseling skills training" (Carkhuff, 1969; Egan, 1975; Ivey & Gluckstein, 1974). These packaged ways of counselor training showed that basic counseling skills could be learned in a relatively short amount of time and that the practice of such skills would positively affect the counseling relationship (Neukrug, 1980).

During the 1980s and into the 1990s, the counseling field continued to expand. To reflect the greater emphasis on counseling and prevention, APGA changed its name to the **American Association for Counseling and Development (AACD).** More recently, AACD underwent another name change to the more streamlined ACA. Today, counselors can be found in almost any setting in which there are mental health professionals. ACA now has nearly 52,000 members and 17 divisions that represent the specialty areas in counseling. Almost 500 graduate programs now train counselors (Hollis & Dodson, 2000). Also, in these decades, certification and state licensure expanded. Currently, there are almost 140,000 credentialed counselors, and almost every state has licensure for counselors (Neukrug, Milliken, & Walden, 2001).

Counseling's Impact on the Human Service Field The counseling field has had a major impact on the human service field. The humanistic approach to the individual, which tends to be the focus of most counseling programs, is also pervasive in human service education. The concept that counseling skills or techniques can be taught in a systematic and focused manner is now a common method of training in most human service programs. In addition, counseling programs and many human service programs have stressed the importance of career as a major life force. Finally, a developmental focus, as well as an emphasis on the importance of support, education, and training can also be found in many human service programs.

The Emerging Need for Human Service Practitioners

In the late 1940s Congress created the **National Institute of Mental Health (NIMH).** This was the first real effort by the federal government to examine mental health issues, and it resulted in a systematic effort to do research and training in the mental health field. On the heels of the creation of NIMH came the **Mental Health Study Act** of 1955, which was a broadly based effort to study the diagnosis and treatment of mental illness. On the basis of the research from this act, Congress passed the **Community Mental Health Centers Act** of 1963. This bill greatly changed the delivery of mental health services in the United States by providing federal funds for the creation of comprehensive mental health centers across the country.

Although mental health centers may seem commonplace in today's society, the concept of having treatment centers available to the general public for mental health concerns is relatively new. Community mental health centers have greatly changed the face of mental health services across the country by supporting the use of paraprofessionals in the delivery of some services, by advocating for deinstitutionalization and the care of the chronically mentally ill within local municipalities, and by supporting the concept of primary prevention, which involves educating the public about mental health problems before they arise. Today, community mental health centers are a common place to find the human service professional.

The 1960s saw great upheaval in American society. There was unrest in the ghettos and a country in bitter turmoil over the Vietnam War. The civil rights movement was growing in momentum. Martin Luther King, Jr., Robert Kennedy, and others were advocating new directions for the country. Both were slain. It is often said that change cannot occur without pain. The death of some of our greatest leaders is perhaps a sad acknowledgment of this truth. Out of the turmoil of the 1960s came landmark civil rights and social change legislation (Diambra, 2001; Osher, 1990). As a result of President Johnson's Great Society legislation, civil rights laws and economic and social laws were passed:

> Service programs were intended to provide the resources and skills that would allow many poor and near poor individuals to compete for jobs effectively. Much of the emphasis was on youth and on education and training programs. Some of the key legislative changes included the Manpower Development and Training Act, Job Corps, Elementary and Secondary Education Act, Head Start, and the Work Incentive Program.
>
> The effort at reshaping the environment extended to the social and economic fabric of the community as well as its physical contours. Various types of discrimination were outlawed. . . . Key legislative actions included the . . . Economic Opportunity Act of 1964, the Public Works and Economic Act of 1965, the Civil Rights Act of 1964, the Voting Rights Act of 1965, and the Model Cities Program of 1966. (Kaplan & Cuciti, 1986, p. 3)

The Reagan administration of the 1980s and into the early 1990s oversaw the elimination or reduction of some human services programs and a move toward federal **block grants.** Instead of the federal government designating which programs states should fund, block grants gave a "block" of money to the states and allowed them to decide which programs to fund. In addition, during this period, there was a stress on volunteerism, and many suggested that business and industry address some of the social woes of the country. The efficacy of this move continues to be in dispute. Despite these efforts to change social policy, many of the programs of the 1960s and 1970s have lasted (Osher, 1990).

The early 1990s were ushered in with promises by President Clinton to "focus like a laser beam" on the economy. And indeed, the economy flourished in the mid- to late-1990s. However, as is evidenced by the continued large number of homeless people, high poverty rates, the lack of or poor health care for a substantial number of citizens, and violence that seems to permeate our society, deep social problems still exist.

Now, as we move into the 21st century, we are faced with a series of new problems. As terrorism strikes the American homeland, President Bush commits himself to the War on Terrorism. Will the effort toward this war deplete resources for human services? Or, might such a war highlight the need that we have as a country, or indeed as a world, for increased services for the poor, desolate, and mentally ill, thus ultimately increasing the need for human service professionals.

The Development of Human Service Programs

Partly because of the social changes that started with the creation of the NIMH and the changes as the result of the turmoil of the 1960s, the human service field emerged (Diambra, 2001; McClam, 1997b). The many federally funded programs and the increased focus on mental health concerns resulted in a need for additional mental health workers and other social service personnel. With this new focus on comprehensive mental health and the diversity of social service agencies, not only was there a need for the highly trained master's- and doctoral-level professionals but there was also a demand for associate's- and bachelor's-level human service professionals. Around this time **Dr. Harold McPheeters** (see Box 2.2) of the Southern Regional Education Board (SREB) applied for and received a grant from NIMH for the development of mental health programs at community colleges in the southern region of the country (McPheeters, 1990). This was the beginning of the associate's-level human service degree in the United States. Therefore, some consider McPheeters to be the "founder" of the human services field.

More recently, we have seen the rise of the bachelor's-level degree in human services (Clubok, 1984, 1997; Diambra, 2001; Fullerton, 1990a, 1990b). These programs were a response to an increased need for professionalism as well as a desire to offer an additional educational path for associate's-level human service majors. With funding from NIMH and SREB, during the mid-1970s several workshops and conferences were offered throughout the country that explored the possibility of offering a bachelor's degree in human services—a degree that would offer professional training in the human services that borrowed from the knowledge base of psychology, social work, and counseling. Although these three fields all explored the possibility of offering a bachelor's-level degree in the mental health professions, ACA and APA ultimately moved toward training graduate-level professionals only, and although NASW developed both bachelor's and graduate programs in social work, the numbers of bachelor's-level social work students did not fill the need that existed for bachelor's-level mental health workers. Thus evolved the human service profession (Fullerton, 1990a, 1990b).

Early in the formation of the human service degree came the establishment of the **Council for Standards in Human Service Education (CSHSE).** Today, this council offers a variety of services for both associate's- and bachelor's-level human service programs. Although a detailed list of some of these services can be found in Appendix C, a summary of the major functions of this council include the following:

- Approving undergraduate human service programs
- Providing directory of human service education programs
- Providing special reports and a monograph series in the human services
- Providing workshops and conferences for human service education
- Advocating for the establishment of standards in the profession

---

BOX 2.2   A Conversation with Dr. Harold McPheeters

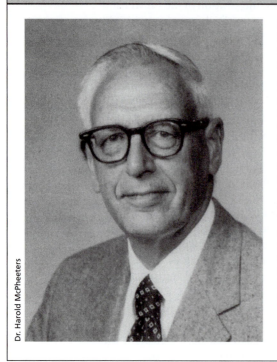

Dr. Harold McPheeters

Question: I think what is particularly interesting is that when the movement started it really was related to several factors that appeared to be unrelated.

McPheeters: Well, there were several things that made it an opportune thing to do. There was rampant professionalism that said "it's got to be done this way or it won't be right." The "great society" with its pressure for more manpower was clearly in conflict with that approach. There were a lot of other things that also came together. The new careers movement, the "hire now, train later" movement, was strong at that point. The movement was seen as a way for minorities and persons from deprived backgrounds to make it into human services. Otherwise, those groups tended to be excluded from the education programs and from the professions. There were civil rights issues that added to the pressure of the development of human services. (McClam & Woodside, 1989, pp. 3–4)

Paralleling the establishment of CSHSE, the National Organization for Human Service Education (NOHSE) was founded in 1975 with its mission being to serve the needs of human service educators and provide a vehicle for the development of local and national organizations for students and human service professionals (Clubok, 1990).

Today, CSHSE and NOHSE work hand in hand to set program standards, develop credentialing processes, to offer workshops and conferences, to provide ethical guidelines, to offer professional journals and newsletters, and to provide an opportunity for networking and mentoring in the field. No doubt, both CSHSE and NOHSE have been setting the standards for professionalism in the human service field (Clubok, 1987; DiGiovanni, 2001; McClam, 1999).

The Human Service Professional Today: A Generalist

The human service professional today is seen as a generalist who draws from all the major mental health fields (McPheeters, 1990; Diambra, 2000, 2001). As defined by McPheeters and King in 1971, this definition still holds:

Works with a limited number of clients or families in consultation with other professionals to provide "across the board" human services as needed; is able to work in a variety of agencies and organizations that provide mental health services; is able to work cooperatively with all of the existing professions in the field rather than affiliating directly with any one; is familiar with a number of therapeutic services and techniques rather than specializing in one or two areas; and is a "beginning professional" who is expected to continue to grow and learn (p. 10). (Clubok, 1984, p. 2)

The human service professional today is a professional who has completed a defined curriculum of study at the associate's or bachelor's level. Drawing from psychology, social work, and counseling, this professional has gained knowledge in an integrated fashion from all three fields. Because of the cross-training that occurs, the human service professional is probably well equipped to work side by side and consult with social workers, counselors, psychologists, as well as other mental health professionals. As a professional with a broad-based background, the human service professional is often the important link between the client and the more highly skilled social worker, counselor, or psychologist.

STANDARDS IN THE PROFESSION

The development of professional standards is an indication that a profession has matured and has taken a serious look at where it's been, where it is, and where it wants to go. As standards evolve, professions can reflect upon, revise, and sometimes even eliminate their standards. Despite the fact that many of the helping professions have been in existence for more than 100 years, the development of standards is relatively new and reflects the fact that the helping professions have only recently moved into the establishment phase of their existence (Bradley, 1991). Standards in the profession can take many forms, with four of the more prominent ones including: (1) **skills standards,** (2) **credentialing,** (3) **ethical standards,** and (4) **program accreditation.** Let's examine how these professional standards in the human services have been established and how they currently affect the delivery of services in the profession.

Skills Standards

The primary purposes of the Skill Standards Project are to foster the adoption of national, voluntary skill standards for direct service workers, to increase both horizontal and vertical career opportunities for human service personnel, and to create a foundation for a nationally recognized, voluntary certification of direct services practitioners. The project is based on the assumption that the development of skill standards in the human service field is a critical step toward strengthening educational and training programs, improving responsiveness to service participants, increasing the marketability of workers, and enhancing the effectiveness and quality of services. (Taylor, Bradley, & Warren, 1996, p. 1)

During the 1990s, a massive effort was undertaken to identify the job characteristics of the human service professional and develop a list of skills that would reflect these job characteristics. To develop these skills standards, an in-depth job analysis was undertaken of human service professionals in four locations across the United States and was validated through a national survey of more than 1,000 individuals involved in human services. The result of this effort was the identification of 12 competency areas that are typically performed by human service professionals, a set of skills or job functions related to each competency, and activity statements or tasks that the human service professional would undertake to fulfill the job functions (Taylor, Bradley, & Warren, 1996).

Competency Areas ⟶ Skills ⟶ Tasks
(Job Functions) (Activity Statements)

As one example, for the competency of "communication," one skill would be to use "effective, sensitive, communication skills to build rapport" (Taylor, Bradley, & Warren, 1996, p. 26) and one activity (task) to accomplish this skill would be to use active listening skills. Table 2.1 defines the 12 competency areas. Can you identify possible skills and tasks that might be used for each of these competency areas?

Credentialing

The credentialing of a professional is one method of assuring minimum competence in a field. Credentialing provides many benefits including

- Increasing the status of those credentialed
- Helping to identify the roles and functions of a profession
- Helping to identify those individuals who are appropriately trained
- Offering a potential avenue for complaints against professionals (Bloom, 1997; Remley, 1991)

Three types of credentialing are **registration, certification,** and **licensure.** Generally regulated by state or national legislation, or by professional association, registration is less restrictive than certification, which is less restrictive than licensure.

Many states register, certify, or license varying professional groups, but requirements differ from state to state. For example, whereas one state might license a psychologist who has two years of postdoctoral experience, another state might only require one year of postdoctoral experience. Although in most states human service professionals are not registered, certified, or licensed, as the profession becomes more solidly defined, we will likely see the beginnings of such a process. In addition, on a state-to-state basis, opportunities may arise for human service professionals to become certified or registered in related fields. For example, in Virginia, as in many other states, the human service professional can become a certified substance abuse counselor if he or she meets the educational and supervisory experience requirements. (For a comprehensive examination of the types of credentialing, see Vroman & Bloom, 1991.)

Table 2.1 Competency Areas for Skills Standards

Competency 1: Participant Empowerment

The competent community support human service practitioner (CSHSP) enhances the ability of the participant to lead a self-determining life by providing the support and information necessary to build self-esteem and assertiveness, and to make decisions. (p. 21)

Competency 2: Communication

The community support human service practitioner should be knowledgeable about the range of effective communication strategies and skills necessary to establish a collaborative relationship with the participant. (p. 26)

Competency 3: Assessment

The community support human service practitioner should be knowledgeable about formal and informal assessment practices to respond to the needs, desires and interests of the participants. (p. 29)

Competency 4: Community and Service Networking

The community support human service practitioner should be knowledgeable about the formal and informal supports available in his or her community and skilled in assisting the participant to identify and gain access to such supports. (p. 35)

Competency 5: Facilitation of Services

The community support human service practitioner is knowledgeable about a range of participatory planning techniques and is skilled in implementing plans in a collaborative and expeditious manner. (p. 40)

Competency 6: Community and Living Skills and Supports

The community support human service practitioner has the ability to match specific supports and interventions to the unique needs of individual participants and recognizes the importance of friends, family, and community relationships. (p. 45)

Competency 7: Education, Training, and Self-Development

The community support human service practitioner should be able to identify areas for self-improvement, pursue necessary educational/training resources, and share knowledge with others. (p. 51)

Competency 8: Advocacy

The community support human service practitioner should be knowledgeable about the diverse challenges facing participants (e.g., human rights, legal, administrative, and financial) and should be able to identify and use effective advocacy strategies to overcome such challenges. (p. 54)

Competency 9: Vocational, Educational, and Career Support

The community support human service practitioner should be knowledgeable about the career and education related concerns of the participant and should be able to mobilize the resources and support necessary to assist the participant to reach his or her goals. (p. 57)

Competency 10: Crisis Intervention

The community support human service practitioner should be knowledgeable about crisis prevention, intervention, and resolution techniques and should match such techniques to particular circumstances and individuals. (p. 60)

Competency 11: Organizational Participation

The community-based support worker is familiar with the mission and practices of the support organization and participates in the life of the organization. (p. 63)

Competency 12: Documentation

The community-based support worker is aware of the requirements for documentation in his or her organization and is able to manage these requirements efficiently. (p. 67)

SOURCE: Taylor, Bradley, & Warren, 1996. Reprinted by permission of the Cambridge Human Services Research Institute.

Registration Registration is the most basic form of ensuring minimum competence for a profession and implies that an individual has met minimum competence, such as having obtained a degree or doing an apprenticeship (Sweeney, 1991). States will often set minimum education or training requirements and will require individuals to register before they can practice within the state.

Certification Certification is considered more rigorous than registration and involves the formal recognition that an individual within a professional group has met certain predetermined standards of professionalism (Forrest & Stone, 1991). States or national organizations usually set the requirements for certification. Besides requiring minimum education or training as in registration, an exam is often mandatory. For example, becoming a National Certified Counselor (NCC) or a member of the ACSW requires obtaining a master's degree in the respective field and passing a national exam. Recently, a movement has been afoot to establish a national certification process for human service professionals that would be based on the Skills Standards just described (Mary DiGiovanni, personal communication, May 31, 2002)

Licensure The most rigorous form of credentialing is licensure. Whereas certification protects the title only, licensure generally defines the scope of what an individual can and cannot do. States generally set the standards for this most rigorous form of credentialing, and it requires a minimum educational level, usually a state or national exam, and additional documentation of expertise such as evidence of posteducation supervision. States may vary considerably on their requirements for licensure. For example, the requirements as a professional counselor will vary from state to state, with some states requiring a national exam, a submission of a case report, and possibly an oral hearing, whereas other states require only an exam. Because of the idiosyncrasies in licensure from state to state, it is best to contact the licensing board of a particular state to determine its requirements.

In reference to registration and certification of human service professionals, McPheeters noted that, although CSHSE has in the past encouraged the registration of human service professionals and at one point attempted to establish a national certification process, there has been little support for their efforts. However, as the human service profession becomes more established, no doubt registration, if not certification, will become inevitable (Clubok, 1990; McClam, 1999).

Ethical Standards

The fields of psychology, social work, and counseling have a long history of fighting social injustices while supporting what some might consider to be "moral correctness." Deciding what is morally correct, however, is not always easy. Consider the varying laws on obscenity around the country. The U.S. Supreme Court stated that local municipalities have the right to set their own standards concerning what is considered obscene (see *Miller v. California,* 1973). Apparently, the Court recognized that the various municipalities around the country might view obscenity differently. Look at how the many religions of the world vary in their stands on such issues as abortion, homosexuality, premarital sex, the right of suicide for the terminally ill, and alcohol consumption. What may on the surface appear to be a matter of black and white or right or wrong is filled with complexities and a lot of gray.

In developing ethical guidelines, those charged with the formation of such standards have likely wrestled with which societal and professional values the guidelines should reflect (see Neukrug, 1996; Neukrug, Lovell, & Parker, 1996). Despite this, it is interesting to note that three of the major helping professions—psychology, social work, and counseling—have developed ethical guidelines that stress similar values while serving a number of other general purposes (Ansell, 1984; Corey et al., 2003; Loewenberg & Dolgoff, 1996; Mabe & Rollin, 1986; VanZandt, 1990):

- They protect consumers and further the professional stance of the organizations.

- They denote the fact that a particular profession has a body of knowledge and skills that it can proclaim and that a set of standards can be established that reflect this knowledge.

- They are a vehicle for professional identity and provide an indication of the maturity of a profession.

- They profess a belief that the professional should exhibit certain types of behaviors that reflect the underlying values considered desirable in the professional.

- They offer the professional a framework in the sometimes-difficult ethical and professional decision-making process.

- They represent, in case of litigation, some measure of defense for professionals who conscientiously practice in accordance with accepted professional codes.

Although ethical guidelines can greatly assist the practitioner's ethical and professional decision-making process, there are limitations to the use of a code of ethics (Mabe & Rollin, 1986):

- Some issues cannot be handled in the context of a code.

- There are some difficulties with enforcing the code, or at least the public may believe that enforcement committees are not tough enough on their peers.

- There is often no way to bring the interests of the client, patient, or research participant systematically into the code construction process.

- There are parallel forums in which the issues in the code may be addressed, with the results sometimes at odds with the findings of the code (for example, in the courts).

- There are possible conflicts associated with codes: between two codes, between the practitioner's values and code requirements, between the code and ordinary morality, between the code and institutional practice, and between requirements within a single code.

- There is a limited range of topics covered in the code. Because a code approach is usually reactive to issues already developed elsewhere, the consensus requirement prevents the code from addressing new issues and problems on the cutting edge.

The establishment of ethical guidelines is relatively new to the mental health professions. For instance, the American Psychological Association (APA) first published its *Ethical Standards of Psychologists* in 1953, the NASW established its guidelines in 1960, and the ACA developed its ethical guidelines in 1961. However, because ethical standards are to some degree a mirror of the values inherent in the culture, they should not be considered static guidelines. Therefore, over the years, the associations' guidelines have undergone a number of major revisions that reflect these ever-changing values (see ACA, 1995; APA, 2002; NASW, 1999). NOHSE, in collaboration with the CSHSE, has always supported the concept of a code of ethics (Linzer, 1990), and in 1995 adopted its *Ethical Standards of Human Service Professionals* (see Appendix B). Although these guidelines have much in common with other codes of ethics, they also reflect the unique perspective and job requirements of the human service professional.

Ethical guidelines are not legal documents. However, as documents that reflect moral positions taken by our professional associations, we are expected to abide by them. Thus, when a professional violates the codes of ethics, some consequences could be removal from a professional association, revocation of one's credential, or even dismissal from a job. In some instances, states have made part or all of a code of ethics into a legal document. In these cases, stiffer penalties such as fines or even imprisonment could result from an ethical violation. Of course, this depends on the seriousness of the violation. Throughout this text, we will raise various professional and ethical issues that relate to the NOHSE codes of ethics.

Resolving Ethical Dilemmas: A Complex Process In view of some of the limitations of ethical guidelines noted earlier, some have suggested that ethical decision making should be based on more than the ethical guidelines (Cottone & Claus, 2000; Cottone & Tarvydas, 1998; Neukrug, 1996). For instance, Corey et al. (2003) developed a practical, problem-solving model that has eight steps in the decision-making process: (1) identifying the problem, (2) identifying the potential issues involved, (3) reviewing the relevant ethical guidelines, (4) knowing relevant laws and regulations, (5) obtaining consultation, (6) considering possible and probable courses of action, (7) listing the consequences of various decisions, and (8) deciding on what appears to be the best course of action.

Although the model of Corey et al. (2003) emphasizes the pragmatic aspects of ethical decision making, other theorists stress the role of moral principles in this process. For instance, **Karen Kitchener** (1984) describes the role of four moral principles in the making of ethical decisions. She states that in working with clients, mental health professionals should promote the autonomy of the client (for example, independence, self-determination, freedom of choice), the beneficence of society (promoting the good of others), the nonmaleficence of people (avoidance of harm toward others), and justice or fairness to all (providing equal and fair treatment to all people).

Some now suggest that ethical decision making may well be influenced by the helper's level of ethical, moral, and cognitive development, such as the kinds of developmental schemes of Perry and Kegan noted in Chapter 1 (Cottone, 2001; Neukrug, 1996). Thus, those who are at the lower developmental levels will view ethical decision making as a black-and-white or right-or-wrong process. Such human service professionals may rigidly rely on the ethical guidelines when making ethical decisions and would suggest there is a "correct" answer to an ethical dilemma. However, those at higher developmental levels would view ethical decision making as a complex process. These individuals will examine the ethical guidelines, will likely use a decision-making model such as that of Corey et al. (2003) and/or a moral model such as Kitchener's (1984), and view the ethical decision-making process as a deep self-reflective and difficult process.

For instance, let's examine two human service professionals, Jason, who is at a lower developmental level, and Jawanda, who is at a higher level. Both are faced with the same dilemma—a client of theirs is smoking crack cocaine and the agency at which they work requires that such individuals be reported to the administration who will then contact the police. Jason examines the ethical guidelines and reads the agency policy guidelines and decides that the "right thing to do" and the only choice he has is to report his client to an administrator. Jawanda, however, views ethical decision-making differently. She also reads the agency policy and reviews the ethical guidelines. In addition, she uses a model such as that of Corey et al. (2003) or Kitchener (1984) in helping her decide what to do. She also consults with others to gain other points of view, and only then carefully deliberates about what would be best for her client, the agency, society, and herself. After careful deliberation, she comes to a conclusion.

The conclusion in this case is really less important than the process, as Jawanda has dealt with the situation in a complex and thoughtful manner compared with Jason's somewhat hasty decision. In fact, although both may come to the same conclusion, I would rather work with someone like Jawanda because she shows thoughtfulness and the ability to self-reflect—qualities I would want in a colleague (and a friend!). Thus, we see that ethical decision making can be, and perhaps should be, a complex process. As you review a number of ethical dilemmas throughout this text, I hope that you will examine the ethical guidelines, use a model such as that of Corey et al. (2003) or Kitchener (1984), consult with others, and consider what is best for the client, the agency, the human service professional, and society when making your decision. You can start this process with the dilemma in Activity 2.1.

Program Accreditation

Another standard that underscores professionalism is program accreditation. There are many benefits to having such a process, including (Altekruse & Wittmer, 1991; Schmidt, 1999):

ACTIVITY 2.1   Becky

As a human service professional for the local department of human services, you have been assisting Becky, a single mother of a 4-year-old daughter, for the past few years as she has attempted to remove herself from the welfare roles, obtain employment, and secure child care. Today, Becky walks into your office and tells you that she has been HIV-positive for the past eight years and that two years ago she developed AIDS. She has not responded well to her recent new regimen of medication. She is clearly despondent, is very concerned for the well-being of her child, and confides to you that she is considering killing herself. She notes that she has few significant people in her life, realizes that it may only be a matter of time before she dies, and is concerned that in the time she has left she will not be able to adequately care for her daughter. She therefore would like your help in finding a good home for her child and in "getting her affairs in order" before she commits suicide. As a helper, as one of her few confidantes, and as someone who cares, what should you do?

- Students who graduate from accredited programs study from a common curriculum, are generally more knowledgeable about core counseling issues, and usually participate in fieldwork experiences that are more intensive and longer in duration.

- Program accreditation often becomes the standard by which credentialing bodies determine who is eligible to become certified or licensed.

- Program accreditation offers the impetus for setting and maintaining high standards.

- Program accreditation almost always results in improved programs.

- Administrators and legislators are often more willing to provide money to maintain the high standards of accredited programs as compared to less rigorous nonaccredited programs.

- Those who graduate from accredited programs generally have better job opportunities.

- Accredited programs will often attract better faculty.

- Accredited programs will often attract better students.

In the human service profession, the CSHSE has developed the national accreditation standards (see Appendix D). These standards delineate general program characteristics and curriculum areas that must be addressed if a program is to be accredited by the Council. If a program values its professional organizations, supports high standards, and wants to develop highly trained students, it should seek program accreditation through CSHSE (DiGiovanni, 2001).

ETHICAL, PROFESSIONAL, AND LEGAL ISSUES

Competence and Qualifications as a Professional

Although human service professionals have generally not obtained registry, certification, or licensure status nationally, the human service professional must be aware of his or her level of competence and training as a professional. The *Ethical Standards of Human Service Professionals* states the following:

> Human service professionals know the limit and scope of their professional knowledge and offer services only within their knowledge and skill base. (See Appendix B, Statement 26)

The ACA (1995), NASW (1999), and APA (2002), codes of ethics make similar statements. In a similar vein, the human service professional must keep abreast of current trends in the field.

> Human service professionals promote the continuing development of their profession. They encourage membership in professional associations, support research endeavors, foster educational advancement, advocate for appropriate legislative actions, and participate in other related professional activities. (See Appendix B, Statement 30)

It is my belief that the human service professional should become a member of his or her professional association(s), subscribe to and read the professional journals, and attend workshops and participate in other continuing education experiences. Excellence as a human service professional means commitment to educational competence.

THE DEVELOPMENTALLY MATURE HUMAN SERVICE PROFESSIONAL

Professionally Committed, Ethically Assured

The developmentally mature human service professional is committed to his or her professional growth and competence. This commitment is not lip service; it is a deeply felt belief that to do one's best in the profession means embracing the field in a professional manner. The developmentally mature human service professional knows the roots of his or her profession and can work in a consultative and mature manner with related professions. This professional knows appropriate ethical conduct because he or she is familiar with the ethical guidelines. Although many ethical decisions are judgment calls, the ethically assured human service professional makes wise decisions because he or she is familiar with the ethical guidelines and has kept abreast of the most recent trends in the field. Finally, the developmentally mature human service professional actively supports standards such as program accreditation, credentialing, and skills standards as he or she understands that such standards ultimately lead to providing the best possible services to clients.

SUMMARY

In this chapter, we were introduced to the notion of "history as knowledge" and the importance of history in helping us understand the concept of paradigm shifts. We then reviewed some of the antecedents to the human service profession and noted that helpers have been around since the dawn of existence. Moving on to the more recent past, we reviewed the rich history of the fields of psychology, social work, and counseling and examined how each of them has affected the profession we call human services. In particular, we noted that the field of psychology has given us an understanding of the process of therapy and a rich appreciation for testing and research, that the social work field brought us a deep caring for the underprivileged and an awareness of the power of social and family systems, and that the counseling profession has brought to the human service field a holistic and wellness approach that attempts to understand the individual within the context of his or her career, love relationships, and group interactions.

This examination of the history of closely related professions was followed by a chronology of the more recent events that brought about the actual emergence of the human service field. We noted that today the human service professional is trained as a generalist and draws from all the major social service fields.

We then went on to note how standards in the profession are a mark of the maturity of the profession. We thus reviewed four important standards in the human service profession including skills standards, credentialing, ethical guidelines, and accreditation. We noted that the recent development of skills standards offers us 12 competencies along with a series of skills and tasks that are a natural outgrowth of these competencies. We highlighted the fact that training in these skills can lead to the strengthening of educational programs. In reference to credentialing, we distinguished among registration, certification, and licensure and discussed the value of each of these credentials. We then examined some of the purposes of ethical guidelines as well as some of their limitations. We noted that making ethical decisions is a complex process that optimally should involve a review of ethical guidelines, an examination of the moral principles behind making the decision, consultation with others, and a self-reflective decision-making process. We suggested that those at higher levels of cognitive development make ethical decisions in a different manner than those at lower levels. Finally, in discussing program accreditation, we highlighted the advantages and noted that the CSHSE has developed the *National Standards for Human Service Worker Education and Training Programs.*

As the chapter ended, we highlighted the importance of keeping abreast of changes in the field and the significance of knowing one's limitations as they relate to the ethical issue of competence. Finally, we pointed out that the developmentally mature human service professional knows his or her roots, can work side by side with other professionals, is committed to the field, and has a strong sense of ethical correctness.

EXPERIENTIAL EXERCISES

1. Important Names and Places

Write a brief statement that defines the term or name listed.

1. Paradigm shift
2. Hippocrates
3. Plato
4. Aristotle
5. Augustine
6. Thomas Aquinas
7. Wilhelm Wundt
8. Sir Francis Galton
9. Alfred Binet
10. Sigmund Freud
11. Franz Mesmer
12. G. Stanley Hall
13. American Psychological Association
14. DSM-IV-TR
15. Poor Laws
16. John Minson Galt II
17. Dorothea Dix
18. Charity organization society
19. Friendly visitors
20. Social casework
21. Settlement movement
22. Jane Addams
23. Hull House
24. Mary Richmond
25. Virginia Satir
26. National Association of Social Workers

27. Academy of Certified Social Workers
28. Frank Parsons
29. National Vocational Guidance Association
30. Carl Rogers
31. National Defense Education Act
32. American Personnel and Guidance Association
33. Great Society
34. American Association for Counseling and Development
35. American Counseling Association
36. National Institute of Mental Health
37. Mental Health Study Act
38. Primary prevention
39. Block grants
40. Dr. Harold McPheeters
41. Southern Regional Education Board
42. Council for Standards in Human Service Education
43. National Organization for Human Service Education
44. Skills Standards
45. Ethical Standards
46. Ethical Decision Making
47. Credentialing
48. Registration
49. Certification
50. Licensure
51. National Standards for Human Service Worker Education and Training Programs
52. Program Accreditation

2. Identifying Positive Qualities

For each of the great historical figures listed here, generate those characteristics that each of them may have embodied that could be considered vital elements to the helping relationship.

Jesus	Moses	Muhammad
Gandhi	Martin Luther King, Jr.	Eleanor Roosevelt
Joan of Arc	Abraham Lincoln	Rosa Parks
Mother Theresa	Malcolm X	

3. Are We Ready for Another Paradigm Shift?

Do you think the mental health professions are "primed" for another paradigm shift? If yes, what direction do you think it would take? If no, why not?

4. Visiting an Institution for the Mentally Ill

Make arrangements to visit a modern mental institution. How does the current mental hospital differ from early institutions as discussed in the text? What similarities do you think exist between today's institutions and those in the 1800s?

5. Discussing the Problems of the Poor and Destitute

Have a discussion with a homeless street person, visit a shelter for the homeless, visit a street-front walk-in center for the underprivileged. Then, in class discuss the problems of the poor and destitute. What solutions do you think would work in today's society? How are your solutions similar to or different from the solutions of the COSs and settlement houses of the 1800s?

6. Skills Standards

Using the competencies identified in Table 2.1, develop a list of five skills that are necessary to implement each competency. Then develop a list of tasks that could be used to develop each skill. Refer to pages 45–47 if you need to review the definitions of competencies, skills, and tasks.

7. Credentialing: Registration, Certification, and Licensure

What are the advantages of registration, certification, and licensure? Are there disadvantages? What might they be?

8. Comparing Credentialing Processes

The following chart lists a number of mental health professionals in the columns and three kinds of credentialing along the rows: registration, certification, and licensing. Following is a list of five questions that are represented in each cell in the chart by their corresponding numbers. By matching up the vertical and horizontal columns, respond to the question that the corresponding numbers represent. For example, in the first cell (psychiatrists/registration), across from number "1," I would want to state whether or not psychiatrists have a credentialing process.

1. Does a credentialing process exist?
2. If a credentialing process does exist, is it regulated by the states, the federal government, or a national professional association?
3. What are the degree requirements for being credentialed?
4. What postdegree experiences, if any, are required for being credentialed?
5. Is a test required to become credentialed?

Comparison of Credentialing Processes Among Select Mental Health Professionals

	Psychiatrist	Psychologist	Mental Health Counselor	School Counselor	College Counselor	Social Worker	Psycho-therapist	Psychiatric Nurse	Human Service Practitioner
Registration									
	1.	1.	1.	1.	1.	1.	1.	1.	1.
	2.	2.	2.	2.	2.	2.	2.	2.	2.
	3.	3.	3.	3.	3.	3.	3.	3.	3.
	4.	4.	4.	4.	4.	4.	4.	4.	4.
	5.	5.	5.	5.	5.	5.	5.	5.	5.
Certification									
	1.	1.	1.	1.	1.	1.	1.	1.	1.
	2.	2.	2.	2.	2.	2.	2.	2.	2.
	3.	3.	3.	3.	3.	3.	3.	3.	3.
	4.	4.	4.	4.	4.	4.	4.	4.	4.
	5.	5.	5.	5.	5.	5.	5.	5.	5.
Licensing									
	1.	1.	1.	1.	1.	1.	1.	1.	1.
	2.	2.	2.	2.	2.	2.	2.	2.	2.
	3.	3.	3.	3.	3.	3.	3.	3.	3.
	4.	4.	4.	4.	4.	4.	4.	4.	4.
	5.	5.	5.	5.	5.	5.	5.	5.	5.

9. Ethical Guidelines

Generate a list of ethical issues you would want addressed by a professional association's code of ethics.

1. Bring your list to class and together generate a class list of items you would want addressed by a professional association's code of ethics.

2. As you read the book during the semester, see whether the items on the list you generated in class have been discussed in the ethics section of the chapters.

3. The instructor should have available a copy of the code of ethics of APA, ACA, NASW, and the *Ethical Standards of Human Service Professionals* listed in Appendix B. Examine all of the guidelines and compare them with the list generated in class.

4. Using the ethical vignettes in Exercise 12, compare and contrast how individuals from different developmental levels might make ethical decisions.

10. Developing Accreditation and Program Accreditation Standards

In small groups, or as a class, consider the kinds of standards you would require if you were an accreditation body charged with developing program standards for human service programs. Specifically, speak to each of the following.

1. What, if any, admissions requirements would you have?

2. What would you include in the curriculum?

3. How many credits in human services would you require?

4. What would you like to see the faculty-student ratio be in your classes?

5. What philosophy would you like to see permeate the program?

6. How many hours would you require for an internship?

7. What activities would you require in the internship?

8. What kind of competency would you require, if any, for a student to graduate with a major in human services?

11. Reviewing CSHSE Program Accreditation Standards

Review the CSHSE summary of program accreditation standards that can be found in Appendix D. After you have completed your review, do the following:

1. Summarize and present various aspects of the standards in class.

2. Using the standards as a reference, critically evaluate your human services program.

3. Based on the program accreditation standards, and what you developed in the previous exercise, make suggestions for change in your human services program.

4. Critically review the standards. What makes sense? What could be changed?

12. Ethical and Professional Vignettes

Discuss the following ethical vignettes in class. In your discussion, decide whether the human service professional acted ethically. If you think that he or she acted unethically, what action might you take?

1. A bachelor's-level human service professional takes some workshops in how to do Gestalt therapy, an advanced therapeutic approach. He feels assured about his skills and decides to run a Gestalt therapy group. The state in which he works licenses psychologists, social workers, and counselors as therapists. Is it ethical for the human service professional to run such a group? Professional? Legal?

2. An associate's-level human service professional, who is planning to return to school to obtain his bachelor's and master's degrees, tells his colleagues that he is a "master's degree candidate" in human services. If this person is not yet enrolled in a graduate program, is he misrepresenting himself? Might clients be confused by the term *master's degree candidate?* Is this ethical? Professional? Legal?

3. You are working with a client who begins to share bizarre thoughts with you concerning the end of the world. You decide that this individual needs special attention, so you decide to spend extra time with him. Is this appropriate? Ethical? Professional?

4. A client tells a human service professional that she is taking Prozac, an antidepressant, and it isn't having any effect. She asks advice regarding taking an increased dosage, and the human service professional states, "If the current dosage isn't working, perhaps you should consider taking a higher dosage." Is it appropriate for a human service professional to suggest that a client change dosage levels? Ethical? Professional? Legal?

5. A human service professional who has received specialized training in running parenting workshops on communication skills decides to run a workshop at the local Holiday Inn. She rents a room and advertises in the local newspaper. The advertisement reads, "Learn How to Talk to Your Kid—Rid Your Family of All Communication Problems." Should she do the workshop? Is this ad ethical? Professional? Legal?

3

Theoretical Approaches to Human Service Work

I have always thought of myself as a kindhearted person. I remember that even as a young child I felt a little different from everyone else—a bit more sensitive, a bit more aware of other people's feelings. For instance, if I were playing ball at the park, I was always worried about the feelings of the kid who was picked last. Similarly, I was worried about the feelings of the kids in class who were overweight, or withdrawn, or "nerdy."

Later, when I was in college, I still was the "nice guy" trying to do what was just and right and to be the caretaker in the crowd. When shifting my major to psychology, I believed that my caring attitude was in and of itself the sufficient tool I would need to be an effective helper. Therefore, I held an attitude that there was little I could learn that would actually benefit me as a helper. As I went on to graduate school, I continued to think I already had the natural skills that alone would make me an effective helper. Basically, I was going to school to get the degree. I believed this so strongly that no one dared tell me how to interact with a client—I knew it all. Just let me at those clients; I could help them. I didn't need any specific training. After all, wasn't I a caring person? Weren't some caring and a little motivation enough?

Well, I do think having a caring attitude is one basic ingredient in being an effective helper. However, over the years I have found that often (if not usually) caring alone is not sufficient to be effective at what you do. Although our clients may appreciate our caring, it is often not enough to assist them in the change process. Thus, I now believe that having a solid theoretical background and clearly defined techniques is essential to being an effective counselor.

In this chapter, we will explore the importance of counseling theory in the helping relationship. We will first examine the differences, if any, between counseling and psychotherapy. Next, we will examine how a theory is developed and review the theoretical underpinnings of four major conceptual orientations: psychodynamic, behavioral, humanistic, and cognitive. We will then review some cross-theoretical approaches to counseling, including theoretical integration or eclecticism, brief treatment, and gender-aware approaches. The chapter will conclude by reviewing important ethical and professional issues related to supervision, confidentiality, dual relationships and the importance of continuing to refine one's approach to doing counseling.

COUNSELING OR PSYCHOTHERAPY?

Before we start examining the theoretical underpinnings to doing counseling or therapy, let's explore the differences, if any, that exist between counseling and psychotherapy.

When I ask my students to make associations with the word *psychotherapy*, I usually get responses that include "long-term, deep personality change," "secrets unveiled," "unconscious," and "focus on past." For the word *counseling*, the responses are usually "short-term," "conscious," "problem solving," and "present focus." In actuality, although dictionary definitions may vary, if you pick up a text on "theories of counseling and psychotherapy" (for example, see Corey, 2001), you would see that both counseling and psychotherapy rely on the same theoretical underpinnings. However, although the theories are the same, how practitioners implement them may vary. Therefore, individuals who see themselves as doing counseling may be applying a theory somewhat differently than do individuals who see themselves as doing psychotherapy. A rule of thumb may be that as you receive more education and training, you are able to move out of a supportive role and become capable of doing counseling and eventually psychotherapy.

Although I would argue that human service professionals do not have the training to do in-depth counseling and psychotherapy, there is no question that they counsel clients. Thus, it is crucial that human service professionals understand the basic theory behind doing counseling.

INDIVIDUAL VERSUS
SYSTEMS APPROACH TO CLIENTS

If caring alone is not enough, what does work? Over the years, a quiet debate has ensued that has pitted the individual approach to counseling against the systems approach to counseling. The individual approach assumes that we are each islands unto ourselves and that, although social forces might influence us, the change process should focus on how the person can change his or her conditions in life. On the other hand, the systems approach assumes that our lives are the result of social conditions such as family dynamics, poverty, crime, racism, and sexism and that it is important to work with the system to effect any significant change in the person (see Box 3.1).

Supporting the individual approach, theorists like Viktor Frankl (1984) and William Glasser (1965, 1999, 2000) strongly make the case that our reality is a construction of internal messages and that we create our attitudes. As evidence of this, Frankl notes that despite the fact that he was a victim of a Nazi concentration camp, he was able to maintain a sense of hope and self-dignity while existing in that hell on earth. He therefore argues that we create our contentment through our search for meaning, and if we have no meaning, we have no contentment: Once an individual's search for meaning is successful, he or she is capable of coping with life's difficulties, even when faced with the worst of life's predicaments. However, if one's search for meaning is unsuccessful, the consequences can be devastating.

> In the concentration camps, [there were] those who one morning, at five, refused to get up and go to work and instead stayed in the hut, on the straw wet with urine and feces. Nothing—neither warnings nor threats—could induce them to change their minds. And then something typical occurred: they took out a cigarette from deep down in a pocket where they had hidden it and started smoking. At that moment we knew that for the next forty-eight hours or so we would watch them dying. Meaning orientation had subsided, and consequently the seeking of immediate pleasure had taken over. (Frankl, 1984, p. 141)

BOX 3.1   Joshua

When Joshua was 5 years old, he lived with his mother, his 15-year-old half brother, and his 20-year-old half sister and her two children. His half sister's children had different fathers. There were no male role models except for periodic boyfriends of his mother and half sister. The family lived in poverty in a three-room apartment in the poor section of town. Drugs and violence were common. Although his mother worked, her income barely made ends meet. Joshua's mother believed that discipline was taught through hitting. Although she might not be considered abusive, she noted that Joshua "got a good whipping when he needed one." She knew little about nutrition, and Joshua grew up on a diet high in fat and carbohydrates and low in protein. Also, it was discovered that the apartment they lived in had lead paint and lead water pipes (ingestion of lead can result in brain damage). When Joshua was older, he became abusive toward his girlfriend, took drugs, and lived on the edge of a life of crime. Has Joshua created this situation or is he the result of situational influences? Is Joshua responsible for his life situation?

In contrast, some systems advocates argue that, to a large degree, social forces determine the ways in which we respond to situations, and we must respond to social concerns with socially oriented actions (Alinsky, 1970, 1971; Voydanoff, 2001). Therefore, the individual who is besieged by poverty, surrounded by drug use, living in a crime-ridden slum, and has been abused, has little chance for survival and little hope for the future. Other systems advocates would contend that there is a complex interaction among one's family members, between families and communities, and between communities and society. This interdependence of systems, they say, can affect the individual in complex and sometimes mysterious ways (see Chapter 6).

Whether you believe that social forces determine your plot in life, or in the complex interactions of systems, it is clear that systems advocates believe that one's fate is controlled by much more than the individual's ability to create his or her own attitudes or choose his or her own behaviors.

Perhaps the truth lies somewhere in between. Maybe the individual is affected both by his or her attitudes and by systems, and changes within the individual or changes in the system can be productive. Theory from an individualistic approach is somewhat different than theory from a systems perspective. Let's examine the importance of theory in individual counseling. Chapter 6 will present a systemic understanding of theory.

WHY HAVE A THEORY?

In theory-driven science, an unending cycle of discovery and testing creates and evolves theories of ever increasing scope that can guide counseling practice. (Strong, 1991, p. 204)

Theory offers us a comprehensive system of doing counseling and assists us in understanding our client, in determining what techniques to apply, and in predicting change. Theories are **heuristic**—they are researchable and testable. Theory comes from practice, is a way of organizing our ideas, and leads to suggested plans of actions. Therefore, regardless of whether you adhere to an individual or systems approach, you must have a theoretical base with which to approach your clients. Otherwise, everyone would be just "doing their own thing," and there would be no rhyme or reason to client interventions (Brammer & MacDonald, 1999; Brammer, Shostrom, & Abrego, 1989). Or, as Hansen, Stevic, and Warner put it, "To try and function without theory is to operate in chaos, for without placing events in some order it is impossible to function in a meaningful manner" (1978, p. 16). All the current, well-known counseling theories have a long history, have gone through revisions, and have been supported to some degree by research. A counseling theory generally arises from a theorist's view of human nature.

Views of Human Nature

Although there are literally dozens of theories of counseling and psychotherapy, most of them can be placed into four major orientations: psychodynamic, behavioral, humanistic, and cognitive. A theory is placed in one of these orientations because it shares key concepts related to its **view of human nature.** Our view of human nature describes how we understand the reasons individuals are motivated to do the things they do.

Our lives would be much easier if we knew which of these broad orientations held "the answer"—that is, which was right. All the approaches, however, seem to have some validity, and all add something to our understanding of the individual. Having a theory that allows us to examine the motivations of individuals is the first step toward developing techniques for working with an individual. For instance, if you think people are inherently evil, you certainly would not encourage your clients to "be all that they can be." Instead, you would be apt to encourage individuals to learn how to place restraints on certain aspects of their behavior—in other words, to help them find ways of controlling their behavior so their evil would not hurt the world. On the other hand, if you think people are born with innate goodness, you would want to allow them the opportunity to express this goodness in the world. You would want to help them get in touch with their goodness and allow it to blossom.

Think about these two polarities in reference to a person like Charles Manson, a sociopath who, during the 1970s, led a cult of young adults who viciously murdered five people. If you believe people are inherently evil, you would want Manson to learn how to place restraints on his evil nature. You might view his past actions as a product of his evil nature taking over. You would probably also believe that we all have such an evil side. On the other hand, the individual who believes we are born with innate goodness would see Manson as a person who had lost touch with his innate loving side—perhaps through a series of horribly abusive experiences in childhood. You would therefore want him to get in touch once again with his caring and loving side, and you would offer him an environment that would allow him to do this.

Deterministic Versus Antideterministic View of Human Nature

Such divergent views of human nature, as noted in the example of Charles Manson, tend to lend themselves to either a **deterministic** or an **antideterministic** view of the individual. A deterministic view asserts that forces such as instincts and early childhood development are so great that there is little ability for the person to change. Those who take a deterministic view of human nature are often adherents of the **medical model,** in that they believe there is most likely a genetic/biological predisposition to mental illness. They postulate that temperament, character, and resulting emotional problems can be viewed as an "illness" and therefore can be diagnosed and managed much like a disease. Proponents of this approach will often use **psychotropic medications** (medications that affect psychological functioning) as an adjunct to therapy.

On the other hand, those who take an antideterministic view use a **wellness approach** and tend to reject the notion that early childhood development and genetic/biological factors determine psychological problems. These theorists have a strong belief in the ability of the individual to change. In highlighting these differences, Glasser, the founder of **reality therapy** and control theory and a strong proponent of the antideterministic approach, proposes that the term *illness* (for example, mental illness) would lend itself to the use of extreme measures to assist an individual—measures that are not necessary if, instead, you view problems as an opportunity for change.

> I contend that we choose essentially everything we do, including behaviors that are commonly called mental illnesses. . . . (2000, p. xv) . . . What is labeled mental illness, regardless of the causation, are the hundreds of ways people choose to behave when they are unable to satisfy basic genetic needs, such as love and power. . . . (2000, p. xvi)

Directive Versus Nondirective Approach to Clients

Regardless of whether one is an adherent of the deterministic or wellness view of human nature, he or she may take a **directive approach** or **nondirective approach** in working with individuals. The helper who takes a directive view believes that clients need direction or guidance in the change process. These individuals tend to teach about and direct the client toward healthier ways of living. On the other hand, the helper who takes a nondirective view has trust in the client's own ability to make change; therefore, he or she attempts to provide a safe, helping environment that enables the client to define his or her own strategies for change. Helpers who adhere to this approach generally rely on the use of empathic understanding and respect for the client's own change process in their facilitation of client growth.

Today, few helpers are strictly deterministic, antideterministic, directive, or nondirective. Instead, most take an eclectic, or integrative, approach toward working with clients. Those who use an **integrative approach** require helpers to reflect on their own views of human nature, with the resulting outcome being a view of human nature that borrows from the varying viewpoints. In this chapter, when you are examining the differing helping theories, think about whether you believe people are determined, whether they need to have problems dealt with from a medical model or wellness orientation, and whether you would have a tendency to be directive or nondirective. Then think about what aspects of the varying theories you like and how you might try to integrate the theories into your own eclectic, or integrative, approach.

MAJOR THEORETICAL ORIENTATIONS

Psychodynamic Approach

It is the latter part of the 19th century. A person walks into a physician's office complaining of melancholia and paralysis of the left arm. No apparent physical problems are found. What does the physician do?

Until this time, symptoms such as these were thought to be organic in nature; that is, they were considered physical in origin. If the physical problem could not be immediately discovered, it was because science had not yet found the physical origins of the problems. Then, in the late 1800s, **Sigmund Freud** developed a comprehensive theory that he applied when doing therapy with individuals. Using hypnosis, he discovered some amazing things. For instance, some patients who had lost the use of a limb or were blind were found not to have symptoms while under hypnosis. Freud had discovered that their illness was not physical but instead had psychological origins **(conversion disorder).** Freud spent years trying to understand the complex intricacies of the mind. Although he later gave up the use of hypnosis for other techniques, he felt strongly that there were **unconscious factors** beyond our everyday awareness that mediated our behavior. In other words, he thought that the reasons we do things are often beyond our understanding and are a function of motivations from the **unconscious.** Freud spent most of his life developing his psychoanalytic theory to explain the causes of human behavior. As the years have gone by, some of Freud's theory has been debunked, other parts have been changed, and still other parts have been accepted as fact. In addition, a number of theorists have borrowed from Freud's original ideas and moved in innovative directions. Freudians and neo-Freudians are often subsumed under the heading psychodynamic theorists.

The Psychodynamic View of Human Nature Although individuals who adhere to a psychodynamic view vary considerably on many points, they do share some basic beliefs concerning their view of human nature. For instance, the **psychodynamic approach** has at its core a belief that drives motivate behavior and

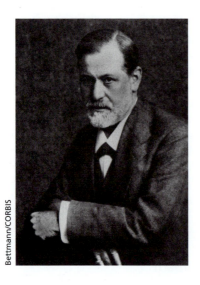

Bettmann/CORBIS

Sigmund Freud (1856–1939)

that these drives are at least somewhat unconscious. Whereas Freud thought that these drives are the instinctual drives of sex and aggression (Appignanesi & Oscar, 1999; Freud, 1947), other theorists like **Alfred Adler** (1890–1937) (1964) and **Erik Erikson** (1902–1994) (1998) believed that people are motivated more by social drives. Still others like **Heinz Kohut** (1913–1981) (1984) played down the effects of sex, aggression, and social forces but highlight the ways we attach and separate from important "others" in our lives. And others, like **Carl Jung** (1875–1961) (1968, 1975), believed that we are motivated by positive unconscious forces that drive us to understand ourselves and our relationships to others. Regardless of which motivating force an individual believes is most important, psychodynamic-oriented individuals believe that childhood events, or perceptions of those events, in combination with our drives, greatly affect our **psyches** and, consequently, our later adult development. Therefore, the purpose of psychodynamic therapy is to help the individual understand his or her early childhood experiences and how those experiences, in combination with the individual's drives, motivate the person today.

Key Concepts of the Psychodynamic Approach Some psychodynamic approaches, such as Freud's psychoanalytic model, tend to specify rather complex developmental stages. These stages describe psychological and physical tasks that must be accomplished throughout the life span. An individual who does not adequately master the tasks of one stage may become **fixated** in that stage; that is, he or she will not successfully pass through later stages because of unresolved issues in the earlier stage. This developmental framework is an important aspect of the psychodynamic approach and has major implications concerning how the human service professional may approach the individual or family. (See Chapter 5 for a more detailed examination of developmental theory as defined by psychodynamic theorists.)

Developmental psychodynamic theorists believe that, as we pass through our developmental stages, repression (putting painful memories out of consciousness) may occur. Therefore, assisting the individual through the change process can be a difficult and long ordeal—a process of peeling back the layers of the person to get to the repressed memories. For instance, the adult who was abused as a child might have repressed early memories, might have learned dysfunctional ways of interacting, and might not be conscious of his or her maladaptive behaviors. One can readily see that "uncovering" the root causes of current behavior might take years. Usually, helpers who are psychodynamically oriented will begin the relationship in a nondirective fashion as they attempt to understand the early root causes of the client's behavior. However, at a later point in the counseling process, the helper will become more directive as he or she attempts to interpret the client's behavior and offer possible avenues for change.

Because of the belief that early childhood experiences together with our instincts affect us in unconscious ways, **psychoanalysis** was originally considered a deterministic approach, which often espoused a medical orientation toward working with clients. However, some of the more recent psychodynamic approaches have placed less emphasis on the long-term effects of early childhood and instincts and have focused more on the conscious process, social causes of behavior, and the ability of the individual to change (DeAngelis, 1996; Dinkmeyer, Dinkmeyer, & Sperry, 1987). Despite some of these modifications, the psychodynamic approach still asserts that the change process can be formidable.

> Now the years are rolling by me[1]
> They are rocking evenly
> I am older than I once was
> Younger than I'll be
> But that's not unusual
> No it isn't strange
> After changes upon changes
> We are more or less the same
> After changes we are more or less the same. (Paul Simon, 1969)

Generally, psychodynamic theorists believe that patterns of behaviors learned in the first few years of life are repeated with our significant others—including the human service professional or therapist with whom the client is working. Called **transference,** this concept can be helpful to understanding the client in that it proposes that although current client behaviors had their origins in childhood, the client may have little or no awareness of this fact. Adherents of the psychodynamic approach try to maintain an emotionally distant relationship with their clients— a relationship where the client expresses his or her feelings but little if any self-disclosure takes place by the helper. This would allow the professional to separate clearly the client's issues from the therapist's issues.

---

[1]Copyright © 1969 Paul Simon. Used by permission of the publisher: Paul Simon Music.

The Human Service Professional's Use of the Psychodynamic Approach
Traditionally, the psychodynamic approach has been used mostly in the intensive psychotherapeutic setting. However, some aspects of this approach can be adapted for the human service professional. First, this approach offers us a developmental model by which we can understand the individual. Understanding that clients may be responding to deep-seated motivations that stem from early childhood and are mostly unconscious helps the human service professional have empathy and patience when working with very difficult clients. Second, this approach helps us to understand deviant behavior. The notion that such behavior is the result of abusive or neglectful early childhood caretaking may help us understand that deviants, perpetrators, criminals, and abusers are also victims. Only with this knowledge can we begin to have the deeper caring and understanding needed to work with such difficult populations.

Finally, the psychodynamic approach has given one other important contribution to the human service field: the concept of **countertransference.** Just as our clients might respond to individuals as if they were significant people from their past, mental health professionals who have not resolved their past issues may do the same. It is important for human service professionals to have worked through their own issues to avoid countertransference with their clients (see Neukrug, Milliken, & Shoemaker, 2001). Countertransference can have negative effects on your relationships with your clients because your own unresolved issues may cause you to respond in unhealthy ways toward your clients.

Behavioral Approach

Around the turn of the century, the Russian scientist **Ivan Pavlov** (1849–1936) found that a hungry dog that salivated when shown food would learn to salivate to a tone if that tone had been repeatedly paired, or associated, with the food. In other words, eventually the dog would salivate when it heard the tone, whether food was present or not. Pavlov discovered what was later called **classical conditioning.**

In the 1920s psychologist **B. F. Skinner** (1909–1990) showed that animals would learn specific behaviors if the target behavior was reinforced. His **operant conditioning** procedures demonstrated that if one presents a **positive reinforcement** (presentation of a stimulus that yields an increase in behavior) or a **negative reinforcement** (removal of a stimulus that yields an increase in behavior), one can successfully change behavior (Nye, 2000). Skinner became so good at changing behavior in animals that during World War II he used his techniques to reinforce pigeons to steer gliders toward enemy targets—gliders that had explosives attached (Skinner, 1960) (see Box 3.2)! Despite great accuracy, the military decided not to use this technique. Significantly, Skinner's approach has also shown that punishing an individual (presenting an aversive stimulus) is a very poor means of changing behavior.

During the 1940s, **Albert Bandura** (1925 to present) discovered another behavioral approach that seemed to hold efficacy for creating change. He had children view a film in which an adult acted aggressively toward a Bobo doll.

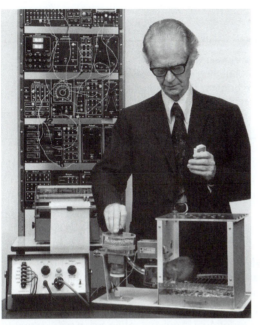

B.F. Skinner Foundation

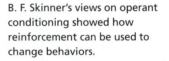

B. F. Skinner's views on operant conditioning showed how reinforcement can be used to change behaviors.

Later, when placed in a room with a Bobo doll, those children acted more aggressively than did children who had not seen the film (Bandura, Ross & Ross, 1963). This **social learning,** or **modeling,** approach has also shown that although we may not always act out behaviors we have viewed, if the behavior is needed later, we have the capacity to act it out.

The three **behavioral approaches** of classical conditioning, operant conditioning, and modeling have similar views of human nature and have been widely applied to the helping professions.

The Behavioral View of Human Nature The behaviorist believes that all behavior is learned and that we are conditioned by reinforcers in our environment. This view does not stress the unconscious and does not place emphasis on gaining insight into our early childhood experiences. Instead, this approach assumes that we have learned our current behaviors and that we could learn new behaviors by applying the principles of behaviorism. Therefore, by using classical conditioning, operant conditioning, or modeling in a scientific and empirical manner, we can explore with our clients the types of behaviors they wish to change and use these approaches to assist them in the change process. Although the past may have been important in conditioning our current behaviors, focusing on the past is not particularly important in the behavioral approach. In its early days, the behavioral approach was seen as a directive approach to working with a client in that the helpee's situation was examined and diagnosed and strategies for

---

BOX 3.2   A Very Bright Pigeon

I walk into a small store in New York's China-town, and I see a sign that says "As Seen on *That's Incredible,* Play Tic-Tac-Toe with the Pigeon." Being a wealthy man, I place a quarter in the slot, then another quarter, then another.

I can't beat the pigeon. Well, I guess operant conditioning really does work or maybe pigeons are brighter than I thought. On the other hand, maybe I'm not quite as smart as I might think.

---

behavior change were made. However, establishing a relationship through nondirective approaches such as the use of empathy and modeling, before suggesting specific behavior changes, has recently become more important (Spiegler, 1998).

Applications of the Behavioral Approach Many behavioral techniques have been very successfully used in a variety of human service, educational, and therapeutic settings (Corey, 2001). For instance, the behavioral technique of establishing a **token economy** has been successfully used with individuals with mental retardation (see Box 3.3). In this case, an individual is given a token for specific targeted behaviors that he or she is asked to exhibit. For example, a person might receive a token for successfully getting dressed in the morning, for exhibiting "appropriate" personal traits, for bathing himself or herself, and so forth. At the end of a specified amount of time, such as a day or a week, the individual can trade in his or her tokens for money or some other reinforcer such as candy or items in a gift shop. On which of the three behavioral approaches is the token economy based?

A second common use of behavioral approaches is in the treatment of phobias. One treatment for phobias includes teaching an individual a series of deep-relaxation exercises and then pairing the feeling of relaxation with the image of the feared object. For instance, suppose an individual had a debilitating fear of cats. A therapist might teach the individual deep-relaxation techniques and then pair the image of a cat with the relaxation. Later, a live cat might be paired with the feeling of relaxation. Techniques like these generally take repeated trials to be successful, and there are often relapses, which are called **spontaneous recovery** of the symptom. On which of the three behavioral approaches is this treatment of phobias based?

One other use of behavioral approaches with which you might be familiar is in the learning of assertive behavior. In this case, individuals who have difficulty asserting themselves are shown effective and nonaggressive ways of stating how they feel and expressing their needs. The facilitator or trainer usually comes up with a situation in which he or she role-plays how to be assertive. Nonassertive individuals can then practice what they just watched. This type of **role-playing** often works well in a group or workshop setting. On which of the three behavioral approaches is this type of training based?

BOX 3.3   The Power of Reinforcement

A friend of mine used to work at a residential home for individuals with mental retardation. One boy who lived there would clap loudly and smile broadly after he successfully urinated in the toilet bowl. For years, human service professionals had reinforced (applauded) him when he successfully urinated in the toilet, and he was responding to their reinforcement. On which of the three behavioral approaches is this example based?

The Human Service Professional's Use of the Behavioral Approach
Unlike the psychodynamic approach, the behavioral approach has been widely applied outside the psychotherapeutic setting. Aside from the preceding examples, behavioral concepts are commonly used in a wide variety of human service settings. For example, reinforcement is used in schools, residential and rehabilitation settings, and day treatment programs, whereas modeling via role-playing is commonly used at employment offices, in educational workshops, and in the training of human service professionals.

Today, finding some behavioral techniques incorporated into the human service professional's repertoire of skills is not unusual. In fact, for some disorders, using behavioral techniques has been shown to be so powerful that it would be unethical for a human service professional not to use them (e.g., alleviation of phobias, assisting individuals with mental retardation to learn new skills) (Plaud & Eifert, 1998). Behavioral techniques are advantageous because, in collaboration with the client, the human service professional can identify client goals, apply specific techniques, and see results in relatively short periods. In residential settings, behavioral techniques are easily understood by clients and help give direction and focus for both staff and clients.

Humanistic Approach

During the 1940s, the mental health field underwent a revolution in its approach to working with people. Individuals like **Carl Rogers** (1902–1987), **Rollo May** (1909–1994), and **Abraham Maslow** (1908–1970) led a reaction against the deterministic flavor of the psychodynamic approach and the scientific reductionistic notions of the behavioral approach. The **humanistic approach** highlights the strengths and the positive aspects of the individual and rejects the concept that people are determined by early childhood experiences or reinforcers in the environment:

> I think it is now possible to be able to delineate this view of human nature as a total, single, comprehensive system of psychology even though much of it has arisen as a reaction against the limitations (as philosophies of human nature) of the two most comprehensive psychologies now available—behaviorism (or associationism) and classical, Freudian psychoanalysis. . . . In the past I have called it the "holistic-dynamic." (Maslow, 1968, p. 189)

The Humanistic View of Human Nature Besides being a reaction to psychodynamic and behavioral theory, this humanistic approach had its origins in **existentialism** and **phenomenology** (Corey, 2001). Therefore, adherents of the humanistic approach believe that we all have choices and that we constantly are making choices that create our existence. Humanists generally think that there is no such thing as an objective reality; instead, they stress the subjective reality of the individual. Trying to understand how the individual constructs his or her reality and helping facilitate the individual's perception of his or her experience is the major goal of this approach. In addition, humanistic theorists generally agree that people are born with some type of **actualizing tendency,** or growth force. This means that individuals have the ability to transcend their current existence and move toward a more fulfilling and harmonious existence. Therefore, although the past may have been important in affecting how we act today, a helping relationship does not have to focus on the past to help a person change and grow. Many approaches to counseling have taken the philosophy of the humanistic approach and applied it to educational, therapeutic, and human service environments. Although techniques might vary among these approaches, all believe in the basic philosophy of this approach (see Box 3.4).

Key Concepts of the Humanistic Approach Probably, the humanistic approaches that have most affected the human service and mental health fields have been the **person-centered** approach of Rogers (1951) and the **hierarchical** approach of Maslow (Maslow, 1968, 1970). Maslow's theory stresses a **hierarchy of needs** in which he stated that a lower-order need would have to be satisfied before the next need on the hierarchy could be approached (Figure 3.1). **Maslow's hierarchy** has great implications for working with individuals. For instance, by examining Figure 3.1, we can see that an individual who is hungry or in need of shelter probably has little ability to focus on the needs of belonging or self-esteem. The highest need to be satisfied is self-actualization. Some of the qualities embodied by the **self-actualized person** are spontaneity, the ability to be in touch with one's feelings, high self-worth, and the development of one's own sense of spirituality.

BOX 3.4   Can a Behaviorist Be a Humanist?

During the defense of my doctoral dissertation, my adviser, who was a behaviorist, asked me if "a behaviorist can be a humanist." I went on to give what I thought at the time to be a rather esoteric response, noting that the basic orientations of the approaches were philosophically different and therefore incompatible with each other. A few years later, I had the opportunity to hear Skinner talk at a church in New Hampshire. Following his talk, I asked him, "Can a behaviorist be a humanist?" Waiting a moment, he turned to me and, with a deeply reflective look, said, "Well, I don't know about that, but he can surely be humane."

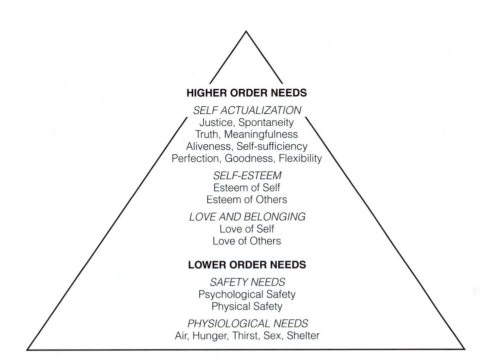

FIGURE 3.1 Maslow's hierarchy

Although Rogers would agree with much of Maslow's philosophy, his approach focuses more on the actual helping relationship. He believed that the conditions of empathy, unconditional positive regard, and genuineness (see Chapter 1) are necessary and sufficient for the growth process of the person (Rogers, 1957). In other words, these personality characteristics alone are enough to facilitate change in the person. In referring to this nondirective approach, Rogers noted that:

> Nondirective counseling is based on the assumption that the client has the right to select his own life goals, even though these may be at variance with the goals the counselor might choose for him. There is also the belief that if the individual has a modicum of insight into himself and his problems, he will be likely to make this choice wisely. (Rogers, 1942, pp. 126–127)

As a humanist, Rogers believed that people are born good with an actualizing tendency. However, such a belief does not negate the fact that individuals do end up with emotional problems. In explaining this, he stated that because significant others in our lives would place expectations and conditions on us, we end up acting as they would have wanted us to be rather than how we actually are—we end up being nongenuine or incongruent. Often, the individual is "out of touch" or not aware of his or her incongruence. Rogers thought that people could get in touch with the natural part of themselves if they were around people who are empathic and who show unconditional positive regard. He used the term **subception** to describe the professional's ability to perceive feelings and deeper meanings beyond what the individual actually experiences within himself or herself. Rogers would certainly have agreed that regardless of where on Maslow's hierarchy of needs we find the person, offering the client empathy, unconditional regard, and genuineness would assist the individual in his or her ability to move up the hierarchy. Later in Rogers's life, he stated that his theory was applicable to all individuals, not just to individuals in the helping professions (Rogers, 1980). He thought that people would live a more peaceful coexistence if they could embody some of the characteristics he deemed important.

The humanistic approach stresses the positive aspects of the individual and displays a belief that the person can change and grow (Corey, 2001). Unlike adherents of the psychoanalytic approach, proponents of the humanistic approach do not state that we are determined by our early experiences and do not stress the role of instincts in our lives. The role of the unconscious is also de-emphasized in the humanistic approach. Instead, humanistically oriented professionals stress the ability to increase awareness. Finally, whereas proponents of the psychodynamic approach stress emotional distance and little use of self-disclosure on the part of the helper and adherents of the behavioral approach stress the ability of the professional to use techniques in a scientific, objective manner, advocates of the humanistic approach stress the personal qualities of the professional in the change process. Helpers using this nondirective approach believe that these qualities alone are the key to client growth.

The Human Service Professional's Use of the Humanistic Approach
Maslow's hierarchy of needs has become an established method of recognizing how to approach the individual initially. In this model, the human service professional who spends the majority of time attempting to raise an individual's self-esteem when that individual is homeless and cold would be doing the client a disservice.

Today, the personal characteristics of empathy, being nonjudgmental, and being genuine have become the essential qualities for mental health professionals to embrace. Along these same lines, stressing the importance of the relationship between the helper and the client has become a key ingredient in the helping relationship. In fact, these qualities have become so important that today, whether the human service professional views himself or herself as psychodynamically, behaviorally, or cognitively oriented, the ability to embody these humanistic personality characteristics and to form a strong relationship has become essential (Neukrug, 2003; Sexton & Whiston, 1994)

Cognitive Approach

The **cognitive approach** stresses how the individual thinks, particularly how cognitions affect our behaviors, and how we feel. Although **Albert Ellis** (1913–present) (Ellis, 1996; Ellis & Harper, 1997) popularized this approach in the 1960s, more recently Aaron Beck's (1921–present) research and treatment applications have gained much prominence (Beck, 1976; Beck & Weishaar, 2000). However, the concept that our thinking process is the root of our personhood can be traced back to early philosophers:

> If you have right opinions, you will fare well; if they are false, you will fare ill. For to every man the cause of his acting is opinion. (Epictetus)

The Cognitive View of Human Nature Cognitive-oriented professionals tend to believe that the individual's thinking is conditioned, starting in early childhood, that our ways of thinking are reinforced throughout our lives, and that these ways of thinking are directly related to how we act and how we feel. They believe that we are not born with innate goodness or evil, as rational or irrational beings, or as individuals who are depressed, happy, angry, or content. Adherents to the cognitive approach propose that we can challenge old, irrational, or dysfunctional ways of thinking and reinforce new, healthier ways of thinking (Corey, 2001). Therefore, what had been learned in childhood can be relearned. They believe that although it might be interesting to understand why we behave the way we do, such understanding is not crucial, and perhaps not even important, to making changes in the way we think. Such changes in our thinking, they believe, will ultimately help us cope with our daily living and will change dysfunctional behavior patterns.

Key Concepts of the Cognitive Approach The cognitive approach can be used with many different client populations. As a teaching approach, it places less emphasis on the qualities of the relationship between the client and the helper and more emphasis on how clients learn about changing the ways in which they think. Proponents of this approach stress the importance of continually evaluating the thinking process and of trying to extinguish past destructive ways of thinking while practicing new, positive ways of thinking. The intent of the cognitive approach, however, is not to change the core values of the individual but to examine how the client's thinking is negatively affecting his or her ability to function in the world. Those who adhere to this approach will usually carefully analyze the way a client thinks to try to understand how a client's thinking is resulting in negative feelings. Once patterns of thinking are identified, clients are challenged to change their thinking and therefore adopt new behaviors and more positive feelings. Some therapists have combined many of the techniques from the behavioral approach with the cognitive approach.

Recently, some cognitive therapists have moved toward a constructivist understanding of how people think and make meaning of the world (Corey, 2001; Mahoney, 1991, 1995). Whereas the rationalist from the traditional schools views cognitive therapy as a logic-oriented process that involves replacing irrational thoughts with rational ones, the constructivist views individuals as complex, perhaps with unconscious motivations, who are continually adapting their cognitions in an effort to make meaning out of the world. **Constructivism** emphasizes how one's construction of reality is based on a complex interaction between our thinking, acting, and feeling worlds, with each individual creating his or her own unique meaning-making system. This approach views the helping relationship as an attempt to understand how the client makes meaning of the world and to find ways of intervening with the individual that will change his or her meaning-making system.

The Human Service Professional's Use of the Cognitive Approach
Although human service professionals have not widely adopted the cognitive approach, professionals in most settings can readily use its basic concepts. Helping clients understand the connection between thinking, feeling, and behaving can dramatically affect how they interact in the world. Understanding that at least to some degree our thinking creates our feelings and actions can give clients hope regarding their future. Perhaps one challenge for human service professionals today is to understand and embrace cognitive theory more fully so they can better help clients take responsibility for their thinking, feeling, and acting.

CROSS-THEORETICAL APPROACHES

In some cases, specific approaches to working with clients can combine or integrate varying theoretical approaches such as those we have already discussed in this chapter. This section looks at three such approaches: eclecticism, brief treatment, and gender-aware counseling.

Eclecticism or Integrative Approaches to Counseling

When using **eclecticism,** mental health professionals draw from a number of different orientations to develop an approach to working with their clients. Professionals using this approach, however, must not shoot from the hip; instead, they must carefully reflect on their views of human nature and draw techniques that fit their ways of viewing the world while meeting the mental health needs of their clients. Unfortunately, my experience has been that many individuals who call themselves eclectic use a hodgepodge of techniques, which may end up being confusing to a client. How many mental health professionals are eclectic? In fact, studies show that between 39% and 70% of counselors and other mental health professionals identify themselves as "Eclectic" (Jensen, Bergin, & Greaves, 1990; Neukrug & Williams, 1993; Norcross, Prochaska, & Gallagher, 1989). And, when human service practitioners and students were asked the orientation of their therapists, 25% stated they were eclectic (Neukrug, Milliken, & Shoemaker, 2001).

Before you borrow techniques from the differing orientations, you must carefully examine your view of human nature. Only after beliefs about the nature of the individual have been established should one choose techniques that will fit that view. In the exercises at the end of this chapter, you will have an opportunity to examine your view of human nature. There are many different ways of developing an eclectic approach (Gilliland, James, & Bowman, 1994; Howard, Nance, & Myers, 1986; Lazarus & Beutler, 1993; Mahalik, 1990; McBride & Martin, 1990; Norcross, 1986); however, all the models tend to address a number of common concerns that lead me to consider the notion that the formation of an eclectic approach is a developmental process that starts with **chaos** and ends with what might be called a commitment to a metatheory (Neukrug, 2002).

Stage 1: **Chaos:** In this initial stage of developing an eclectic approach, the human service professional has no theory, is sloppy, bases his or her responses on moment-to-moment subjective judgments, and can be harmful to clients. Beginning students who are just starting to understand counseling theory and are attempting to haphazardly combine theories may be at this chaos stage.

Stage 2: **Coalescent Stage:** As theory is learned, many mental health professionals drift toward adherence to one approach. As they begin to feel comfortable with this approach, they may begin to integrate different techniques from other approaches into their theoretical style.

Stage 3: **Theoretical Integration Stage:** During this stage, mental health professionals have thoroughly learned one theory and have successfully integrated one or more other theories into their approach. The professional mental health worker in this stage is becoming "seasoned" and feels comfortable with his or her unique integrative approach.

Stage 4: **Metatheory Stage:** As mental health professionals develop a full appreciation of many theories, they begin to wonder about underlying commonalities and themes among the varying theories. This leads some helpers to develop or take on what some have called a metatheory. For instance, two mental health professionals with very different eclectic approaches may realize that an underlying theme of all clients is how family and social systems affect them (see Chapter 6). Thus, this "systemic understanding" is seen as common to all clients and must be addressed, regardless of the eclectic approach used.

If you are just beginning your journey as a human service professional, you might expect to pass through these stages as you begin to sort through the various theoretical approaches and develop your own unique integrative style of counseling.

Brief Treatment Approaches

With HMOs overseeing the number of sessions individuals can have with their therapists, and with cutbacks in funding for agencies, **brief treatment,** which has been defined as anywhere from 2 to 50 sessions, has become increasingly popular in the past 15 years. With brief treatment possibly being as effective as longer-term counseling, brief treatment approaches seem an important and practical approach in today's world (Carlson & Sperry, 2000; Gelso, 1992; Gingerich & Eisengart, 2000; Koss & Butcher, 1986).

Because human service professionals are generally not doing in-depth therapy, and because they tend to work on very-focused problems, brief treatment approaches have a home with the human service professional. What is the difference between brief treatment and longer-term approaches? Budman and Gurman (1988) offer some comparisons (see Table 3.1).

Table 3.1 Comparison of Long-Term and Short-Term Treatment Approaches

Long-Term Approach	Short-Term Approach
1. Seeks change in the basic character.	1. Prefers pragmatism, parsimony, and least radical intervention and does not believe in notion of "cure."
2. Believes that significant psychological change is unlikely in everyday life.	2. Maintains an adult developmental perspective from which significant psychological change is viewed as inevitable.
3. Sees presenting problems as reflecting more basic pathology.	3. Emphasizes patient's strengths and resources; presenting problems are taken seriously (although not necessarily at face value).
4. Wants to "be there" as patient makes significant changes.	4. Accepts that many changes will occur "after therapy" and will not be observable to the therapist.
5. Sees therapy as having a "timeless" quality and is willing to wait for change.	5. Does not accept the timelessness of some models of therapy.
6. Unconsciously recognizes the fiscal convenience of maintaining long-term patients.	6. Fiscal issues often muted, either by the nature of the therapist's practice or by the organizational structure for reimbursement.
7. Views psychotherapy as almost always being useful.	7. Views psychotherapy as being sometimes useful and sometimes harmful.
8. Sees patient's being in therapy as the most important part of patient's life.	8. Sees being in the world as more important than being in therapy.

SOURCE: *Theory and Practice of Brief Therapy* by Budman & Gurman. 1988. Reprinted by permission of Guilford Publications

Brief treatment can be used across different therapeutic approaches (see Garfield, 1989; Steenbarger, 1992). Garfield (1989) suggests that all brief treatment approaches pass through four stages that include (1) building the relationship and assessing the problem; (2) developing a plan for the client, encouraging homework assignments, and working on the problem; (3) following through on treatment plans and reformulating treatment plans based on new information and client feedback; and (4) termination, in which the client's feelings concerning progress are assessed, future plans discussed (for example, follow-up, referral, ways of continuing progress), and closure accomplished. These stages can be applied in many human service settings and the human service professional should pay particular attention to brief treatment approaches (see Box 3.5).

Gender-Aware Approaches

In recent years, some have argued that because gender biases exist in helpers (Seem & Johnson, 1998), when working with women or with men, there should be specific guidelines that address differences in gender. Called **feminist therapy** and **men's issues therapy** by some, each of these approaches are unique and focus on specific tasks to be achieved in the helping relationship (see Fitzgerald & Nutt, 1995; McNamara & Rickard, 1989; Osherson, 1986; Williams & Myer, 1992).

Some suggest that all mental health professionals should be actively involved in doing **gender-aware therapy** (Good, Gilbert, and Scher, 1995). Such treatment

---

BOX 3.5   A Cure in One Session?

Brief therapy is one thing, but can clients be cured in one session? Well, perhaps sometimes. For instance, I was once working with a family that consisted of a mother, her daughter, and the new stepfather. The family came in to see me, very distraught. During the one-hour session, I explained to the family how they were dealing with new ways of relating, being a new family. I made some suggestions about how the stepfather and stepdaughter could spend more time together (both had a desire to deepen their relationship). And, I suggested that the mother might want to slowly give her daughter a little more space. At the end of the session, they were all smiling. They said they were "cured" and did not need to come back. A one-month follow-up revealed a happy family. A six-month follow-up did the same. They insisted that this one session was all they needed!

---

approaches consider gender central to the helping relationship, view problems within a societal context, encourage helpers to actively address gender injustices, encourage the development of a collaborative and equal relationship, and respect the client's right to choose the gender roles appropriate for himself or herself regardless of their political correctness (Chapter 7 will present an outline of suggestions when working with women and with men). Finally, we must always keep in mind that as many differences as there are between men and women, there is still much that we share in common. We must not overemphasize the differences, as we all swim in the sea of humanity.

> In general it is imperative that researchers learn to conceive of sex differences dialectically, constantly balancing the tendency to overemphasize differences with the tendency to underemphasize differences. (Horst, 1995, p. 276)

ETHICAL AND PROFESSIONAL ISSUES

The Importance of Supervision
for the Human Service Professional

To become a better human service professional, it is important to constantly examine your view of human nature, your theoretical approach, and, ultimately, your effectiveness with your clients. One way of accomplishing this is through the supervisory relationship (Bernard & Goodyear, 1998). **Supervision** should start during one's training program, to "serve as a unique link between preparation and skilled service" (Cogan & O'Connell, 1982, p. 12), and should continue as long as one is working with clients in the human service field. There is nothing better than a good supervisory relationship that is based on trust, mutual respect, and understanding to help us take a good look at what we are doing (Sadow, Ryder, Stein, & Geller, 1987).

The supervisor has a number of roles and responsibilities including ensuring the welfare of the client; making sure that ethical, professional, and legal standards are being upheld; overseeing the clinical and professional development of the supervisee; and evaluating the supervisee (ACES, 1995). Like the effective helper, the good supervisor is empathic, flexible, genuine, and open (Borders, 1994). In addition, the good supervisor is able to be an evaluator of the **supervisee** and is comfortable with being an authority figure (Bradley & Gould, 1994). Good supervisors know counseling, have good client conceptualization skills, and are good problem solvers.

Unfortunately, all too often I have seen professionals avoid supervision because of fears about their own adequacy. These fears can create an atmosphere of isolation for the human service professional, an isolation that leads to rigidity and an inability to examine varying methods of working with clients. It is important that we as professionals face our own vulnerable spots—to look at what we do not do well. A good supervisory relationship can help us look at issues such as when to break confidentiality or when we might be losing our objectivity because of a dual relationship.

Confidentiality and the Helping Relationship

Regardless of the theoretical approach to which one adheres, keeping client information confidential is one of the most important ingredients in building a trusting relationship. However, is **confidentiality** always guaranteed or warranted? For instance, suppose you encounter the following situation: A 17-year-old client tells you that she is pregnant. Do you need to tell her parents? What if the client was 15 or 12? What if she was drinking while pregnant, or using cocaine, or . . . What if she tells you she wants an abortion? What if she tells you she is suicidal because of the pregnancy? Although most of us would agree that confidentiality is an important ingredient in the helping relationship, it might not always be best to keep things confidential. Although all ethical decisions are to some degree judgment calls, we can follow some general guidelines when making a decision to break confidentiality (always check local laws, however, to see if there are variations). Generally, you can break confidentiality in these situations:

1. If a client is in danger of harming himself or herself or someone else

2. If a child is a minor and the law states that parents have a right to information about their child

3. If a client asks you to break confidentiality (for example, your testimony is needed in court)

4. If you are bound by the law to break confidentiality (for example, a local law requires human service professionals to report the selling of drugs)

5. To reveal information about your client to your supervisor to benefit the client

6. When you have a written agreement from your client to reveal information to specified sources (for example, other social service agencies that are working with the same client)

Now that we have looked at when it is all right to break confidentiality, let's examine times when it is not usually permissible:

1. When you're frustrated with a client and you talk to a friend or colleague about the case just to "let off steam"
2. When a helping professional requests information about your client and you have not received written permission
3. When a friend asks you to tell him or her something interesting about a client with whom you are working
4. When breaking confidentiality will clearly cause harm to your client and does not fall into one of the categories previously listed

Confidentiality is an ethical guideline, not a legal right. The legal term that ensures the right of professionals not to reveal information about their clients is **privileged communication** (Glosoff, Herlihy, & Spence, 2000). In fact, the privilege actually belongs to the client and can only be waived by him or her (Attorney C. Borstein, personal communication, May 1, 2002; Swenson, 1997, p. 464). Generally, this means that, if called to court, these professionals do not have to reveal information unless the client allows them to. In many states, lawyers, priests, physicians, and licensed therapists have been given privileged communication with their clients, but other mental health professionals, including human service professionals, have not. Thus, they cannot ensure confidentiality in some cases.

The ethical guidelines of the American Counseling Association (ACA, 1995), the American Psychological Association (APA, 2002), and the National Association of Social Workers (NASW, 1999), as well as the *Ethical Standards of Human Service Professionals* (see Appendix B), ensure the right to confidentiality, usually with some limitations, as listed earlier. More specifically, the *Ethical Standards of Human Service Professionals* states

> Human service professionals protect the client's right to privacy and confidentiality except when such confidentiality would cause harm to the client or others, when agency guidelines state otherwise, or under other stated conditions (e.g., local, state, or federal laws). Professionals inform clients of the limits of confidentiality prior to the onset of the relationship. (See Appendix B, Statement 3)

Dual Relationships and the Human Service Professional

Is it all right to have as a client a friend, relative, or lover? Most professional groups like ACA (1995), NASW (1999), and APA (2002) have taken clear stands that this is not ethical (Cottone & Tarvydas, 1998). Similarly, the *Ethical Standards of Human Service Professionals* strongly discourages **dual relationships:**

> Human service professionals are aware that in their relationship with clients power and status are unequal. Therefore they recognize that dual or multiple relationships may increase the risk of harm to, or exploitation of, clients, and

may impair their professional judgment. However, in some communities and situations it may not be feasible to avoid social or other nonprofessional contact with clients. Human service professionals support the trust implicit in the helping relationship by avoiding dual relationships that may impair professional judgment, increase the risk of harm to clients or lead to exploitation. (See Appendix B, Statement 6)

Because human service professionals are not involved in intensive psychotherapeutic relationships, the relationship with their clients differs from those of counselors and psychologists. I believe, however, that it is the responsibility of each human service professional to decide whether his or her objectivity and professional judgment are impaired by having a dual relationship with a client. Generally, it is not wise to have a dual relationship, especially because, in almost every case, another human service professional can help that individual.

THE DEVELOPMENTALLY MATURE HUMAN SERVICE PROFESSIONAL

Committed to a Counseling Approach and Willing to Change

Remember Perry and the concept of commitment in relativism (Chapter 1)? Well, effective human service professionals have reflected on the various approaches to counseling and have made a commitment to that approach. This commitment includes learning more about the approach, reading current research about that and other approaches, being open to the supervisory process, and, most important, changing the approach if evidence indicates that it is ineffective. Human service professionals who are committed in relativism are willing and eager to explore new theories and to adapt their theories as evidence accrues that a newer approach is more effective. These are human service professionals who are truly dedicated to growth in the field, in the self, and in their clients.

SUMMARY

This chapter began by contrasting the words *counseling* and *psychotherapy*. We noted that although a text on counseling theories would be indistinguishable from a text on theories of psychotherapy, how a mental health practitioner applies these theories often distinguishes whether he or she is practicing counseling or psychotherapy. We also noted that although human service professionals do not do in-depth counseling or therapy, they do counsel clients, and thus it is crucial that they have a basic understanding of the theory behind what they do. We then discussed the importance of having a theoretical approach drive the way in which one does counseling, and that theory tends to be an outgrowth of one's view of human nature. In reference to views of human nature, we discussed the difference between a deterministic and antideterministic approach to counseling, and a direct versus a nondirective approach.

In reference to theory, we first contrasted the individual approach to counseling with a systemic approach and concluded that both have some value. The individual approaches to counseling we examined in this chapter included psychodynamic, behavioral, humanistic, and cognitive approaches to working with the individual. Each approach is distinguished by its unique view of human nature, which emphasizes beliefs about the nature of the person. We learned that the psychodynamic approach stresses unconscious factors, early childhood development, and instincts, whereas the behavioral approach focuses on how the individual was conditioned and what types of models were prominent in an individual's life. Whereas both approaches were originally considered to be deterministic, modern versions focus more on the ability of the individual to change. We learned that the humanistic approach was originally a reaction to the deterministic views of the psychodynamic and behavioral approaches and that this approach, along with the cognitive approach, has a strong belief in the ability of the individual to make choices that can positively affect the individual's functioning in the world. Whereas the humanistic approach stresses the importance of increased self-awareness for the client in making effective choices, the cognitive approach stresses being able to alter our thinking process in making changes in our lives.

In addition to looking at specific theoretical orientations, we also examined cross-theoretical approaches, or approaches that might use one or more of the theoretical orientations when working with clients. Thus, we briefly reviewed eclecticism or integrative approaches to counseling, brief treatment approaches, and gender-aware counseling.

As the chapter continued, we examined the ethical and professional issues of supervision, confidentiality, and dual relationships. The supervisory relationship is particularly important because that relationship can help us understand how we interact with our clients, provides feedback when we might be losing objectivity, and can help us make difficult decisions related to breaking confidentiality. We concluded the chapter by noting that the developmentally mature human service professional is committed to a counseling approach yet willing to change as new concepts become known.

EXPERIENTIAL EXERCISES

1. What Is Your Theoretical Approach?—A Checklist to Determine Your Theoretical Approach

To the left of each statement listed below, place the appropriate number. Then, when you are finished, follow the directions for scoring the inventory.

    0 = Strongly disagree
    1 = Mildly disagree
    2 = Mildly agree
    3 = Strongly agree

1. ___ People can go beyond their early childhood experiences and make major personality changes in their lives.

2. ___ Effective counseling can take place in a relatively short period.

3. ___ People are born with a tendency to actualize their real self. This tendency will be squashed if placed in a dysfunctional environment but can re-emerge if the individual is once again introduced to a nurturing environment.

4. ___ Reinforcements in the environment greatly affect how we act.

5. ___ We are born with drives that greatly affect how we live our lives. Oftentimes these drives are unconsciousness; that is, we behave in ways to get our drives met yet we don't realize that this is the underlying reason why we're doing what we're doing.

6. ___ My sexual urges greatly affect my behavior in mysterious and unknown ways.

7. ___ My thinking affects my feelings.

8. ___ My behaviors affect my feelings.

9. ___ I have a number of instincts that may affect my behavior in mysterious and known ways.

10. ___ Although some change is possible, much of my life is predestined due to my early childhood experiences.

11. ___ I know that if I can change the way I perceive the world and the way I think, I can live a well-adjusted life.

12. ___ Understanding a client's personality formation from a critical and objective standpoint is probably the most crucial factor in helping a client manage his or her problems.

13. ___ Long-term counseling is a waste of time and money as the same kinds of changes can take place in a brief amount of time.

14. ___ My early childhood may have affected me greatly, but it does not determine my present-day behavior.

15. ___ My early childhood affected me greatly, continues to affect how I live; I have only a limited amount of power to change.

16. ___ Unconditional positive regard is an essential element in the counseling relationship.

17. ___ By controlling the environment, one can help a person feel good about who he or she is.

18. ___ It is not events that cause me to feel bad; it is what I believe about those events.

19. ___ The bottom line is that things outside of me greatly control my life; I have little ability to change how I feel about myself if events around me are horrible.

20. ___ The change process should be focused on the future, not on current problems.

21. ___ How I act is the major force in creating my mental health.

22. ___ How I feel is the major force in creating my mental health.

23. ___ My behavior affects my thinking.

24. ___ The most crucial aspect for effective counseling is the relationship between the counselor and client.

25. ___ I am in control of most of my behaviors.

26. ___ My unconscious controls most of my behaviors.

27. ___ My early childhood probably affected my way of thinking, but I can change the way I think and live a healthier life.

28. ___ A positive attitude toward life and belief in the ability of people to change are the most crucial aspects of helping a client work through his or her problems.

29. ___ How we make meaning in the world is complex and can best be understood through the stories clients tell.

30. ___ Long-lasting change is affected by my ability to "catch" and change my "automatic" thoughts.

31. ___ It is important that I maintain certain defenses to live reasonably in this world.

32. ___ The most crucial aspect of the counseling relationship is the ability to be empathic with the client.

33. ___ My theoretical orientation is not as important as my ability to help the client focus on the future and his or her change process.

34. ___ My feelings affect my behavior and cognitions.

35. ___ If placed in a nurturing environment, I will be able to get in touch with my true self.

36. ___ If we can understand the types of parenting that occurred through predictable stages of child development, we can understand the problems faced by individuals later in life.

Scoring the Inventory

For each item in the inventory, place the number that you wrote for that item number in the space provided on the following scoresheet. For instance, if you placed a "3" under item "5," a "3" should be written for the first item under "psychodynamic." Note that some items are used for more than one approach (e.g., item number "1" is used for humanistic, behavioral, cognitive, and brief approaches). Because there are fewer items for "Brief/Solution Focused Counseling," you need to multiply your total for that category by the correction factor of 1.4. Some theorists might differ with my categorization of items on the inventory; however, your results should give you an approximation of the theoretical orientation to which you lean.

Psychodynamic	Humanistic	Behavioral	Cognitive	Brief/Solution Focused
5. ____	1. ____	1. ____	1. ____	1. ____
6. ____	2. ____	2. ____	2. ____	2. ____
9. ____	3. ____	4. ____	7. ____	13. ____
10. ____	14. ____	8. ____	11. ____	14. ____
12. ____	16. ____	13. ____	13. ____	20. ____
15. ____	22. ____	14. ____	14. ____	28. ____
19. ____	24. ____	17. ____	18. ____	33. ____
26. ____	32. ____	21. ____	27. ____	Total = _____
31. ____	34. ____	23. ____	29. ____	Total × 1.4 = _____
36. ____	35. ____	25. ____	30. ____	
Total = _____	Total = _____	Total = _____	Total = _____	Total = _____

2. Understanding Your View of Human Nature

For each of the four statements below, circle all items that best describe your view of the person. When you are finished, take all of the circled items, and using them as a guide, develop a paragraph describing your view of human nature. (Note: each statement represents a particular perspective on the view of human nature; that perspective is italicized).

1. *Innate at Birth.* I believe people are born
   a. good
   b. bad
   c. neutral
   d. with original sin
   e. restricted by their genetics
   f. with a growth force that allows them to change throughout life
   g. capable of being anything they want to be
   h. with sexual drives that consciously and unconsciously affect their lives
   i. with aggressive drives that consciously and unconsciously affect their lives

    j. with social drives that consciously and unconsciously affect their lives

    k. other attributes _____

2. *The Developing Person.* Personality development is most influenced by

    a. genetics

    b. learning

    c. early child-rearing patterns

    d. drives

    e. values that are taught

    f. environment

    g. relationships with others

    h. biology

    i. conscious decisions

    j. the unconscious

    k. instincts

    l. modeling the behavior of others

    m. relationships we form

    n. developmental issues (e.g., puberty)

    o. other

3. *The Change Process.* As a people grow older, I believe they are

    a. capable of major changes in their personality

    b. capable of moderate changes in their personality

    c. capable of minor changes in their personality

    d. incapable of change in their personality

    e. determined by their early childhood experiences

    f. determined by their genetics

    g. determined by how they were conditioned and reinforced

    h. determined by unconscious motivations

    i. able to transcend or go beyond early childhood experiences

4. *How Change Occurs.* Change is likely to be most facilitated by a focus on

a. conscious mind	h. the past
b. unconscious mind	i. the present
c. thoughts	j. the future
d. behaviors	k. biology (e.g., the use of medications)
e. feelings	l. unfinished business and repressed memories
f. early experiences	m. getting in touch with the "true" self
g. biology	n. other

3. Applying Differing Theoretical Orientations

Read the description of each of the following clients and think about how each theoretical orientation listed in this chapter would describe the origins of this person's current situation. Then discuss how you might apply each orientation.

The story of Jill. Jill is a 32-year-old married mother of two children, ages 7 and 2. She states that, before getting married 6 years ago, she drank heavily, smoked pot, and "hung out with bikers and slept with a lot of guys." She has settled down since then but has started hanging out with her neighbor Steven, is drinking again, and is thinking about having an affair with Steven. She says that she loves her husband, but he has not been paying attention to her lately. She is angry at him but reports that she and her husband rarely talk about their feelings. Although she maintained average grades in school, she never completed high school and would like to obtain her GED. She reports having frequent anxiety attacks and rarely leaves her house other than to go to her part-time job in a factory.

Jill, the second child in a family of four, states that her father was verbally abusive, drank a lot, and generally didn't pay attention to her. Since he stopped drinking a few years ago, however, he has become closer to her. She reports her childhood as being chaotic because she never knew whether her father would blow up at her or at other members of her family when he was drunk. No one in her family has ever received a high school diploma.

The story of Harley. Harley was recently released from the state mental hospital where he spent most of his adolescence. Harley has a history of being psychotic; that is, he has periodically been out of touch with reality. His parents abandoned him when he was 9 years old, and he has lived in foster homes and at state hospitals since that time. He just turned 18 years old. Harley is currently taking antipsychotic and antianxiety medications and is in the day treatment program at the local community mental health center. At day treatment, he spends the day attending support groups, doing vocational skills training, and socializing. He has little memory of his childhood, but what he can remember is very painful. For instance, he does have vague memories of verbal and sexual abuse, and he thinks there were older siblings in his home. Harley's lifelong dream is to own a motorcycle, and he seems to talk about a motorcycle as if it were his lover. Confidentially, he reports having had sexual feelings toward a motorcycle.

Harley has few friends and has an impulsive temper; that is, he periodically just blows up. Although he generally does not act out physically toward people, on rare occasions he has been known to attack someone in an impulsive rage. His medication seems to help him with his outbursts.

4. The Human Service Professional's Implementation of Varying Theoretical Approaches

Describe how a human service professional in each of the following occupations might apply the theoretical orientations discussed in this chapter.

1. A human service professional who helps at a shelter for the homeless

2. A human service professional who helps the mentally retarded at a residential home

3. A human service professional who helps the mentally ill at a day treatment program in a mental health center

4. A human service professional assisting poor women at a problem-pregnancy counseling center

5. A human service professional who helps the poor at an unemployment office

5. Eclecticism or Integrative Approaches to Helping

1. Using Exercises 1 and 2 as a resource, make a list of items that reflect your view of human nature.

2. Based on this list, begin to develop your own theory of counseling.

3. What "techniques" are natural outgrowths of your theory?

4. Do you think your theory will change over time?

6. Ethical and Professional Issues: Supervision

1. Discuss the qualities you would want in a supervisor.

2. Have one person role-play a supervisor and one person role-play a human service professional and then discuss the case of Harley or Jill in Exercise 3.

   a. What theoretical approach do you think would work best with your client? Discuss with your "supervisor" what you think you might want to do to assist your client.

   b. Did the "supervisor" offer a supervisory environment that was conducive to you talking about your client? What supervisory qualities were helpful? Unhelpful?

7. Ethical and Professional Vignettes: Confidentiality and Dual Relationships

A. Refer to Harley and Jill in Exercise 3 to discuss the following vignettes.

   1. While you are helping Jill find study classes for the GED exam, she reveals that sometimes when she's drinking she takes the belt out and "whacks my kids good—they just won't shut up." Do you break confidentiality and tell Child Protective Services?

   2. While driving to work one day, your car breaks down. Harley sees you and says, "I'm good with mechanical things, let me help for a small fee— besides, I could use a little money for buying my bike." You want to get your car fixed, and you want Harley to have his bike. Do you let him help you?

3. One day Jill tells you she is pregnant by Steven. She's going to have an abortion. Your state has a law requiring women to tell their spouses if they're to have an abortion. She refuses. What do you do?

4. Jill's husband shows up at your office demanding information about his wife. You tell him things are confidential. He tells you that he'll sue you and the rest of this "fleabag" operation. What do you do?

5. You've been encouraging Jill for months to get involved in more social activities to get out of the house more. One day in your art class, Jill shows up saying that she signed up for the same class. What do you do?

6. Jill tells you that from time to time, usually when she's drinking, she gets severely depressed and thinks about killing herself. You ask her if she has a plan, and she says, "Well, sometimes I think about just doing it with that gun my husband has." One day she calls you; she's been drinking, and she tells you she's depressed. She hangs up saying, "I don't know what I might do." What do you do?

7. Harley stops taking his medication, stops by your office, and seems pretty angry. He says, "That cheating Harley dealer, he's trying to rip me off. He told me I could have that bike at a discount and went back on his word." You try to talk with Harley, but he storms out of your office saying, "I'm going get that man!" What do you do?

B. Other Ethical Vignettes

1. Your supervisor tells you that he is going to have to report your client to social services for possible child abuse. You believe that he has broken the confidentiality of your relationship with your client. Is what he's doing ethical? Professional? Legal?

2. A colleague of yours who works with female clients who have been abused encourages all of her clients to leave their husbands and states that this is the "right thing to do" from a feminist perspective. Does she have a point? Is what she's doing ethical? Professional? Legal?

3. A fellow student of yours tells you that being eclectic is the way to go because then you can pretty much pull any techniques you like from the different theories and combine them into your own approach. When working in an internship, you discover that this student is counseling clients without a solid theoretical base—just using techniques she likes. What is your responsibility to this student? To the clients? What is your ethical obligation?

4. After obtaining your first job you discover that many of your human service colleagues have forgotten the theories they have learned in school and do not feel obligated to continuing education. What is your responsibility in this situation? What is your ethical obligation?

5. You discover that a colleague of yours is seeing clients for extended periods to "pad" his contact hours. Many of these clients could have been worked with in a brief treatment mode, but your colleague has continued with them regardless of this fact. What is your responsibility to the clients? To the colleague? To the agency? To your profession? What should you do?

4

✠

The Helping Interview:
Skills, Process,
and Case Management

The first time I did counseling, I was a volunteer at the drug crisis clinic at my college. I had no training, but somehow I instinctively knew that it was probably best to listen a lot and be kind. Having been a psychology major, I never had a course in counseling theories or counseling methods. I knew little about the "correct" way to respond to a drop-in at the center. I hope I did more good than harm as I tried to help students who had overdosed or were "bumming" from doing hallucinogens.

Immediately following receipt of a bachelor's degree, I went on to obtain my master's degree in counseling. I then spent a few months painstakingly looking for employment. I obtained my first real job at "The Rap House." A drug and alcohol government-funded agency, this storefront drop-in and crisis center was the place where many of the street alcoholics could stop in, get a cup of coffee, and, if need be, talk to a counselor or get a referral to a detox center. These were my first clients.

Now that I had a graduate degree, I at least had some training in appropriate ways to respond to a client. At that time, my theoretical approach was humanistically based, and I felt it was good if people could express their feelings and let things out. Although my counseling approach had become somewhat focused, my old untrained self, which sometimes would get very advice oriented, periodically raised its ugly head.

From these experiences, I have come to learn that one is not born with an ability to counsel. Counseling skills can be learned. However, one need not have an advanced degree to become a fairly effective helper (Barz, 2001; Neukrug, 1987, 2002). What is important is learning the skills and practicing them. Much like riding a bicycle or putting on in-line skates for the first time, learning counseling skills feels awkward at first. However, you will find that the more you practice, the more natural and at ease you feel. In my own life, I now approach the learning and refinement of my skills as a never-ending process. One never "gets there"; instead, we hope to get better as we learn new and more effective ways of working with our clients. Some of us are lucky because we had good modeling from our parents or other significant people and thus we have a head start in learning skills. Unfortunately, I have found that most of us have not been so blessed, so practicing tried-and-true techniques becomes extremely important.

More than any other area in the human services, I have found that learning skills is the most sensitive and awkward area for many students. This part of the curriculum is where students often feel that they are putting themselves "out there," showing their capabilities to their peers. Unfortunately, because students often feel so vulnerable in front of their peers, I find many protect themselves and partially shut out this important learning experience. If you are apprehensive, that's normal. However, if you find that this fear prevents you from taking an active role in learning these important skills, then reflect on what you are doing and see whether you can take a more open approach.

In this chapter, we will examine the importance of creating a conducive atmosphere for the helping relationship and examine techniques that over the years have been shown to be effective in working with a wide range of clients. Some of these include listening, empathy, silence, encouragement, affirmations, modeling, self-disclosure, the use of questions, giving information, advice giving, offering alternatives, information giving, and confrontation.

We will also examine the structure of the interview, or the predictable manner in which the interview flows and how to develop problem-solving strategies as we pass through these stages. In addition to responding effectively to your clients and knowing the predictable stages of the interview, good case management is critical to successful work with clients and will be examined in this chapter. Case management involves a myriad of tasks including treatment planning; diagnosis; monitoring the use of psychotropic drugs; case report writing; managing and documenting client contact hours; monitoring, evaluating, and documenting progress toward client goals; making referrals; follow-up; and time management. The chapter will conclude with an examination of ethical, professional, and legal issues as they relate to these important matters.

CREATING THE HELPING ENVIRONMENT

Office Environment

I'm sure you've had the experience of walking into someone's office and finding it cold and inhospitable. How one arranges one's office can be crucial to eliciting positive attitudes from people and gives a message to our clients about whether they are welcomed (Pressly & Heesacker, 2001). Although all human service professionals may not have their own offices, wherever we meet our clients, we should attempt to make the environment as conducive as possible to a positive working relationship. If we are lucky enough to have an office, simple things like nonglare lighting, comfortable seating, and not having obstructions (for example, large desks) between ourselves and our clients can be helpful in creating a comfortable helping environment. You may want to review Exercise 1 at the end of this chapter to determine how you might arrange an office.

Personal Characteristics of the Helper

Whether the human service professional is found doing one-to-one counseling within an office or chatting with clients in a group home, the attitudes he or she brings can help to create a facilitative helping relationship. Therefore, it is important that we bring with us some of the attitudes noted in Chapter 1—that we are empathic, open minded, accepting, cognitively complex, psychologically adjusted, genuine, capable of building meaningful helping relationships, and competent. These characteristics allow our clients to feel a sense of safety and trust with us. If you find a client who is particularly nasty or angry, first examine your attitudes to see how you bring yourself to the session. If you are not embodying the characteristics of the effective helper, perhaps your attitude is feeding the client's anger.

Importance of Nonverbal Behavior

Yet when humans communicate, as much as eighty percent of the meaning of their messages is derived from nonverbal language. The implication is disturbing. As far as communication is concerned, human beings spend most of their time studying the wrong thing. (Thompson, 1973, p. 1)

The importance of our **nonverbal** behavior with clients is vastly underrated. How we present ourselves nonverbally can greatly add to or detract from our overall relationship with our clients. Posture or tone of voice that says "don't open up to me" will obviously affect our clients in very different ways than will the helper who is nonverbally conveying, "I'm open to hearing what you have to say." We tell our clients that we are there for them through our body posture, how we make eye contact, and in the types of verbal responses we make. In the next section, "Listening Skills," you have an opportunity to do some role-playing. As you do this, give one another feedback on how your body language is or is not facilitative for the other person.

Personal space and touch are two other areas of nonverbal behavior important to the helping relationship. Touching at important moments, of course, is quite natural. For instance, when someone is expressing deep pain, it is not unusual for us to hold a hand or embrace a person while he or she sobs. Or, when a client is coming to or leaving a meeting with a human service professional, many find it natural to place a hand on a shoulder or maybe even give a hug. However, in today's litigious society, touch has become a particularly delicate subject, so it is important for each of us to be sensitive to our clients' boundaries, our own boundaries, and limits as suggested by our professional ethics (Gabbard, 1995). Some have become so "touchy" over this issue that a therapist in Massachusetts, branded "the hugging therapist," was fired from his job at a mental health agency because he hugged his clients too much. Brammer and MacDonald (1999) suggest that whether or not one has physical contact with a client should be based on (1) the helper's assessment of the helpee, (2) the helper's awareness of his or her own needs, (3) what is most likely to be helpful within the helping relationship, and (4) risks that may be involved as a function of "agency policy, local custom, professional ethics, and the age, sex, culture, and attitude of the helpee" (p. 159).

Finally, it is now suggested that helpers be acutely sensitive to nonverbal differences that may be a function of culture (Morse & Ivey, 1996; Sue & Sue, 1999). The human service professional must understand that some clients will expect to be looked at, but others will be offended by eye contact; that some clients will expect you to lean forward, whereas others will experience this as an intrusion; and that some clients will expect you to touch them, and others will see this as an invasion of privacy. In respect to nonverbal behavior, effective helpers must keep in mind what works for the many and be sensitive to what works for the few.

COUNSELING TECHNIQUES

Listening Skills

First there is the hearing with the ear, which we all know; and the hearing with the non-ear, which is a state like that of a tranquil pond, a lake that is completely quiet and when you drop a stone into it, it makes little waves that disappear. I think that [insight] is the hearing with the non-ear, a state where there is absolute quietness of the mind; and when the question is put into the mind, the response is the wave, the little wave. (Krishnamurti, cited in Jayakar, 1986, p. 325)

Assuming we have created an environment conducive to a positive client/helper relationship, we are now ready to assess the client situation. Usually, our first step is to understand the issues our clients bring with them. This means being able to hear our clients—good listening. Effective listening helps to build trust, convinces the client you understand him or her, encourages the client to reflect on what he or she has just said, ensures that you are on track with your understanding of the client, and can facilitate gathering information from your client (Scissons, 1993).

Webster (2002) defines *listen* as "to hear something with thoughtful attention." Whenever I have taught **listening skills,** I like to stress that good listening involves keeping one's mouth shut. Although these definitions seem basic, I have found that too many people confuse listening with advice giving. It's almost as if we have learned that if someone is in distress or has a problem, we should tell them what to do. Although advice giving has its place (we will talk more about this later), my experience has been that, more often than not, most people want to be heard rather than being given advice.

> When I ask you to listen to me and you start giving me advice,
>   you have not done what I asked.
> When I ask you to listen to me and you begin to tell me why I shouldn't
>   feel that way, you are trampling on my feelings.
> When I ask you to listen to me and you feel you have to do something to
>   solve my problem, you have failed me, strange as that may seem.
> Listen: All that I ask is that you listen, not talk or do—just hear me.
> When you do something for me that I can and need to do for myself,
>   you contribute to my fear and inadequacy.
> But when you accept as a simple fact that I do feel what I feel, no matter
>   how irrational, then I can quit trying to convince you and get about this
>   business of understanding what's behind these feelings.
> So, please listen and just hear me.
> And, if you want to talk, wait a minute for your turn and I'll listen to you.
>
> (AUTHOR UNKNOWN)

Hindrances to Listening Even when we know how to listen, we are often blocked in our ability to do so. Our own prejudices and issues tend to interfere with our ability to hear the other person. Therefore, to effectively hear another person, we need to be aware of the unique prejudices or blocks that we might have to opening our inner selves to the helpee. Activity 4.1 helps point out some of these blocks. Knowing the blocks and prejudices you hold is crucial to effective listening. However, it is also helpful to have some useful techniques such as the following (Egan, 1994; Ivey & Ivey, 1999; Neukrug, 2002, 2003):

1. *Calm yourself down.* Before meeting with your client, calm yourself down—meditate, pray, jog, or blow out air, but calm your inner self.

2. *Stop talking and don't interrupt.* You cannot listen while you are talking.

3. *Show interest.* With your body language and tone of voice, show the person you are interested in what he or she is saying.

4. *Don't jump to conclusions.* Take in all of what the person says and don't assume you understand the person more than he or she understands himself or herself.

5. *Actively listen.* Many people do not realize that listening is an active process that takes deep concentration. If your mind is wandering, you are not listening.

6. *Concentrate on feelings.* Listen to, identify, and acknowledge the person's feelings to him or her.

7. *Concentrate on content.* Listen to, identify, and acknowledge what the person is saying.

8. *Maintain appropriate eye contact.* (Be sensitive to cultural differences.)

9. *Have an open body posture.* (Be sensitive to cultural differences.)

10. *Be sensitive to the amount of personal space.*

11. *Don't ask questions.* (Except to clarify the client's content.)

Empathy: A Special Kind of Listening

Many of the early Greek philosophers noted the importance of listening to another person from a deep inner perspective (Gompertz, 1960). In the 20th century, Lipps (1935) is given credit for coining the word *empathy* from the German word **Einfühlung,** "to feel within." The person who probably had most impact on our modern day understanding and usage of empathy was Carl Rogers (1959):

> The state of empathy, or being empathic, is to perceive the internal frame of reference of another with accuracy and with the emotional components and meanings which pertain thereto as if one were the person, but without ever losing the "as if" condition. (pp. 210–211)

Since Rogers originally defined empathy, others have attempted to **operationalize** the concept. This means that they have taken Rogers's definition and developed a method to measure one's ability to make empathic responses. For instance, **Robert Carkhuff** (1969) developed a five-point scale to measure empathy (see Figure 4.1). He notes that Level 1 and Level 2 responses in some ways detract from what the person is saying (for example, advice giving, not accurately reflecting feeling, not including content), with a Level 1 response being way off the mark and a Level 2 only slightly off. For instance, suppose a client said, "I've had it with my dad; he never does anything with me. He's always working, drinking, or playing with my little sister." A Level 1 response might be, "Well, why don't you do something to change the situation, like tell him what an idiot he is?" (advice giving and being judgmental). A Level 2 response might be, "You seem to think your dad spends too much time with your sister" (does not reflect feeling and misses some important content).

ACTIVITY 4.1 Hindrances to Effective Listening

In class, break into triads (groups of three). Within your group, each person takes the number 1, 2, or 3. With the three topics listed below (or other topics of the instructor's choice), have the instructor assign one of the topics to persons 1 and 2. Number 1, you be "pro" the situation, and, number 2, you be "con" the situation. Now, one of you start debating the situation while the other listens. When the first person is finished, the second person should repeat back verbatim what he or she heard. Then, debate back and forth, taking turns listening and repeating verbatim until the instructor tells you to stop. Number 3, you are an objective helper, to give feedback if needed. As the objective person,

don't forget also to give feedback concerning each person's body language. When you have finished this first situation, have numbers 2 and 3 do the second situation, and then numbers 3 and 1 do the third situation with the third person being the objective helper.

When you have finished, the instructor will ask for feedback concerning what things prevented you from hearing the other person. Make a list on the board, and in particular make sure you discuss some of the following items: preoccupation, defensiveness, emotional blocks, and distractions.

Situations: Abortion, torturing suspected terrorists to gain information, capital punishment

---

On the other hand, a Level 3 response accurately reflects the affect and meaning of what the helpee has said. Using the same example, you might say, "Well, it sounds as if you're pretty upset at your dad for not spending time with you."

Level 4 and Level 5 responses reflect feelings and meaning beyond what the person is outwardly saying and add to the meaning of the person's outward expression. For instance, in the example, a Level 4 response might be, "It sounds like you're pretty hurt because your father seems to ignore you" (expresses new feeling, hurt, which client did not outwardly state). Level 5 responses are usually made in long-term therapeutic relationships by expert therapists. They express to the helpee a deep understanding of the pain he or she feels as well as recognizing the complexity of the situation.

Usually, in the training of helpers, it is suggested that they attempt to make Level 3 responses because such responses have been shown to be effective for clients (Carkhuff, 2000). Using the Carkhuff (1969) operational definition of empathy, an enormous body of evidence indicates that making good empathic responses (Level 3 or above) can be taught in a relatively short amount of time and that such responses by both paraprofessionals and professionals are beneficial to clients (Carkhuff, 2000; Neukrug, 1980).

Over the years, good empathic responses have been sometimes confused with active listening or reflection of feeling. Although Rogers was instrumental in encouraging the use of empathy, he warned against a mechanistic and wooden response to clients:

Although I am partially responsible for the use of this term [reflection of feelings] to describe a certain type of therapist response, I have, over the years, become very unhappy with it. A major reason is that "reflection of feelings" has not been infrequently taught as a technique, and sometimes a

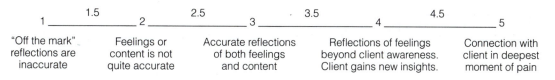

FIGURE 4.1 The Carkhuff Scale

very wooden technique at that. Such training has very little to do with an effective therapeutic relationship. (Rogers, 1986, p. 375)

As Rogers alluded to, although it is important to learn this new skill of empathy, sometimes making such responses will feel stilted and mechanistic. With practice, your responses to clients will become naturally empathic. Activity 4.2 gives you an opportunity to practice this important skill of empathy.

Silence

When   is   empty   space   facilitative,   and

when   does   it   become   a   bit   much?

Silence is a powerful tool in the helping relationship that can be used advantageously for the growth of the client (Hutchins & Cole, 1997; Kleinke, 1994). Silence allows the client to reflect on what he or she has been saying and allows the helper to process the session and to formulate his or her next response. Silence says to the client that communication does not always have to be filled with words, and it gives the client the opportunity to look at how words can sometimes be used to divert a person from his or her feelings. Silence is powerful. It will sometimes raise anxiety within the client, anxiety that on the one hand could push the client to talk further about a particular topic, and on the other hand could cause a client to drop out of treatment.

A former professor of mine used to suggest waiting 30 seconds before making a response. Thirty seconds during a helping relationship is a VEEEEEEEEEERY LOOOOONG TIIIIIIIIIIIIME. There have been times when I've had a student role-play a client, and I've waited 30 seconds before responding. Trust me, this is a VERY LONG TIME. I would have difficulty waiting this long during a helping relationship. However, others may feel comfortable with this amount of silence. For instance, my former professor could do this. During these 30 seconds you could SEE him moving in his chair, SEE him thinking about the last client statement, and SEE him thinking about what he was to say next. This worked for him. Silence is powerful.

Finally, silence by the helper or client may be somewhat culturally determined. For instance, some research has found that the pause time for different cultures varies. Therefore, one's natural inclination to talk—to respond to another—will vary as a function of culture (Tafoya, 1996). As a human service professional, you may want to consider your pause time to discover your comfort level with silence. When working with clients you might consider a client's pause

---

ACTIVITY 4.2   Making Empathic Responses

In class, break up into triads. Two students role-play a helping relationship, trying to make Carkhuff Level 3 responses, while the third student rates the responses of the helper. Then switch roles, giving each student the opportunity to be the helper. After a few minutes, give one another feedback concerning your nonverbal behavior and the ability to make Carkhuff Level 3 responses. Then discuss the level of comfort (or discomfort) you felt with this activity. Do you feel natural in your ability to make empathic responses? If not, how can you work to make it more natural?

---

time. In fact, Tafoya (1996) notes that Native Americans have at times been labeled reticent to talk and resistant in the helping relationship when in fact they have long pause times. If they had been treated by Native American therapists, they most likely would not have been labeled in this fashion.

Encouragement and Affirmation

> The need for supporting core self-esteem doesn't end in childhood. Adults still need "unconditional" love from family, friends, life partners, animals, perhaps even an all-forgiving deity. Love that says: "no matter how the world may judge you, I love you for yourself." (Steinem, 1992, p. 66)

Many of the clients with whom you will be working are coming in with hurts from the past that continue to infiltrate their lives and cause low **self-esteem.** These hurts create depression and anger that sometimes seem to have lost their origins. Such feelings can create negativity and sometimes an "attitude" toward the world that can make these clients some of the most difficult clients with whom we will work. In fact, sometimes our inclination may be to tell these clients to "cut it out" or "pick yourself up off your duff." However, this is the last thing they need. In fact, such clients have generally been so abused and put down throughout their lives that unconsciously, they may be expecting to be treated this way from everyone, even the human service professional. Carrying around this attitude in life rarely, if ever, brings them what they really need—affirmation of self and an attitude that says "you can do it."

Human service professionals must be able to see beyond the hurts, the depression, the anger, and the attitude. They need to believe that clients have potential—can "do it." Human service professionals can express this positive attitude toward clients through encouragement and affirmations. Affirming a client is reinforcing a client's existing way of being, whereas encouragement is reinforcing a client's ability to perform a task. For instance, affirming a client by saying, "good job," "I know you are lovable and capable," or "You are a good person inside" helps the client feel supported and worthwhile. Similarly, encouraging a client by saying, "I know you can do this," or "I'm confident of your ability to change," can help build a client's sense of self-worth. Ultimately, clients need to internalize, or believe that they possess these feelings on their own. Encouragement and affirma-

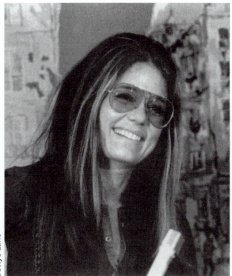

Bettye Lane

Gloria Steinem believes that our need for high self-esteem continues throughout adulthood. Fulfilling that need starts with our ability to love ourselves.

tion can be an important aspect toward helping the client integrate a more positive attitude toward life.

Modeling One time I was asked to talk to a large family reunion about the importance of education. School always came easy for me, but I knew that this was not the case for the audience to whom I was giving my talk. For them, finishing high school was very difficult, and going on to college was rarely considered. I decided instead to model the importance of working hard for a goal. I did not, however, talk about my various degrees; I felt this might be demeaning. Instead, I talked about the time I ran the New York marathon. I was never very athletic, and for me, running the marathon was more difficult than obtaining my doctorate. I worked and trained hard. It took perseverance, and I used this model as an analogy for the importance of working hard for something you really want.

We are constantly **modeling** for our clients, sometimes in intentional ways, as in the previous example, and sometimes, in very subtle ways (Brammer & MacDonald, 1999). Because our clients look up to us, and sometimes even idealize us, the ways in which we model behaviors can have a powerful effect on our clients and dramatically affect our clients in their change process.

When modeling occurs in very subtle ways, clients learn new behaviors simply as a by-product of being in a helping relationship with us. If we are empathic, then they may learn how to listen to loved ones more effectively. If we are assertive, they may learn how to positively confront someone in their lives. And, if we can show them that we can resolve conflict, then they may learn new ways of dealing with conflict in their lives.

When modeling occurs in an intentional manner, the helper deliberately assists the client in establishing new behaviors. For instance, a former client of mine wanted to work on how he could become more assertive with his peers. Thus, he described certain situations with his peers in which he was passive. I then modeled ways in which he could have been assertive. After watching me as a model, he practiced similar behaviors in the office, then at home, and finally with his peers. Now, he did not miraculously become assertive, but with time and patience, he slowly changed some behaviors that he did not feel good about.

Self-Disclosure

A former student once shared with me that her psychiatrist had recently committed suicide. She told me that for the couple of months before his suicide, during her sessions, he was revealing more and more about himself and listening to her less. She now was feeling guilty about his death, thinking that she should have been attending to his needs. What a terrible legacy to leave her! We are helpers, caregivers. We are not in this business to take—to have our needs met. Therefore, keeping a check on when and why we are self-disclosing is extremely important.

Although self-disclosure, as in the previous case, has the potential for harm, certain amounts may facilitate a client's openness and may model positive behaviors for clients (Thompson, 1996). However, if self-disclosure is to be practiced, it must be done gingerly, at the right time, and only as a means for client growth, not to satisfy our needs: "A good interviewer discloses if it appears that it will help the client" (Evans, Hearn, Uhlemann, & Ivey, 1998, p. 150). One general rule of thumb I have is, if it feels good to self-disclose—don't. Probably you're meeting more of your needs than the needs of your client.

> I try not to make a foolish fetish out of not talking about myself. If a client, on the way out the door, asks in a friendly and casual way, "Where are you going on your vacation?" I tell where I'm going. If the client were then to probe, however ("Who are you going with? Are you married?") I would likely respond, "Ah . . . maybe we'd better talk about that next time." (Kahn, 1997, p. 150)

Self-disclosure can be important and helpful for clients (Kleinke, 1994; Pennebaker, Colder, & Sharp, 1990; Pennebaker & Susman, 1988); however, as a counseling skill, it is at best a mixed bag (Donley, Horan, & DeShong, 1990; Doster & Nesbitt, 1979).

The Use of Questions

In his classic book *The Helping Interview,* Benjamin (1987) notes that the use of questions can be detrimental. He states that the overuse of **questions** can set up an atmosphere in which the interviewee "submits to this humiliating treatment only because she expects you to come up with a solution to her problem or because she feels that this is the only way you have of helping her" (p. 135).

Generally, asking a question is not as facilitative to a client as making an empathic response. This is because a good empathic response is empowering—it allows the client to feel as if he or she is discovering answers on his or her own—whereas questions can lead to an authoritarian atmosphere that fosters dependency (Byrne, 1995; Cormier & Cormier, 1998). Most questions that are asked come from a "hunch" and could easily be turned around and made into an empathic response. For instance, suppose the client said the following:

Client: You know, I'm a bit disturbed that my parents never taught me how to be more in charge of my life.

A human service professional could respond by saying something like this:

HSP: Do you feel angry at your parents for not teaching you how to take charge?

However, probably a more effective response would be:

HSP: I get a sense that you're angry at your parents for not teaching you how to take charge.

The empathic response is more focused and to the point, and the client can respond in the affirmative if you are on target or deny your response if you are off the mark. However, sometimes it may be important to ask questions. Obviously, if you need to know specific information like medical history or employment history, you will probably need to ask specific questions. Questions are also useful if you want to probe more deeply into a specific area.

Open versus Closed Questions If you ask a question, an **open question** is generally more facilitative than a **closed question.** An open question such as "How do you feel?" allows a wide variety of responses by the client. A closed question such as "Did you feel angry or sad?" may elicit a yes or no response. This type of question clearly lessens the likelihood of the client disclosing something other than the choices you gave.

Direct versus Indirect Questions Benjamin (1987) notes that a question can be made even more open if it is asked indirectly. For instance, a helper can ask a **direct question** in an open manner:

HSP: How did you feel about your parents divorcing?

To make the question even more palatable to the client, however, you might ask it in the following manner:

HSP: I would guess you had a lot of feelings about your parents divorcing?

The **indirect question** is hardly a question at all; it clearly borders on being an empathic response. Open questions that are indirect tend to "sit well" with clients. They are easier to hear and therefore easier to respond to in an open way.

Use of "Why" Questions Generally, asking a **"why" question** is not recommended. Although, ideally, asking why seems to make sense, people often feel interrogated and put on guard when asked why they felt or did something. Usually, "what" or "how" questions are more palpable for clients. For instance, compare the following "why" and "what" questions:

HSP: Why did you feel depressed and angry at your parents' divorce?

In this case, it is almost as if the interviewer is challenging the helpee about how he or she felt. Look at the following question, but this time start the question with "what"

HSP: What was it about your parents' divorce that made you feel depressed and angry?

In this case, the helpee is not being put on the defensive. Although much more can be said about the different uses of questions in the interviewing process, for now, suffice it to say that one should always be careful whenever questions are being used. Keeping this in mind, Benjamin (1987) suggests the following when asking questions:

1. Are you aware of the fact that you are asking a question?
2. Have you weighed carefully the desirability of asking specific questions and have you challenged their usage?
3. Have you examined the types of questions available to you and the types of questions you personally tend to use?
4. Have you considered alternatives to the asking of questions?
5. Are you sensitive to the questions the interviewee is asking, whether he or she is asking them outright or not?
6. Will the question you are about to ask inhibit the flow of the interview?

Giving Information, Advice, and Offering Alternatives Have you ever been in a situation where you have had someone try to give you advice and you felt like telling him or her to mind his or her own business? Unfortunately, I have seen this happen all too often. Most of us want to be (or at least feel) independent in our decision making, and when someone tries to tell us how to live our lives, we may get defensive sometimes even if his or her advice is good. Therefore, like confrontation, advice should only be given once you have established a relationship; even then, some better ways of facilitating change for the client might be available. For instance, **offering alternatives** might make more sense.

Usually, providing clients with a few options to consider is better than just offering advice or making a suggestion. Offering alternatives can help clients feel empowered because they can choose the alternative rather than feeling as if you told them what to do. Don't be surprised, however, if the client has already thought about some of the alternatives you offer.

Sometimes we may have some valuable objective information to offer our clients. For instance, suppose a client is eligible for Social Security disability and you have information on how he or she might apply for it. Obviously, you would not want to just sit there and reflect back the client's feeling—you would want your client to know about the information. Information should be given when you have some vital objective piece of knowledge that you believe will help the client in some manner. **Information giving,** however, is very different from **advice giving:** "Presenting information is not the same as giving advice, suggestions, or directives; it is not value-laden material, but rather objective and accurate factual material about people, places, or things" (Doyle, 1998, p. 191).

Although offering alternatives, information giving, and advice giving are similar in the sense that they all move the focus of the session from the client to the helper, each has a different potential for being destructive to the helping relationship. Table 4.1 shows the differences between these types of responses, and Box 4.1 gives an example of when these responses might be used.

Clearly, of the three possible leading responses, offering alternatives would be least likely to have destructive influences in the helping relationship. As we move toward advice giving, the helper becomes more value laden in his or her response mode and more helper centered (Doyle, 1998).

Confrontation: Support with Challenge

When hearing the word **confrontation,** many people think of someone yelling at another or telling another person how to live his or her life. Along these lines, I have found that some clients "hook" me, and I start to argue with them about how to live life. This is rarely if ever helpful to the client and is almost always a result of some unfinished business of my own. In fact, trying to get another person to change if he or she is not ready is nearly impossible. Confrontation that is facilitative is usually very different from this; instead, facilitative confrontation is the ability to give feedback to others without being judgmental, critical, or aggressive (Thompson, 1996).

If you have built a solid relationship with a person and gently challenge him or her, the individual will more likely hear what you are saying and will consider

Table 4.1 Comparison of Leading Responses and Their Potential for Harm

Response	Definition	Potential for Harm
Offering Alternatives	A response that suggests to the client that there may be a number of ways to tackle the problem and suggests a variety of alternatives from which that client can choose.	Has the least potential for harm because it does not presume there is one solution to the problem. Does not set up the helper as the final expert, and to some degree, allows the client to pursue various options while maintaining a sense that he or she is directing the session. Least value-laden response.
Information Giving	A response that offers the client valuable "objective" information of which the client is unaware, which will facilitate client understanding and client growth.	Assumes that the helper has some valuable information that the client needs and sets up the therapist as the expert, thereby increasing the potential for the client to become dependent on the relationship. Attempts, sometimes not successfully, to not be value laden. Often the client already knows the information given.
Advice Giving	A response that suggests to the client that the helper is the expert and that he or she may hold the solution to the problem.	Sets up the therapist as expert. Assumes the therapist has the solution and carries with it the potential for developing a dependent relationship. May mimic control issues from family of origin (for example, parents giving advice). Is a value-laden response.

BOX 4.1   A Scenario

You work at a problem-pregnancy clinic and a 17-year-old woman comes in seeking information about birth control. She has been sexually active for two years, has not used any birth control, and knows little about sexually transmitted diseases (STDs). When she comes into your office, you affirm her decision to come to the clinic. You then listen carefully and try to understand her situation. After you spend some time listening, you tell her about the various types of birth control, suggest that she may not want to have unprotected sex, and give her information about AIDS and other STDs. You also suggest that she might want to consider being tested for STDs. You then ask her if she has any thoughts about what she would like to do. She thinks a while and then says that she will try to use condoms but also thinks it might be smart if she is on the Pill. She thinks she would like to be tested for STDs but would like more information on the testing process. After you explain the testing process to her, she agrees to come back to the clinic for the tests. You then thank her for coming in and schedule another appointment.

In this short scenario, one can easily see how a human service professional can be affirming, empathic, an information giver, an advice giver, a person who offers alternatives, and a problem solver. What do you think would be most effective for this 17-year-old? How might you work with her fears of having an STD? Are there other techniques that we have talked about that might be helpful for this young woman?

---

your suggestions. To build this kind of relationship, spend some time trying to understand the life circumstances of the client. The best way to do this is to make sure you have listened and have used empathy. Once you have this supportive base, confrontation becomes much easier (Byrne, 1995).

One way of gently confronting a client is to make a higher-level empathic response, such as a Level 4 response. These very effective responses reflect back feelings that you sense from the person, feelings of which the client is not quite aware. Therefore, when you tell the client that you hear some deeper feelings underlying what he or she is saying, and if you have that base of caring, the client might better be able to hear this kind of feedback.

Another way of gently confronting a client is to suggest alternatives. Offering alternatives challenges the client to look at new ways of viewing the world. Like the case of high-level empathy, such a confrontation should only be done if there is a base of caring; otherwise, the client may respond defensively.

Pointing out discrepancies is a third way of confronting the client (Hackney & Cormier, 2001). In this case, you carefully highlight that there is some type of incongruence in what the client is saying. As before, the key to effective use of this technique has to do with your ability to develop a trusting relationship (see Box 4.2). If you have such a relationship, the client is more likely to let you challenge his or her perception of the world. Point out a discrepancy before building a solid relationship, and the client may walk out on you. For instance, I have seen numerous clients who drink heavily, perhaps the equivalent of five or more beers a night, yet state they do not have a drinking problem. I have learned that unless I have an alliance with these clients through having established a relationship, they will not be able to examine the discrepancy between how much they drink and the statement about not having a drinking problem.

Whether you use higher-level empathic responses, the offering of alternatives, or pointing out discrepancies, using confrontation can be a very powerful technique in the helping relationship.

PROBLEM SOLVING
AND THE STRUCTURE OF THE INTERVIEW

An effective human service professional has learned to integrate listening skills, empathic responses, the use of silence, questioning, confronting, advice giving and offering alternatives, information giving, encouragement, and self-esteem building to facilitate the client's **problem solving.** Although all these techniques may be used during the various parts of an interview, some are used more at certain stages than at others, and all are useful in the problem-solving process. Therefore, understanding the **structure of the interview** is essential. Because the roles and functions of the human service professional can vary considerably, many different types of interviewing can occur. Some human service professionals may do more information gathering, others may do more supportive work, and others may be doing mostly counseling. Some may be seeing clients for 15 minutes, others for a couple of hours. Regardless of the kind of interviewing you're doing, be cognizant of the process of the interview. Although the outline that follows might not apply to the roles and functions of all human service professionals, it does provide a general framework.

Opening the Interview

When beginning an interview, clients today are often handed a **professional disclosure statement** that describes the following items and helps the client understand the counseling process (AMHCA, 2000; Corey et al., 2003):

1. Limits of confidentiality
2. Length of the interview

BOX 4.2 Confronting Sally

One time I worked with a client who was making almost $60,000 a year, was in an abusive relationship, had no major bills, and insisted that she could not leave the relationship because she could not afford to live on $60,000. Clearly, her verbal statement that she could not leave the relationship did not match the reality that one could live on this amount (certainly, most of us would be happy to live on this amount). After building a relationship using empathy, I gently challenged this perception by pointing out the discrepancy between what she earned and her statement that she did not earn enough to live on her own. This allowed her to examine the real reasons she was not leaving—reasons that had more to do with low self-esteem and fears of being alone.

3. Purpose of the interview

4. Your credentials

5. Limits of the relationship

6. Your theoretical orientation

7. Legal issues of concern to you and your client

8. Fees for services

9. Agency rules that might affect your client (e.g., reporting a client's use of illegal drugs)

After providing the professional disclosure statement to the client, it is important to obtain **informed consent** from the client that indicates that the client has been given this information and agrees to participate in the helping relationship. Although informed consent can be obtained verbally, it is always best to have clients sign a statement noting that they gave their informed consent.

Following an explanation of these basic issues, building a facilitative helping relationship is particularly important. You can accomplish this by using your listening skills and empathy. These skills allow you to build trust, and they also help the client get oriented to the interview.

Information-Gathering Stage

After trust has been built, it is important to make sure that you have all the information needed to assist you in the planning phase of the interview. Therefore, if empathy and listening alone have not been enough to help you gather all the necessary information, then use your questioning techniques at this time. Sometimes, it is important to have a series of standard questions to ask the client. Many agencies actually have developed standard questionnaires that help them in this information-gathering phase. This reduces the possibility of not obtaining important information from the client that could affect the goals that you are setting.

Goal-Setting Stage

After you have gathered information, it's time for you and your client to set goals. Whether of a general nature (e.g., increase in self-concept), or focused and specific (e.g., losing five pounds), these goals should be attainable and measurable and based on the information gained thus far in the interview. In addition, goal setting should be a collaborative process; that is, you and your client mutually decide on the goals.

As you are deciding which goals are appropriate, this may be an opportunity for giving information to the client, offering suggestions, using mild confrontation (for example, higher-level empathy), or offering advice. Effective listening is also important during this stage because it allows the client to feel empowered as he or she decides which goals to set. Although affirmation and encouragement can be done at any stage, affirming the client's ability and encouraging the client to meet his or her goals is particularly important in this stage.

Closure Stage

After you and your client have determined goals, to ensure accuracy, it is critical that they be reviewed. Then, it is often advisable to summarize what you did during the interview. You can do this by listing the highlights of the interview. It is then important to determine whether you are going to meet again and, if so, when the meeting will take place. For any goals that have been set, make sure the client is aware of his or her tasks. Finally, it is important to ensure there are no loose ends and that there is a sense that you and the client are finished for that session. If this is the only time you will meet with the client, some kind of follow-up would be helpful so you can evaluate the success of your meeting.

CASE MANAGEMENT

Managing a caseload of clients can be tedious and time-consuming and involves a myriad of activities collectively called **case management.** Although definitions of case management have varied, generally, case management has been viewed as the overall process that is involved in maintaining the optimal functioning of clients (Sullivan, Wolk, & Hartman, 1992; Woodside & McClam, 1998b). Thus, case management involves such things as: (1) treatment planning, (2) diagnosis, (3) monitoring the use of psychotropic drugs, (4) case report writing, (5) managing and documenting client contact hours, (6) monitoring, evaluating, and documenting progress toward client goals, (7) making referrals, (8) follow-up, and (9) time management. The following is a quick overview of the case management process. However, you are encouraged to look at the literature for a more in-depth understanding of this important process (e.g., see Neukrug, 2002).

Treatment Planning

Treatment planning involves the accurate assessment of client needs leading toward the formation of client goals. As the helper increases the ways to assess the client, the ability to develop accurate goals is increased (Drum, 1992; Goldman, 1992; Hohenshil, 1993). Thus, ideally, assessment involves a myriad of information-gathering activities that can include (1) the clinical interview, (2) testing, (3) observation, (4) client self-assessment, (5) assessment of the client by others, and (6) review of past records (Harrington, 1995).

The actual development of client goals should be a relatively easy process if the helper has completed a thorough assessment of the client. As noted earlier, goal setting should be a collaborative process, goals need to be attainable, and progress toward goals should be monitored and changed if necessary.

Diagnosis

A diagnosis is a natural outgrowth of the assessment process and can occur in many ways. For instance, one can make an informal diagnosis to be used in goal setting, a rehabilitation diagnosis for physical problems, a vocational diagnosis for career planning, a medical diagnosis, and a mental health diagnosis, such as those made from the *Diagnostic and Statistical Manual-IV-Text Revision* (DSM-IV-TR) (APA, 2000). DSM-IV-TR deserves some special attention because it has become the most widespread and accepted diagnostic classification system of emotional disorders and has become increasingly important. Although many clinicians do not use all five axes, many will find two or more of the axes useful. Axis I describes "Clinical Disorders and Other Conditions That May Be a Focus of Clinical Attention." Axis II delineates "Personality Disorders and Mental Retardation." Axis III explains "General Medical Conditions." Axis IV describes "Psychosocial and Environmental Problems," and Axis V offers a "Global Assessment of Functioning Scale," which helps determine the client's current level of functioning and can be used to assess if progress is being made (see Appendix E).

Psychotropic Medications

Today, a host of medications can be used as an adjunct to counseling in the treatment of many disorders (Kalat, 2001; Schatzberg & Nemeroff, 1998). In fact, it is now common for helpers to consult or refer to a physician, generally a psychiatrist, who can assess the client and prescribe appropriate psychotropic medications. Therefore, it is important for human service professionals to have a basic working knowledge of psychopharmacology, more than can be offered in this brief overview. For the treatment of a wide array of emotional disorders, psychotropic medications are generally classified into five groups: antipsychotics, antimanics, antidepressants, antianxiety agents, and stimulants (Donlon, Schaffer, Ericksen, Pepitone-Arreola-Rockwell, & Schaffer, 1983; National Institute of Mental Health, 1995).

Case Report Writing

> Problems associated with writing and reading mental health records are well worth our attention. . . . more and more people are entering in an increasing number of mental health care delivery systems. . . . Consequently, an increasing number of people are writing and reading mental health records for an increasing number of purposes. (Reynolds, Mair, & Fischer, 1995, p. 1)

Changing times have brought a greater emphasis on the importance of accurate record keeping. Personally, I think that this sometimes goes to extremes; however, good case records can (Kleinke, 1994; Neukrug, 2002, 2003) do the following:

1. Be used in court to show adequate client care took place
2. Assist helpers in conceptualizing client problems and making diagnoses
3. Help determine whether clients have made progress
4. Be useful when obtaining supervision

5. Assist the helper in remembering what the client said

6. Be part of the process for insurance companies and government agencies to approve the treatment being given to clients

7. Be a determining factor, in this age of accountability, for which agencies will receive funding

Today, depending on the agency, the many kinds of case report writing include daily case notes, intake summaries, quarterly summaries, and summaries for companies, students' individual education plans, vocational rehabilitation planning, referrals to other clinicians, and termination, to name just a few.

Managing and Documenting Client Contact Hours

Human service professionals are increasingly being asked to find ways to meet with all their clients on a consistent and continual basis. For accountability, it is essential that human service professionals find a credible way of doing this. This sometimes means using some creative activities, such as running special groups (e.g., medication review groups), and working additional evening hours to meet with clients who cannot meet during the day.

In addition to how the helper manages to meet with all of his or her clients, the documentation of these contact hours has become crucial because reimbursement by insurance companies, as well as local, state, and federal funding agencies is often based on the clear documentation of contact hours. Thus, most agencies today have some mechanism for documenting these hours. Often, this is done on a simple grid, but increasingly, documentation can be completed using computer software specifically developed for this purpose.

Monitoring, Evaluating, and Documenting Progress Toward Client Goals

The documentation of progress toward goals is increasingly being reviewed by funding agencies. In fact, some funding agencies today will not renew funding if documentation and progress are not shown. The simplest way to document progress toward goals is to make a note in the client's chart. Innovative human service professionals can also create charts and graphs to visually document client progress. Finally, the GAF scale of DSM-IV-TR is increasingly being used as one measurement of progress toward goals and treatment success (see Appendix E).

Making Referrals

There are many reasons to refer a client to another professional. For instance, a client may be referred as a part of the treatment plan, because the professional is leaving the agency, because the professional feels incompetent to work with the client, or because the client has reached his or her goals and is ready to move on to another form of treatment. In any case, the manner in which the referral is made is crucial, and in this process the human service professional should do all of the following:

1. Discuss the reason for making the referral with the client and obtain his or her approval.
2. Obtain, in writing, permission to discuss anything about the client with another professional, even if one is simply sharing the client's name with another professional.
3. Monitor the client's progress with the other professional.
4. Ensure that confidentiality of client information is maintained in the referral process.

Follow-up

Follow-up, another important function of case management, can be completed in many ways. Some helpers follow up by a phone call, others send a letter, and still others may do an elaborate survey of clients. Follow-up can be done a few days to a few weeks after the relationship has ended and serves many purposes (Hutchins & Cole, 1997; Kleinke, 1994; Neukrug, 2002):

1. Functions as a check to see if clients would like to return for counseling or be referred to a different helper
2. Allows the helper to assess if change has been maintained
3. Gives the helper the opportunity to look at which techniques have been most successful
4. Offers an opportunity to reinforce past change
5. Offers a mechanism whereby the helper can evaluate services provided

Time Management

With ever-increasing case loads and demands placed on the helper, time management, the last aspect of case management, has become crucial if the helper is to avoid burnout. Time management strategies serve a number of purposes. They are useful in planning activities and can help a human service professional ensure that all clients are seen within a reasonable period. They are also useful in helping professionals remember meetings, appointment times, and other obligations. Today, there are a number of time management systems. Although this text will not delve into these different systems, suffice it to say that addressing time management concerns is paramount in today's world.

ETHICAL AND PROFESSIONAL ISSUES

Primary Obligation: Client, Agency, or Society?

Think about the following scenario:

In building your relationship with a 17-year-old client, you discover that she is using crack cocaine, possibly selling drugs to friends, and involved in gang violence including looting. Your agency has a policy to report any illegal acts to the "proper authorities."

What is your responsibility to this client? What are the limits of confidentiality with her? If you are primarily responsible to your client, what are the implications of being required to report her to the proper authorities? If you do not report her to the proper authorities as you are supposed to do, what implications might this have for your employment? What responsibility do you have to protect society from the illegal activities in which she is involved? What liability concerns do you have if you do not report the illegal acts in which she is participating? These are some of the tough ethical and professional questions human service professionals sometimes have to face.

If this were a dualistic world, there would be an easy answer to these tough ethical and professional dilemmas. The world is fortunately (unfortunately?) more complex than this. Although most ethical guidelines, including the *Ethical Standards of Human Service Professionals* (1996; see Appendix B), imply that the mental health professional has a primary responsibility to the client, we all must acknowledge legal and moral responsibility toward others. Therefore, ethical guidelines usually include a statement that requires the mental health professional to take responsible action if a client's behavior is perceived as potentially harmful to the self or others. For instance, the *Ethical Standards of Human Service Professionals* has such a statement and suggests that the human service professional seek consultation or supervision if a client's actions might harm self or others (see Box 4.4). The same standards also require that the human service professional follow agency guidelines, whenever reasonable, as well as local, state, and federal laws. With these guidelines in mind, it is prudent to be clear about the limitations of the helping relationship before starting your work with clients. Probably the best way to do this is by using a professional disclosure statement.

Case Records

Confidentiality of Case Notes Generally, clients should have the expectation that information they share with the helper be kept confidential. However, there are some exceptions to this rule, such as (1) if an employer requests information from a helper concerning a client, (2) if a helper shares client information with a supervisor as a means of assisting the helper in his or her work with the client, (3) if the court subpoenas a helper's records, or (4) if a client gives permission, in writing, to share information with others.

You should also remember that human service professionals do *not* have the legal protection afforded to licensed professionals through **privileged communication** (see Chapter 3). Privileged communication is the legal right that clients have to not have information shared with third-party sources, especially the court. Thus, if a client asks that a human service professional *not* share information requested from the court (e.g., case notes), the practitioner will probably have to go against the client's wishes. In fact, there is a good chance that a human service

---

BOX 4.4   The Tarasoff Case

The case of *Tarasoff et al. v. Regents of University of California* (1976) set a precedent for the responsibility that mental health professionals have regarding maintaining confidentiality and acting to prevent a client from harming self or others. This case involved a client who was seeing a psychologist at the University of California–Berkeley health services. The client told the psychologist that he intended to kill Tatiana Tarasoff, his former girlfriend. After the psychologist consulted with his supervisor, the supervisor suggested that he call the campus police. Campus security subsequently questioned the client and released him. The client refused to see the psychologist any longer, and two months later, he killed Ms. Tarasoff. The parents of Ms. Tarasoff sued and won, with the California Supreme Court stating that the psychologist did not do all that he could to protect Tatiana Tarasoff.

Although state laws vary on how to handle confidentiality, this case generally is seen as signifying to mental health professionals that it is their responsibility to protect the public if serious threats are made.

---

professional who does *not* share requested information with the courts would be found in contempt of court.

Security of Case Notes Written client records need to be kept in secured places such as locked file cabinets and nonaccessible computer disks. Clerical help needs to understand the importance of confidentiality when working with records. Some agencies have clerical staff members sign statements acknowledging that they understand the importance of the confidentiality of records.

Access to Case Notes One should expect that clients might request to see their records. Keep this in mind when you are writing case notes. Legally, although it seems to be a gray area, clients probably have a right to view their records; along these same lines, parents probably have the right to view records of their children. You should be aware of any specific local or state laws that might set standards for access to client records.

The federal **Freedom of Information Act** of 1966, and subsequent amendments allow individuals to have access to any records maintained by a federal agency that contain personal information about the individual. Similarly, the **Buckley amendment** of 1974, otherwise known as the **Family Educational Rights and Privacy Act (FERPA),** grants parents the right to access their children's educational records (Committee on Government Operations, 1997). Of course, any records not protected by privileged communication can be subpoenaed by a court (see Chapter 3).

On a more practical level, a client rarely asks to see his or her records. However, if a client did make such a request, I would first attempt to talk with the client about what is written in the records. If this was not satisfactory to the client, I would suggest that I might write a summary of the records. However, if a client steadfastly states a desire to view his or her records, I believe that this is his or her right.

BOX 4.5   How Secure Are Records?

When I worked as an outpatient therapist at a comprehensive mental-health center, a client of another therapist had apparently appropriated his records that had been left "lying around." Because the therapist's records tended to be written in "psychologese" using diagnostic language, the client was understandably quite upset by what he found. He would periodically call the emergency services at night and read his records over the phone to the emergency worker while making fun of the language used in the records.

Another time, when I was in my doctoral program, we were reviewing an intellectual test assessment of an adolescent that had been done a number of years earlier. Suddenly, one of the students in the class yelled, "That's me!" Apparently, although there was no identifying name on the report, he recognized it as describing him (he had been given a copy of the report previously). These two examples show the importance of keeping client information confidential and secure.

THE DEVELOPMENTALLY MATURE HUMAN SERVICE PROFESSIONAL

Looking for Feedback from Others

Developmentally mature human service professionals are open to hearing both positive and negative feedback about their helping skills. They want to "stretch" and are willing to take a critical look at how they interact with clients. They want to try out new approaches to working with clients and are willing to feel vulnerable in the learning process. Finally, such professionals actively seek out supervision and consultation from experts in the field, and view the learning of counseling skills as a process in which one continually grows and adapts his or her approach.

SUMMARY

This chapter presented an overview of the basic helping skills used for working effectively with clients. We first noted that a conducive environment for the helping relationship includes the physical comfort of the surroundings, positive personality characteristics of the human service professional, and appropriate nonverbal behaviors. This was followed by a discussion concerning the foundations of good helping skills, which include effective listening; the use of empathy, where we examined the Carkhuff scale; the importance of silence; the effective use of encouragement and affirmation; and how to intersperse modeling and self-disclosure into the helping relationship. We then examined how and when one might use questions and specifically discussed open versus closed questions, direct versus indirect questions, and the use of "why" questions. From there we moved on and compared information giving, advice giving, and offering alternatives and noted that offering alternatives has the least potential for harm. We next discussed confrontation and noted that the gentlest and probably most effective type of confrontation is a higher-level empathic response such that the client feels supported while perceiving new feelings. We also suggested that offering alternatives and pointing out discrepancies are two other means of confronting the client.

We next discussed the structure of the interview and noted that a number of stages are typically passed through in an effective interview. The stages included the opening of the interview, information gathering, goal setting, and closure. We noted that some of the counseling skills are used more at some stages than at others.

We explained that case management is a broad term that includes such things as (1) treatment planning, (2) diagnosis, (3) monitoring the use of psychotropic drugs, (4) case report writing, (5) managing and documenting client contact hours, (6) monitoring, evaluating, and documenting progress toward client goals, (7) making referrals, (8) follow-up, and (9) time management. We briefly reviewed these important areas of managing cases, and highlighted the importance of needing to examine these areas in more detail to be effective at the case management process.

As we neared the end of the chapter, we discussed ethical and legal issues related to case ownership and security. We also discussed the human service professional's responsibility to his or her client, to the agency at which he or she works, and to society. Finally, we noted that developmentally mature human service professionals are those who see their helping skills as continually in process; that is, mature human service professionals are always willing to adapt their skills to become better helpers.

EXPERIENTIAL EXERCISES

1. Arranging Your Office

The instructor will distribute a number of magazines and some scissors. From these magazines, cut out pieces of furniture that you like and create your own office the way you would like it to be. Compare your office to the office of other students. What makes your office more or less conducive to the counseling relationship? Come up with a justification for your office arrangement based on your counseling style.

2. Listening Quiz

Next to each item below, place an "X" in the appropriate space to represent how you *generally* respond to someone to whom you are attempting to listen. Then, go through the list again and this time place an "O" next to each item to represent how you think you *should* listen to another. Look at the end of the chapter for the optimal answers. U = Usually, S = Sometimes, R = Rarely

U　　S　　R
_____ _____ _____　　　1. I try to determine what should be talked about during the interview.

___ ___ ___   2. When listening to someone, I prepare myself physically by sitting in a way that I can make sure that I hear what is being said.

___ ___ ___   3. I try to be "in charge" and lead the conversation.

___ ___ ___   4. I usually clear my mind and take on a nonjudgmental attitude when listening to another.

___ ___ ___   5. When listening to another, I try to tell the other my opinion of what he or she is doing.

___ ___ ___   6. I try to decide from the other's appearance whether or not what he or she is saying is worthwhile.

___ ___ ___   7. I attempt to ask questions if I need further clarification.

___ ___ ___   8. I try to judge from the person's opening statement whether or not I know what is going to be said.

___ ___ ___   9. I try to listen intently to feelings.

___ ___ ___   10. I try to listen intently to content.

___ ___ ___   11. I try to tell the other person what is "right" about what he or she is saying.

___ ___ ___   12. I try to "analyze" the situation and give interpretations.

___ ___ ___   13. I try to use my experiences to best understand the other person's feelings.

___ ___ ___   14. I try to convince the other person of the "correct" way to view the situation.

___ ___ ___   15. I try to have the last word.

After finishing the listening quiz, define the term *listening* as a small group or as a class. You may want to use the following definition in developing your group definition. After you have defined *listening,* see if the answers you gave on your quiz reflect this definition. Webster (2002) asserts that to listen means:

1. To pay attention to.
2. To hear something through thoughtful attention: To give consideration.
3. To be alert, to catch an expected sound.

3. Affirmation and Encouragement

Make a list of times in your life when you have been affirmed or encouraged. What did that do to improve your self-esteem?

4. Making Empathic Responses

A good empathic response accurately reflects to the client the feelings and the meaning of what the client has said (Carkhuff's Level 3 response). For the following situations, write the feeling in the spaces provided, followed by the meaning of what the client has said. Follow this by writing another statement that again reflects the feelings and meaning of the client, but this time in your own words.

In small groups in class, share some of your responses and get feedback from others about the accuracy of what you wrote. For example, wife to human service professional:

Client: I don't know what's wrong with my husband. Since he lost his job, he just sits around all day and does nothing, doesn't look for a job, doesn't cook, just does nothing. He seems worthless.

Next is an example of a feeling word ("angry") followed by the client's meaning ("husband doesn't do anything all day long") in response to the preceding client statement:

HSP: You feel <u>angry</u> because your <u>husband doesn't do anything all day long.</u>

The following is an example of a response to the same client, but this time in one's own words, again reflecting feeling and meaning:

HSP: I guess I hear you're disappointed and upset at your husband for not taking charge of his life.

Respond to the following scenarios:

1. Teenager to human service professional:

   Client: Why should I use condoms? I'm not going to get AIDS or nothing like that. Only fags get AIDS. Don't you agree?

   HSP: You feel _____ because _____

   HSP: _____

   _____

2. Abused wife to human service professional:

   Client: I don't know why I keep going back to him. He just keeps beating on me. But afterward, he always tells me he loves me. I think he loves me, but he just drinks too much sometimes.

   HSP: You feel _____ because _____

   HSP: _____

   _____

3. Pregnant teenager to human service professional:

   Client: I want this baby; I don't care what my parents say about an abortion. I can bring this baby up by myself. I'll quit school and get a job and bring the baby to work with me.

   HSP: You feel _____ because _____

   HSP: _____

   _____

4. Disabled enlisted person to human service professional.

   Client: Even though I lost my leg, I have lots to live for. I have a good family, and I know I'm employable. I just hope I can get through rehab quickly.

   HSP: You feel _____ because _____

   HSP: _____

   _____

5. Older person to human service professional:

   Client: Since I moved to this retirement home, I have nothing to live for. I can't drive any more, and I know nobody here.

   HSP: You feel _____ because _____

   HSP: _____

   _____

6. Minority person to human service professional:

   Client: I think I'm getting the shaft with my realtor. I keep telling her I want to move to this one community, and she can't find anything for sale there. I don't believe it!

   HSP: You feel _____ because _____

   HSP: _____

   _____

7. Pro-life person to human service professional:

   Client: I refuse to let any more babies die. I'll do anything to close down those murdering abortion clinics.

   HSP: You feel _____ because _____

   HSP: _____

   _____

8. Pro-choice person to human service professional:

   Client: I believe a woman has a right to choose what to do with her body, and I'm sick and tired of these pro-lifers interfering with other people's right to choose!

   HSP: You feel _____ because _____

   HSP: _____

   _____

9. Estranged husband to human service professional:

   Client: So I wasn't faithful to my wife. So what? I loved her. She didn't have to leave me. I still was good to her despite my failings. I miss her so much!

HSP: You feel _____ because _____

HSP: _____

_____

10. Estranged wife to human service professional:

    Client: I loved my husband, but I couldn't put up with his unfaithfulness any longer. He just couldn't give me the love I needed in a relationship. I'm sorry he is so depressed now, but I can't go back to him.

    HSP: You feel _____ because _____

    HSP: _____

    _____

5. An Interview with a Client

The following is an interview between a client and human service professional who is employed at an employee assistance program for a large business. Go through the interview and identify the type of response being made by the helper (empathy, advice giving, information giving, offering alternatives, confrontation, self-disclosure, modeling, open questions, closed questions, affirmation or encouragement, referral, and/or summarizing). Each response may have more than one answer. Check the end of this chapter for the answers.

1. **Client/employee:** I woke up this morning feeling depressed. My life is out of sorts, and I'm not sure why. Do you think this is something that will pass?

   HSP: So, it seems as if your depression just came out of nowhere, and you're not sure what's causing it.

2. **Client:** Well, yeah. I guess I haven't been real happy at work lately. I've been at this same job for 20 years, and it seems like I never get promoted. All my friends get promoted, and I just make my little yearly salary increases but never move up. Maybe I'm just no good.

   HSP: Well, I hear how you're not feeling real good about yourself and it seems to be at least partly related to the fact that things haven't worked out at your job as you thought they might.

3. **Client:** That's true. You know, maybe I should take some courses and that would help me do better at work. What do you think?

   HSP: I'm not sure. But it seems as if you've had some ideas about how to change your life.

4. **Client:** Yeah, I've thought about going back to school, quitting my job, looking for another job, and even just storming into my boss's office and telling her what I think.

   HSP: What do you think about all these different options?

5. **Client:** Well, I guess I have thought about at least talking to my boss and asking her what she thinks I might do. That would be at least a beginning.

   HSP: Do you feel good or bad about your relationship with your boss?

6. **Client:** Well, I don't know if it's either. Perhaps more neutral. I don't really know her real well. She is not approachable, but on the other hand, maybe I'm not either.

   HSP: So on one hand it might be difficult to talk with her, but on the other hand, you also see that maybe you haven't made it easy for her to approach you.

7. **Client:** Kind of. Maybe I need to talk with her to see what the different options are for me.

   HSP: When you say "options," I'm unclear what you mean. Can you explain that to me?

8. **Client:** Well, I guess I mean whether I should take a course for credit, do some in-house workshops, or maybe something else. . . . like, like talk to my supervisor more and get feedback from her, or become more active in the employees' association, or something.

   HSP: Well, it seems as if you have a lot of ideas that you can approach your boss with.

9. **Client:** Yeah, I guess I do. I hope I can do it. You know, I get pretty nervous talking to her.

   HSP: I know you can do it if you want to. I know you're capable of lots!

10. **Client:** Yes! I can do it. But you know, this fear I feel with her, that's something I feel with a lot of people in positions of authority. Like, take my church. You know, I've been on this fund-raising committee now for a number of years and I've had a lot of ideas, but I never tell them to the chair because I think he's going to put me down.

    HSP: So, you see this as a pattern in your life; that is, this fear you have expressing yourself with people in positions of authority.

11. **Client:** Yeah, I think it goes back to the fact that my parents, particularly my father, were really strict and always told me how to live my life. I get so scared sometimes around authority figures that I just don't know what to say or do.

    HSP: Well, you're bringing up some really important issues for yourself. What are your thoughts about seeking out counseling for this?

12. **Client:** It had crossed my mind. Especially because I believe this issue is something that prevents me from getting ahead in my life. What do you think?

    HSP: I know of some good counselors, and I know of an assertiveness-training group. I think considering some counseling might be really good for you.

13. **Client:** Yes, I think so.

    HSP: I admire your wanting to work on this issue. Here, let me give you the names of some counselors and a couple of groups. [HSP gives the names.]

14. **Client:** I really appreciate this. Sometimes I think I'm never going to get through this problem I have. I guess I think that change is really not possible.

    HSP: You know, I had some problems once in my life that were really difficult for me, and I saw a counselor. It really helped me get through it, and I feel much better about me now.

15. **Client:** Really?

    HSP: Yeah, it was really helpful. I know you can move on in your life in a positive way and feel good about you. You have all the ingredients in you to make this work.

16. **Client:** I hope so. I think this is a really good start. Can I talk about one other thing?

    HSP: Sure.

17. **Client:** I notice that on some nights, not all nights mind you, I seem to drink a lot. I wake up in the morning feeling terrible. I wonder if this affects my work performance. I've been thinking about maybe trying out an AA meeting. What do you think?

    HSP: I hear your concern about your drinking and the fact that you have been giving some serious thought to doing something about it.

18. **Client:** To be honest, sometimes I really think I go overboard with my drinking.

    HSP: Well, it sounds to me as if you might have a problem with alcohol and perhaps you should do something about it.

19. **Client:** Do you know of any AA meetings?

    HSP: Yep, let me give you a list I have right here. You know AA meetings usually last a couple of hours and one's anonymity is ensured. I have heard that people who go to AA meetings are usually accepting of one another.

20. **Client:** Well, you've been helpful. I appreciate all of what you've done for me.

    HSP: Well, thanks. I hear that you are ready to do some important things for yourself. For instance, today you talked about some concerns you were having at work relative to getting promoted as well as how this might relate to both issues with authority figures and your drinking. You've gotten some referrals from me, and it sounds as if you're seriously thinking about following up on them. I think that it's great that you're so motivated, and I know you can make great strides. Maybe next week you can touch base with me to let me know what you've done to follow up.

6. Writing Case Notes

Using the interview in Exercise 5, and following the guidelines in this chapter, write case notes that have the following information:

1. Reason for referral

2. Summary of contact with client

3. Recommendations for client

7. Writing Case Reports

Meet with someone in class and have each student role-play a problem situation. Then write a two- to three-page case report that addresses the following categories:

1. Client Information

   Name

   Address

   Email Address

   Date of Birth

   Date of Interview

2. Reason for interview

3. Background information about person that is relevant to interview (for example, family background, educational background, work background)

4. Assessment of client problem

5. Summary and recommendations

6. Signature with credentials

8. Ethical and Professional Vignettes

For the following vignettes, write some possible solutions and be prepared to discuss them in class.

Case note security

1. A client who is coming to your agency demands to see her case notes. In them, you have noted that you suspect she may be lying about her Social Security eligibility and that you also suspect she might be paranoid. What do you do?

2. A client you have been seeing at a crisis center comes in and asks to see all records pertaining to him. These include crisis logs that have information in them about other clients, as well as case notes you have made concerning his contacts. What do you do?

Confidentiality and primary obligation: client, agency, or society?

3. You're working for social services, and in the course of a conversation with a client, you discover that she has been using heroin. An agency dictate states that any client suspected of using illegal drugs must be immediately referred

to rehabilitation, and if he or she refuses, you can no longer see the client at your agency. You explain this to her, she gets angry, walks out, and states she'll "blow this place up." What do you do?

4. In your conversation with a client at the homeless shelter, you discover that he is drinking and taking quaaludes in amounts that you believe could kill him. You mention this to him, but he tells you to mind your own business. What do you do?

5. In the course of working with a client, she expresses her concern about her grandmother who, she states, lives by herself, is depressed, has stopped eating, and has lost a considerable amount of weight. You contact the grandmother, but she refuses services. What do you do?

6. While talking with a 15-year-old male client, he informs you that on a recent vacation he was sexually molested by an uncle. He asks you not to tell his parents. What do you do?

7. A 15-year-old client tells you he is having sexual relations with his 14-year-old stepsister. What do you do?

8. An adult client informs you that he wants to kill his ex-girlfriend and her new boyfriend. He denies that he actually will act on these feelings but says that he just "thinks about it a lot." What do you do?

Answers to Exercises

Exercise 2: Usually: 2, 4, 9, 10; Sometimes: 7, 13; Seldom: 1, 3, 5, 6, 8, 11, 12, 14, 15. *Exercise* 5: 1. empathy; 2. empathy; 3. empathy; 4. open question; 5. closed question; 6. empathy; 7. open question; 8. empathy, affirmation; 9. encouragement; 10. empathy; 11. empathy, open question, referral; 12. offering alternatives, advice giving, referral; 13. referral, affirmation; 14. modeling, self-disclosure; 15. affirmation, encouragement; 16. not ratable; 17. empathy; 18. confrontation; 19. referrals, information giving; 20. summarizing, affirmation, encouragement.

5

Development
of the Person

With each passage from one stage of human growth to the next we, too, must shed a protective structure. We are left exposed and vulnerable—but also yeast and embryonic again, capable of stretching in ways we hadn't known before. These sheddings may take several years or more. Coming out of each passage, though, we enter a longer and more stable period in which we can expect relative tranquility and a sense of equilibrium regained. (Sheehy, 1976, p. 29)

In my senior year in college, I was staying with my girlfriend, and in the middle of the night I began to have what I now would call a panic attack. I walked the campus the rest of the night trying to calm myself down. I thought I had lost it. The next day I went to the college counseling service and saw a psychologist who reassured me that I was not "crazy." I was soon referred to a group at the center for what became my first therapeutic experience. Subsequently, I have participated in different groups and in individual counseling. Through these experiences, I have had the opportunity to examine some of my life events that have dramatically affected my development. Some of these experiences, such as a childhood heart disorder and the death of my father, might be considered situational, in that they were unexpected events in my life that had a dramatic effect on me. Other experiences, however, such as developing a sense of my own values or belief system, going through puberty, entering the world of work, and dealing with how I create intimacy in my life are considered developmental, in that they are issues we all deal with at around the same times in our lives.

This chapter will examine the developmental process, from birth through death. Whether it is the physical changes, the psychological seesaw, or moral growth, theories have been developed to explain the natural progression of the person over the life span. These theories are particularly important to help us, as helpers, understand some of the reasons why people act the way they do, and these theories can provide a knowledge base to help us ease people through these natural transitions.

DEFINING DEVELOPMENT

The development of a person is complex and occurs on many levels. Although developmental models differ, they tend to share common elements. For instance, most hold the belief that development is (Neukrug, 2003a, b):

- *Continual:* It starts at birth and we continue to develop until we die.
- *Orderly, sequential, and builds upon itself:* Models that describe human growth have a predictable pattern of development from earlier to later stages in which the latter stages build on what has already been experienced and integrated into our lives.
- *A change process:* By its very nature, development means that we are constantly changing, moving on to different life phases and stages. Our core remains the same but like a piece of clay we can be molded, sometimes torn apart and

then put back together, but we are always clay. Each piece has a different shape, and it can come in different colors, different weights, and different consistencies, but it is all clay.

- *Painful yet growth producing:* Because development implies giving up past ways of behaving or perceiving the world, it is painful because we have to let go of something that is familiar. On the other hand, it is growth producing, as we move on to newer ways of being in the world that will, by their very nature, help us adapt more easily to the world.

- *Hopeful:* "[M]ost modern developmental theories are optimistic. They see growth and development as the natural tendency of the organism" (Wallen, 1993, p. 1). Thus, all individuals have the ability to understand where they are developmentally and how they can optimize their growth as they move to higher stages of development.

Developmental counseling offers the human service professional a unique perspective when working with clients. The developmentally astute helper knows the (1) characteristics that are commonly displayed by clients at different developmental stages, (2) types of social issues and personal problems often experienced by clients as they pass through specific developmental stages, (3) reasons why such problems occur, and (4) techniques that might work with clients who have similar developmental concerns (Thomas, 1990). Clearly, knowledge of human development can go far in assisting the human service professional in his or her work with clients.

Many theories of human development have been identified over the years. For instance, some developmental approaches have helped us understand the unique problems of students as they pass through school (Dahir, Sheldon, & Valiga, 1998; Neukrug, Barr, Hoffman, & Kaplan, 1993), the lifelong process involved in choosing and maintaining contentment in one's career (for example, Super, 1990), the maturation of faith experiences over the life span (for example, Fowler, 1995), and the process toward self-actualization (for example, Maslow, 1968). An in-depth examination of developmental theories would require a separate course. Therefore, in this chapter, we will focus only on some of the more prevalent theories of child development, personality development, and life-span development.

CHILD DEVELOPMENT

The developing child offers many challenges for the human service professional. As the child grows, understanding his or her physical, cognitive, and moral development is crucial to our successful work with young people.

Physical Development of the Growing Child

As the child develops, major physiological changes take place (see Rice, 2001). Although the rate of children's physical development is fairly consistent, the scope of a specific child's development is based on the genetic predisposition of the child in interaction with the environment. For instance, although most children will be ready to learn multiplication in third grade, the rate and depth of learning will vary based on genetics and environment. Along these lines, a brilliant child is at a major disadvantage if he or she is brought up in a home that has lead paint and lead in the water or in an environment that does not nurture the child's innate intelligence. On the other hand, a child who is less able can shine if placed in a stimulating and nurturing environment.

The importance of a nurturing environment can be seen through the success of the **Head Start Program.** This federally funded program, which was started in the 1970s, places disadvantaged preschool children in intellectually stimulating and nurturing environments before they enter public school. On average, these children have done noticeably better academically and socially than have children of similar backgrounds who have not received such opportunities (Lee, Brooks-Gunn, Schnur, & Liaw, 1990; Schweinhart, 2001).

Because most children will develop at fairly predictable rates, if a child specialist is aware of the expected physiological timetable that is *normed* for the majority of children, he or she can determine whether a child is on target for his or her physiological development (Gesell & Ilg, 1943; Rice, 2001). Sometimes, lagging behind in physical development can be a first indication of a physiological, emotional, or intellectual impairment. For instance, a friend of mine has a daughter who could not crawl at age 1. Because most children are beginning to walk at this time, my friend was concerned that this might be an indication of a developmental disability. In this case, the child had a rare but harmless form of hypertrophy of the muscles and was walking within a few months of being tested. If tests had revealed a developmental disability, however, early diagnosis could have been crucial to optimizing the skills that the child does possess.

Typically, child specialists will examine age-appropriate milestones in the areas of motor development, speech development, sensory development, and the development of secondary sex characteristics (breast development, pubic hair, and so on) in determining what may be considered normal compared with what could be a deviation from the norm (Sprinthall & Sprinthall, 1998). A course on human growth and development will help familiarize human service professionals with many of these expected developmental milestones.

Cognitive Development: Jean Piaget

Probably the person who most helped us understand the intellectual or cognitive development of children is Jean Piaget (Flavell, 1963). Piaget stated that as the child grows, he or she takes new information into an already existing view of the world. Known as **assimilation,** this process refers to incorporating new information within the framework that the child already has for understanding the world. For instance, my daughter, Emma, is 3 years old, and recently she asked me for some M&M's. I gave her two, and she told me she wanted five more. So I then gave her five more of the miniature M&M's (which are equivalent to about two regular size ones). She was very pleased, not realizing that five of the small ones were not the same as five of the larger ones. Emma had not yet learned the con-

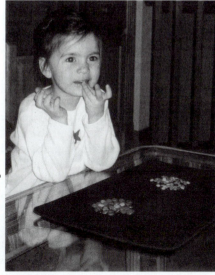

Kristina Williams-Neukrug

Three-year-old Emma does not realize that five small M&M's are not more than two large M&M's, thus supporting Piaget's theory on conservation.

cept of **conservation,** or the "notion that liquids and solids can be transformed in shape without changing their volume or mass" (Mussen, Conger, & Kagan, 1969, p. 452). As Emma grows older, she will clearly understand this difference in mass. As she learns the concept behind this, she will **accommodate** to this way of knowing. In other words, she will change her previous way of understanding the world and adapt a new method. Piaget stated that in accommodating to the world, certain **schemata** or new cognitive structures (new ways of thinking) are formed that allow an individual to adapt and change his or her view of the world. The processes of assimilation, forming new schemata, and eventual accommodation occur throughout the life span.

Through his research on child cognitive development, Piaget determined that as children grow they pass through predictable periods, which he called the sensorimotor, preoperational, concrete-operational, and formal-operational stages. The **sensorimotor stage,** birth through 2 years, is when the infant responds totally to physical and sensory experiences. Because the child hasn't acquired full language ability, he or she cannot maintain mental images and responds only to the here and now of experience. Thus, trying to have a logical and reasoned conversation with a child at this age would make little sense because he or she cannot yet make rational sense out of the world. For instance, imagine a parent saying to a 2-year-old child who just reached out for candy at a checkout counter, "Let's sit down and talk about this when we get home so you'll understand why you shouldn't take candy without asking." Unfortunately, some parents try to make children understand this logic. Can you consider other options to a reasoned approach that can change this child's behavior without using anger or punishment?

As the child moves into the **preoperational stage** (ages 2–7 years), he or she is developing language ability and can maintain mental images. This *intuitive* way of being in the world is when the child responds to what seems immediately obvious rather than the child having the ability to think logically. When this child sees a tall glass of water, he or she assumes that it has more volume than a smaller but wider glass of water (or the piece of toast cut in two is more than the one piece of toast). Because children at this age have not yet adopted logical thinking, trying to explain such logical principles would be difficult, if not impossible (unless the child is on the verge of entering the concrete-operational stage). Imagine trying to explain to 3-year-old Emma why five small M&M's are the same as two large M&M's. She just won't get it!

From age 7 through 11 years, the child enters the **concrete-operational stage** in which he or she can begin to "figure things out" through a series of logical tasks. Children in this stage often are very adamant about their logical way of viewing the world. For instance, when helping a friend's son figure out a math addition problem, I suggested to him a new way of doing it. However, because my method did not follow his "logical" way, he became very angry and told me I was wrong, even though the answer was the same. I was wrong because I didn't do it the way he learned, and he did not yet have the flexibility to examine other ways of problem solving. Children in this stage will have difficulty with metaphors or proverbs because they have not developed the capacity to think abstractly. However, when children move into Piaget's final **formal-operational stage** (ages 11–16) they can begin to think abstractly and apply more complex levels of knowing to their understanding of the world. A child in this stage can understand how objects might have symbolic meaning (for example, the Liberty Bell is more than just a bell), test hypotheses, understand proverbs, and consider more than one aspect of a problem at one time.

Piaget's research on child development has greatly helped us understand how children learn and the limitations on their abilities based on their age and developmental stage. Such knowledge has greatly affected styles of teaching, ways to parent effectively, and methods of counseling children.

MORAL DEVELOPMENT

Lawrence Kohlberg

By having children respond to **moral dilemmas** (problems of a moral nature that have no clear-cut answer), Lawrence Kohlberg (1969) discovered that moral understanding and reasoning develop in a predictable pattern. He identified three levels of development, each containing two stages. The first level, **preconventional** (roughly ages 2–9 years), is based on the notion that children make moral decisions out of fear of being punished or out of desire for reward. In Stage 1 of this level, moral decision making is based on perceived power that others hold over them and the desire to avoid punishment from these individuals in authority. In Stage 2, decisions are made with an egocentric/hedonistic desire to satisfy one's own needs and in hopes of gaining personal rewards. Imagine a 6-year-old wanting to watch her favorite video during dinner. A parent might say, "No, you can't watch that now, but after dinner we'll make special time to do whatever you want." A child might initially say, "Sure Mom" (not wanting to get punished for doing the wrong thing), but then, when Mom is not watching, secretly put the video in the VCR.

In Kohlberg's **conventional level** (9–18), moral decisions are initially based on social conformity and mutualism; in an effort to gain approval from others (Stage 3), whereas later the accent is on adhering to rule-governed behavior—that we have a duty to society to avoid guilt and dishonor (Stage 4). In this level, children respond less to punishment or reward and more to avoid displeasing others and out of a sense of right and wrong as defined by rules of law and order.

In Stage 3 of this level, the child responds to what he or she believes significant others would view as morally correct in hopes of avoiding their disapproval and of gaining their acceptance. Most children will reach Stage 3 by age 13 (Gerrig & Zimbardo, 2002). For example, my 9-year-old daughter has a strong need to be approved by my wife and me so she acts in a manner that she feels will not disappoint us. When she does "go against the rules," she will often feel guilty as she feels that she has not lived up to our expectations. As she grows older, approval from her parents will take a back seat in her moral decision making and a rigid adherence to societal rules of law and order will take precedence (Stage 4). Then she will be living by the adage, "It is important to follow the law if we are going to have a moral society that functions adequately."

Kohlberg noted that many individuals will never reach the final **postconventional level** of moral development. If postconventional thinking comes at all, it comes only at or after age 13. It is based on acceptance of a social contract that is related to democratically recognized universal truths (Stage 5) or on individual conscience based on universal principles and moral values that are not necessarily principles or values held by others (Stage 6).

In Stage 5 of the postconventional level, the individual now believes that laws can be examined, interpreted, discussed, and changed. Although an individual in this stage would generally be law abiding, this individual is no longer rigidly adhering to the law, as was the case of the Stage 4 individual. Instead, this individual would reflect on a law to consider whether it makes sense at all times and might attempt to change the law when the law did not seem justified (for example, perhaps stealing would be allowed if it meant the survival of a child—if the parent of a starving child stole food for the child).

In Stage 6, the final stage of the postconventional level, moral decisions are based on a sense of universal truths, personal conscience, individual decision making, and respect of human rights and dignity (Rice, 2001). Here an individual would consider moral truths in his or her decision-making process and, after deep reflection, might choose to break a law, deciding that such an action is taken out of respect for the dignity of people and for the betterment of society (Sprinthall & Sprinthall, 1998). For instance, during the civil rights movement of the 1960s, some individuals broke laws to advance the cause of civil rights for all people.

Carol Gilligan

In 1982, Carol Gilligan wrote *In a Different Voice,* a book that questioned some of Kohlberg's assumptions. Gilligan, who had worked with Kohlberg, points out that most of his research had been done on a small group of boys and proposes that moral reasoning for females might be based on a different way of knowing or understanding the world. She notes that Kohlberg's theory stresses the notion that high-stage individuals make choices autonomously, whereas her research seems to indicate that women value connectedness and interdependence and view the relationship as primary when making moral decisions. In describing the differences between men and women, Gilligan observes the responses of one of Kohlberg's subjects and compares him with a woman she interviewed: "Thus while Kohlberg's subject worries about people interfering with each other's rights, this woman worries about 'the possibility of omission, of your not helping others when you could help them'" (1982, p. 21).

Gilligan states that in the development of moral reasoning, especially in Stages 3 and above, women will emphasize a "standard of care" as they move toward self-realization. Also, she notes that women are more likely to be concerned about the effect their choices have on others, whereas men are more concerned about a sense of justice being maintained (Gerrig & Zimbardo, 2002). Noting these male and female differences, Gilligan states, "Given the differences in women's conceptions of self and morality, women bring to the life cycle a different point of view and order human experience in terms of different priorities" (1982, p. 22).

More specifically, the Level 1 preconventional girl is not dissimilar to Kohlberg's Level 1 boy, in that her moral reasoning is narcissistic—she reasons from a survival, self-protective perspective. For Gilligan, the Level 2 conventional female shows a concern for others and feels responsible for others compared with Kohlberg's Level 2 person who is concerned about pleasing others or following the rules. Gilligan's Level 3, postconventional woman is a complex thinker who recognizes the interdependent nature of humans and who knows that every action a person takes affects others in deeply personal ways.

In thinking about the examples given to clarify Kohlberg's theory, you might consider how a woman's decisions might differ from a man's if her decision-making process takes into account how a person's decisions affect others and the interconnectedness of people. Gilligan has added a unique perspective to the concept of moral development and may be bringing to the forefront major differences that men and women hold toward moral reasoning. Understanding such differences is crucial in helping us comprehend why the different sexes make certain choices.

Although there is not a direct relationship between cognitive development and moral development, it is clear that one cannot be at the upper levels of moral development if he or she cannot think abstractly. Also, evidence indicates that our actions are not always in sync with how we think, in that most individuals prefer the reasoning of a moral development stage one level above where they actually are.

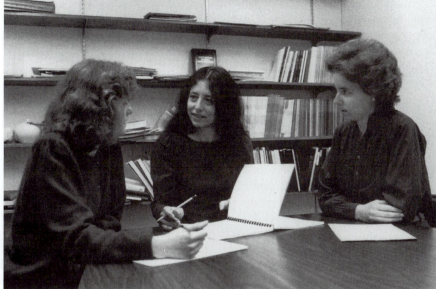

Carol Gilligan, center, states that women's moral development is different from men's in that women tend to stress interdependence rather than autonomy.

Knowledge of Child Development:
Applications for the Human Service Professional

Although the human service professional is not necessarily an expert in child development, knowledge of such development can help one understand whether the child is developing within normal rates. If the human service professional can recognize physical problems or delays in social, cognitive, or moral reasoning, then appropriate referrals can be made to medical, psychological, or educational sources that can assist the child in his or her development. Early identification of such problems can greatly help to ameliorate these concerns.

PERSONALITY DEVELOPMENT

How are our personalities formed? This question has intrigued philosophers for centuries. In the last 100 years, psychologists have attempted to answer this question through a number of theories that seek to explain the personality development of the individual. Paralleling the counseling theories discussed in Chapter 3, theories of personality development, based on views of human nature of the major counseling theories, describe a system for the developing person and explain the underlying beliefs that result in a specific counseling approach.

Although many theories of personality development have been developed over the years, we will examine Freud's theory of psychosexual development, learning theorists' views on development, and Rogers's humanistic understanding of growth and development. These represent three of the more prevalent views concerning personality development of the individual.

Sigmund Freud's Psychosexual Model of Development

Sigmund Freud viewed individual personality as forming within the first five years of life. As noted in Chapter 3, he believed that the person is born with sexual and aggressive instincts that are regulated as a function of parenting received in early childhood. Freud stated that the child is born all **id;** that is, he or she responds only to instincts in an effort to satisfy his or her needs. As the child develops, the type of parenting he or she receives greatly affects the formation of the **ego,** or the ways in which the child deals with reality. As the ego is developing, the formation of the **superego** begins to occur. The superego represents the formation of the child's morality and values and is greatly affected by the values of parents and society. Freud thought the individual passes through five **psychosexual stages of development,** each of which affects the formation of the id, ego, and superego, which he collectively called the **structures of personality** (Appignanesi & Oscar, 1999; Corey, 2001).

Stating that sexual satisfaction and resulting psychosexual development is centered on **erogenous zones,** Freud presented a unique view of the developing individual. During the **oral stage,** the first stage of psychosexual development, the infant receives pleasure through feeding. The major developmental task of this stage, which occurs between birth and age 1 year, is how the child becomes attached to the mother (or the major caretaker). Therefore, the relationship between caretaker and infant is extremely important. Clearly, a child who goes hungry or is physically abused will have difficulty successfully passing through this stage. Invariably, Freud stated, this child would develop trust problems as an adult.

During the **anal stage,** Freud stated that the child receives pleasure from bowel movements. During this stage, which occurs between ages 1 and 3 years, the child becomes physiologically ready to be toilet trained. How parents assist with the child's newfound ability to control his or her bodily functions greatly affects the child's ability to be independent, feel powerful, and express negative feelings. Think about the parent who demands the child "sit on the potty" versus the parent who encourages and supports the child's newfound control of his or her bodily functions. These two types of parenting will affect the child's sense of autonomy very differently.

In the third stage of development, the **phallic stage,** which occurs between ages 3 and 5 years, the child becomes aware of his or her genitals as well as of the genitals of the opposite sex. Now the child receives pleasure from self-stimulation. How parents respond to a child in this stage can greatly affect the child's attitudes and values. The parent who consistently tells his or her child that it is sinful to touch the genitals will affect the child's values very differently than will the parent who allows the child to touch his or her genitals and self-stimulate.

The **latency stage,** occurring between ages 5 years through puberty, is a period of relative relaxation for the child, in which he or she replaces earlier sexual feelings with a focus on socialization. Here, the child becomes more aware of peers and increased attention is placed on peer-related activities. Freud's final stage of development is the **genital stage,** which begins at puberty and continues through the life span of the individual. Here, we see the emergence of unresolved issues that were raised in the first three stages of development, and sexual energy is focused on social activities with peers and on love relationships.

Freud believed that becoming **fixated,** or having problems with maturing and developing and dysfunctional patterns of relating as the result of incomplete development during a stage, is often the result of inadequate parenting or caretaking. These dysfunctional ways of being, Freud stated, generally occur *unconsciously;* that is, outside of our awareness. This means that we respond to situations in ways for which we have no deep understanding. For instance, the child who is sexually abused at age 5 might have repressed these memories, yet Freud would say that the abuse still would affect the child's behaviors in unconscious ways. Therefore, it is not uncommon to see an adult who was sexually abused find ways to avoid dealing with his or her sexuality (for example, becoming obese, becoming a workaholic, or, in an extreme case, taking on multiple personalities).

Typically, to avoid and protect the individual from the anxiety that unresolved issues might arouse, the individual develops **defense mechanisms.** For instance, the sexually abused child might develop defenses as an adult to protect the ego that became so fragile as a result of the abuse. Although there are many defense mechanisms, some of the more common ones are **repression,** pushing out of awareness threatening or painful memories; **denial,** distorting reality to deny perceived threats to the person; **projection,** viewing others as having unacceptable qualities that the individual himself or herself actually has; **rationalization,** explaining away a bruised or hurt ego; and **regression,** reverting to behavior from an earlier stage of development that is a less demanding way of responding to anxiety (for example, sucking one's thumb).

Freud's psychoanalytic model of personality development has added much to our understanding of the complexity of the individual and why there is such a variety of ways in which people respond. His stage theory and the concepts of the structures of personality, the unconscious, and defense mechanisms represented the first comprehensive approach to our understanding of the development of personality.

Learning Theory and the Development of the Person

B. F. Skinner and other learning theorists hold the belief that individuals are born a blank slate, or **tabula rasa,** and that personality development is based on the types of conditioning that have affected us throughout our lifetime (Bandura, Ross, & Ross, 1963; Skinner, 1971). Drastically differing with Freud's notion of instincts, Skinner believed that *"the most important causes of behavior are environmental and it only confuses matters to talk about inner drives"* (Nye, 1996, p. 71).

As noted in Chapter 3, learning theorists believe that one adapts behaviors through **operant conditioning, classical conditioning,** or **modeling (social learning).** Learning theorists do not view personality development as a function of developmental stages as in the psychoanalytic model. Although behaviorists do not deny that a person's genetics or biology can affect behavior, they emphasize how positive or negative reinforcement, social learning, and the pairing of an unconditioned stimulus with a conditioned stimulus affect our personality development.

Operant conditioning is generally considered to be the most common type of conditioning and occurs when behavior that is emitted is reinforced, thus increasing the probability of that response occurring again. Over the years, through rigorous research, Skinner and others delineated many principles of operant conditioning, each of which is crucial to the shaping of behaviors and the development of personality. A small portion of these include the following:

1. *Positive Reinforcement:* Any stimulus that, when presented, increases the likelihood of a response.

2. *Negative Reinforcement:* Any stimulus that, when removed, increases the likelihood of a response.

3. *Schedules of Reinforcement:* The numerous ways in which a stimulus can be arranged to reinforce behavior. Based on elapsed time and frequency of responses.

4. *Discrimination:* The ability of a person to respond selectively to one stimulus but not respond to a similar stimulus.

5. *Generalization:* The tendency for stimuli that are similar to a conditioned stimulus to take on the power of the conditioned stimulus.

6. *Extinction:* When a behavior ceases because it is not reinforced.

7. *Spontaneous Recovery:* The tendency for responses to recur after they have been extinguished.

8. *Punishment:* Applying an aversive stimulus following a behavior in an effort to decrease a specific behavior. Punishment is often an ineffective method of changing behavior as it can lead to undesirable side effects (e.g., counteraggression).

Learning theorists believe that personality development is generally shaped by the significant people in one's life. This is because those individuals are most readily available to apply these principles, although such application is rarely, if ever, done in a purposeful way. Skinner and other learning theorists believe that reinforcements from significant others often occur very subtly, in ways that we do not immediately recognize (Nye, 1996; Skinner, 1971; Wolpe, 1969). Therefore, changes in voice intonation, subtle glances, or body language could subliminally affect one's personality development. Learning theorists note that if a situation is examined closely enough, one could attain an understanding of the types of **reinforcement contingencies,** or modeling, that were instrumental in shaping behavior.

Because reinforcement contingencies are so powerful, behaviors are generalized to other situations. This is why an individual's behavior will be relatively consistent from situation to situation. Extinguishing behaviors that have been continually reinforced is difficult, and a major task of helpers who work with maladaptive personality formation is to use counterconditioning (conditioning new adaptive behaviors) so the individual can learn more effective ways of living in the world.

Recently, many learning theorists have included a cognitive framework within their conceptualization of development. Such cognitive therapists as **Albert Ellis** (1997), **Donald Meichenbaum** (1977), and **Aaron Beck** (1976; Beck & Weishaar, 2000) believe that it is not only the behavior of the individual that becomes reinforced, but the ways in which the individual thinks. Therefore, thinking can dramatically affect behavior, and behavior can dramatically affect thinking in a complex interaction. Cognitive-behaviorists have challenged the beliefs of the original behavioral purists and have changed the manner in which most learning theorists conceptualize the development of the individual.

Because development is seen as a result of reinforcement contingencies, learning theorists believe that change can occur at any point in the life cycle. Therefore, one can identify dysfunctional behaviors and irrational thinking, determine the reinforcers that continue the dysfunctional ways of living in the world, and devise a method of reinforcing new behaviors and different cognitions.

Learning theory has had a great impact on our ability to change maladaptive behaviors (see Chapter 3). We owe much to Skinner and his colleagues for adding this important dimension to our understanding of personality development.

The Humanistic Understanding of Personality Development

As noted in previous chapters, **Carl Rogers** greatly affected our understanding of the person. His thoughts on personality development starkly contrast with the views of Freud and Skinner. Although representing just one of the many humanistic approaches to understanding personality development, Rogers's ideas embody many of the key concepts put forth by the humanistic theorists.

Rogers believed that individuals are born good and have a natural tendency to actualize and obtain fulfillment if placed in a nurturing environment that includes **empathy, congruence,** and **positive regard** (see Chapters 1 and 3). In contrast with Freud, Rogers did not emphasize the importance of instincts, the unconscious, or developmental stages in the formation of personality development. In contrast with Skinner, Rogers did not place much value on reinforcement contingencies as creating the personality of the individual. Instead, he viewed the relationship between the child and his or her major caretakers as the most significant factor in personality development (Rogers, 1951, 1957, 1980).

Rogers believed that we all have a need to be loved. He stated that significant people in our lives often set up **conditions of worth,** or ways we should act so we can receive their love. Therefore, as children we will sometimes act in ways to please others so we obtain a sense of acceptance—even if the pleasing self is not our **real self.** At this point, the child has learned that if he or she practices

---

BOX 5.1   The Story of Ellen West

This story, so eloquently told by Rogers (1961), describes the history of a famous psychotherapy client (a client Rogers knew about but never saw himself). Rogers described the estrangement of this person from her feelings—how she felt obligated to follow her father's wishes and not marry the man she loved, how she disengaged herself from her feelings by overeating, how a few years later she again fell in love but instead married a distant cousin according to her parents' wishes. Following this marriage, she became anorexic, taking 60 laxative pills a day, again as an apparent attempt to divorce herself from her feelings. She saw numerous doctors, who gave her differing diagnoses, treated her dispassionately, and generally denied her humanness. Eventually, disenchanted with her life, Ellen West committed suicide.

This story, Rogers noted, gives a poignant view of what it is like to lose touch with self—to be incongruent. Because Ellen West felt she needed to gain the conditional love of her parents, she gave up the most valuable part of self—her real self. Losing touch with self led to a life filled with self-hate and a sense of being out of touch. Eventually, therapists viewed her as being mentally ill, which Rogers implied might have added to her feelings of estrangement and her eventual suicide.

---

incongruity, or not being real, he or she will receive acceptance (see Box 5.1). This nongenuine way of living then becomes our way of relating to the world and prevents us from becoming self-actualized—becoming our true selves. Often this is seen through our **introjection** (swallowing whole) of the values of others without ever giving ourselves the opportunity to reflect and decide whether we truly adhere to these values. This is when our self-actualizing tendency is squashed. The helper who works with an individual who is incongruent attempts to set up an environment in which the client feels safe enough to get in touch with his or her true self. Only when one realizes his or her true self can one become self-actualized, as noted by Abraham Maslow in his hierarchy (see Chapter 3).

The humanistic approach downplays, and in many cases challenges, the concept of abnormality. Instead, so-called abnormal behavior is seen as an attempt by reductionistic and dispassionate clinicians to objectify and isolate the client. If we call the individual "abnormal," we take away his or her humanness and no longer need to deal with this person as a human being. In fact, humanists would say, abnormal behavior can be seen as a healthy response to an unhealthy situation. The individual's attempt to survive in a world places conditions of worth on the person and makes life untenable. What is abnormal, say the humanists, is the attempt to call something abnormal that is actually natural.

The humanistic approach to personality development represents a departure from the deterministic views of Freud and the reductionistic ideas of the learning theorists. The humanists' stress on the importance of significant relationships has added an important dimension to our understanding of personality development.

Knowledge of Personality Development:
Applications for the Human Service Professional

When we initially meet clients, we are sometimes bewildered by their actions. Why does a rapist rape? Why does a parent abuse his or her child? Why does an adult who seemingly has everything live in a state of depression? Why does an able-bodied, intelligent person end up on the streets as a homeless person? Understanding the personality development of the individual can give us insight into the client's world. Such insights into the developing world of the person as offered to us by psychoanalysts, humanists, and learning theorists can assist us in our ability to empathize with our clients, help us in treatment planning for our clients, and give us the knowledge base to help us make appropriate referrals. If we did not have this basic understanding of personality development, we could be left without a clue to the makeup of the person or how to work with the individual (see Box 5.2).

LIFE-SPAN DEVELOPMENT THEORIES

Some models of understanding the development of the person have taken a life-span approach; those who adhere to this approach believe that the individual continues to grow over the life span, with development *not* suddenly ending in childhood. One of the more prevalent **life-span development theories** has been Erik Erikson's **stages of psychosocial development.** More recently, Robert Kegan's **subject/object theory** has gained some prominence. In Chapter 1, we viewed the adult stages of Kegan's model; here we will view the whole model, from birth through adulthood.

Erik Erikson's Stages of Psychosocial Development

Although Erikson started out studying Freud's psychoanalytic approach, he later developed a model that rejected many of Freud's original tenets. Contrary to Freud, Erikson believed that the individual is not determined by instincts, early childhood development, and the unconscious but instead that psychosocial forces are major motivators in the development of the individual over the life span. As opposed to Freud's deterministic philosophy, Erikson had faith in the ability of the individual to overcome many of his or her problems. Erikson believed that as the individual passes through life, he or she has specific age-related developmental life tasks to overcome. If the individual successfully masters these developmental milestones, a strong ego is formed, a positive identity is created, and the individual is ready to move on to the next level. On the other hand, if the individual cannot cope with the developmental tasks, then he or she develops a low self-image and bruised ego and carries these dysfunctions into the next levels, making it difficult to successfully complete later developmental tasks. Erikson's eight life-span stages

---

BOX 5.2   A Psychotic Relative

When I was about 10 years old, I had a favorite relative named Joyce with whom I loved to play. Suddenly, she no longer came to visit. I heard rumors that Joyce's father, David, had had a "nervous breakdown" and that his wife had divorced him. The families became estranged at that point. David, who was college educated, never seemed the same after his nervous breakdown. He rarely bathed, wore dilapidated clothes, and often would come up with delusional and grandiose ideas about life. When I was older, I realized that David had been psychotic. He had lost touch with reality, was paranoid, and had been hospitalized in a large, city psychiatric hospital. Since his hospitalization, he would often stay in sleazy apartments and at times was a homeless "Bowery bum." What had happened to David?

Recently, when I asked my mother about David, she stated that he had at times seemed different, even before the hospitalization. I often wonder about David's personality development. What kinds of early childhood development affected his personality? What kind of parenting did he receive? Were there genetic or biological factors that affected his mental health? Unfortunately, much of David's life is masked in mystery. Perhaps with early intervention and knowledge of personality development, the tragedy that befell him and his family would never have occurred.

---

offer a means of helping us understand the typical developmental tasks of the individual (Erikson, 1968, 1998).

* **Trust versus mistrust** *(ages birth to 1 year)*. During this first year of life, the infant develops a sense of trust or mistrust based on the type of caretaking received from significant individuals in his or her life.

* **Autonomy versus shame and doubt** *(ages 1–3 years)*. During these years, the child begins to gain control over his or her body and explore the environment. Significant caretakers can either promote autonomy or thwart it, leaving the child feeling ashamed or doubtful of self.

* **Initiative versus guilt** *(ages 3–5 years)*. As the child continues to explore the environment and gains an increased sense of independence, how caretakers encourage exploration can greatly affect the child's sense of self.

* **Industry versus inferiority** *(ages 6–12 years)*. In this stage, the child begins to examine what he or she does well. The testing ground for this stage is often with peers at school where the child begins to compare his or her skills with those of others. The ability of the child to feel a sense of self-worth through his or her interaction with others is crucial in this stage.

* **Identity versus role confusion** *(adolescence)*. As adolescents begin to identify the temperament, values, interests, and abilities they hold, they are able to recognize the specific attributes that define their personality. Significant others such as caretakers, peers, teachers, and school counselors can assist in such development. Lack of role models and lack of experiences that encourage such self-understanding can lead to a lack of identity and confusion about self.

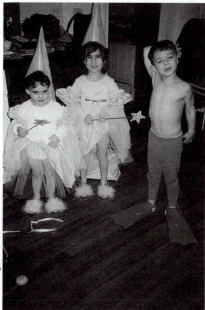

Ed Neukrug

As Erikson suggests, here Sarah, Hannah, and Joe are exploring their environment and trying out new behaviors. How they get reinforced for these behaviors will affect their self-esteem. Notice how they gravitated to traditional sex-role stereotyped behaviors. Nature, nurture, or both?

* *Intimacy versus isolation* *(early adulthood/adulthood)*. Once the young adult has achieved a sense of self, he or she is ready to develop intimate relationships with others. Lack of self-understanding leads to isolation from others or an inability to have mutually supporting relationships that encourage individuality with interdependency (see Box 5.3).

* *Generativity versus stagnation* *(middle/late adulthood)*. The healthy adult in this stage is concerned about others and about future generations. This individual has a life that is productive and responsible and can find meaning through such activities as work, volunteering, parenting, or community activities.

* *Integrity versus despair* *(later life)*. In this last stage of development, the older person examines his or her life and may feel a sense of fulfillment or despair. Successfully mastering the preceding developmental tasks will lead to a sense of integrity for the individual.

Erikson's life-span model is often used as a cornerstone for helping individuals understand expected crises through which they may pass. Such understanding can sometimes help normalize problems that may feel unbearable in the moment.

Robert Kegan's Constructive Model of Development

Kegan (1982, 1994) believes that our understanding of the world is based on the ways in which we construct reality as we pass through life. His subject/object theory states that individuals pass through specific developmental stages that reflect a meaning-making system. Movement from a lower to a higher stage necessitates a letting go of the earlier stage. This is not done easily, and Kegan (1982) suggests

---

BOX 5.3   The Case of Miles

I once saw a 32-year-old client who was having trouble with intimacy. Miles was engaged despite the fact that he had rarely dated, had very poor interpersonal skills, and was quite fearful of having a sexual relationship. He was a virgin when he eventually married, and he soon found that he could not maintain an erection and have intercourse with his wife. Although he was dealing directly with Erikson's intimacy versus isolation stage, it became evident that he had never successfully passed through earlier stages. He had been verbally abused as a child, which resulted in his having difficulty building trust and being fearful of the world. This gave him an inferiority complex, which made him want to hide from people. He therefore was unable to interact successfully with his peers and generally felt lost in the world. He never discovered what he was good at, what he liked, or what he valued. Clearly, he had a very poor identity formation. His problems with intimacy seemed closely related to not successfully completing earlier stages of development.

As Miles and I worked on his concerns related to intimacy, we also spent much time examining issues related to earlier stages of development. As he reflected on his life and as he worked through his issues, he eventually was able to have a closer, more intimate relationship with his wife. This ultimately also led to their having a satisfactory sexual relationship.

---

that movement occurs most successfully if there is challenge to one's existing view of the world within a supportive environment.

Being born into the **incorporative stage,** Kegan states, the self-absorbed infant is all reflexive and has no sense of self as separate from the outside world. However, as very young children begin to experience the world, reflexes are no longer the primary focus; instead children attempt to have their needs met through attainment of objects outside of self: "In disembedding herself from her reflexes the two-year-old comes to have reflexes rather than be them, and the new self is embedded in that which coordinates the reflexes, namely, the 'perceptions' and the 'impulses'" (Kegan, 1982, p. 85). In this **impulsive stage,** children have limited control over their actions and act spontaneously to have needs met. No wonder the second year of life is often called the "terrible twos."

As children gain control over their impulses, they move into the **imperial stage** where needs, interests, and wishes become primary and impulses can begin to be controlled. For instance, children begin to recognize what they want, can begin to reflect on such needs, and can control impulses to meet the needs (see Box 5.4). The child who wants a new toy, perceives the toy, and recognizes the desire for it now has some control over how to obtain the toy.

The last three stages occur primarily in adulthood and were noted in Chapter 1. Briefly, during the **interpersonal stage,** the individual is embedded in relationships: relationships become primary, and needs and wishes are met through the relationship. In this stage, there is a beginning awareness of other people's feelings. This is manifested by the ability of individuals to show empathy because it helps them understand the other with whom they are embedded. The Stage 3 need for relationships is highlighted by many of the songs of this and past generations, songs that say, "Without you, I can't go on living."

As the individual moves out of embeddedness in other, he or she moves into the **institutional stage** where a sense of autonomy and self-authorship of life is

---

BOX 5.4   Garrett: Responding from the Imperial Stage

Garrett is a 12-year-old son of a friend. Recently, when wanting to spend time with a friend of his, he was told that this friend had already made plans to spend time with another boy. Garrett felt rejected and left out. If Garrett had still been in the impulsive stage, he might have thrown a temper tantrum. Instead, having passed into the imperial stage, he had control over his impulses and devised a way to have his needs met. He manipulated a way to spend time with both of them, disregarding their need to be with each other. In the imperial stage, one can control impulses and develop plans to have one's needs met. However, in this stage, there is little empathy for other people's desires. Therefore, Garrett did not yet have the ability to talk over his feelings with his friends. I suspect that when he is a little older, he will be able to share his feelings of being left out and understand his friends' desire to be with each other.

When his father was explaining this situation to me, he said that at first he was going to try to talk to his son about the other boys' feelings, but then he realized that Garrett just could not hear that yet. If someone is in the imperial stage and not yet ready to give it up, there is little you can do to make that person move to the interpersonal stage.

---

acquired. Relationships in this stage are still important but no longer seem to be the essential ingredient for living. In this stage, the individual's understanding of his or her values and interests becomes important. Here the individual may *choose* a partner because this person shares similar values; however, the person in this stage does not *need* the partner as he or she does in the interpersonal stage.

Kegan's final stage, the **interindividual stage,** highlights mutuality in relationships; that is, the individual can share with others and learn from others in a nonembedded, nondependent way. Here there is a sharing of selves without a giving up of self. In this stage, differentness is tolerated and even encouraged at times.

Kegan's model offers an important departure from the other life-span developmental models in that it stresses the interpersonal nature of development. Growth is based on our ability to interact with others and to let go of past, less effective types of relating. Although Kegan gives some general timelines for when movement into higher levels could occur, it is not unusual to find older adults who have not moved out of the interpersonal and sometimes even the imperial stages. Knowing the developmental stage of a person can help human service professionals provide an environment conducive to the personal growth of the client.

Knowledge of Life-Span Development:
Applications for the Human Service Professional

Whereas knowledge of child development and personality development can be crucial to understanding the person, these views tend to stress early development instead of changes in the individual *throughout* the life span. On the other hand, the life-span approach acknowledges that growth and struggles continue after puberty and on through older age in a predictable manner. Knowledge of some of the life-span stages can help the human service professional facilitate the expected transitions through which the individual will pass. Therefore, the human service professional is better able to make appropriate referrals, counsel adequately, and provide educational materials to help the client.

COUNSELING ACROSS THE LIFE SPAN

Life-span development is more than linear growth over time. We do not just move through a series of events in our lives. Our early individual and family experiences remain with us. The manner in which we have connected with others in the past provides us with resources as we move toward autonomy and individuation (Ivey, 1993, p. 120).

Allen Ivey (1993) developed a process for helping professionals use their knowledge of human development in the helping process. He states that understanding the developmental level of the client is crucial to working effectively toward client goals. Therefore, key components to Ivey's approach include assessing developmental level, devising developmental-based strategies to working with the client, and supporting yet challenging the client toward growth. Ivey believes that it makes no sense to try to assist a client toward growth if we cannot meet the immediate needs of the client. For instance, it would make no sense to be working on a client's sense of self-esteem if he or she is in physical danger from an abusive spouse. First, help the client be safe, then later worry about sense of self. Therefore, Ivey's model necessitates knowledge of the different developmental levels before the helper can aid the client.

Human service programs are now acknowledging the importance of the developmental perspective for their students (McAuliffe & Eriksen, 2000; Petrie, 1984). As ways of infusing human development theory into human service programs become more common, we hope to see new means of applying such knowledge to the work with our clients (McAuliffe & Eriksen, 2000; Neukrug, 1996; Neukrug & McAuliffe, 1993; Petrie, 1987).

COMPARISON
OF DEVELOPMENTAL MODELS

The varying models of development discussed in this chapter offer differing dimensions to our understanding of the person. Figure 5.1 outlines the varying stages of the theories we examined. Keep in mind that many individuals become fixated in stages. This will hinder their passage through the later stages.

NORMAL AND ABNORMAL DEVELOPMENT

While employed as an outpatient therapist at a mental health center, I was working with a 35-year-old married woman who had a history of several **acute psychotic episodes.** This meant that for short periods she lost touch with reality, had auditory hallucinations, and her thinking process became disorganized, or not clear. I saw her for a few months and she seemed rather coherent, warm, and relatively normal. One day I received a call from her panicked husband who stated

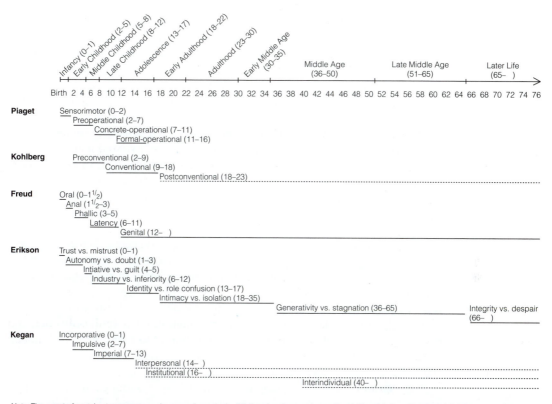

FIGURE 5.1 Varying models of human development offer different ways of understanding the person through the life span.

his wife was "out of control." He brought her to the mental health center, and I was startled to see a woman I hardly recognized. She thought she was possessed by the devil, was in a panicked state, and was screaming about some unusual sexual acts in which she stated she had participated. It was difficult to follow her line of reasoning. In fact, little of what she said seemed to make sense. This once warm, coherent, lucid woman seemed like a different person. She was placed on medication to calm her and to help her regain stability and lucidity.

As a young therapist, I wondered how much of what she stated was real, how much was fantasy, how a seemingly "together" person suddenly lost it, and what I could do to help her get back in touch with reality. This woman was *very scared* and desperately wanted help. To this day, this woman represents to me the difference between what we call "normal" and "abnormal," as well as how fragile that line can sometimes be.

Mental health professionals have for years struggled with the concepts of normal and abnormal. When do people cross the line to abnormality? Some individuals like **Thomas Szaz, William Glasser,** and **R. D. Laing** do not believe in the traditional views on mental illness and abnormal behavior. For instance, Szaz believes that abnormal behavior is a function of **power dynamics** in relationships. He believes that individuals, institutions, or society places undue demands on some individuals, and these demands push an individual into behaviors that many people call abnormal (Davison & Neale, 2001; Szaz, 1961, 1990). Glasser (1961, 2000) believes that abnormal behavior is a function of irresponsible behavior, and if you can help identify and change such behaviors, the person can then show responsible or normal behaviors. Laing (1967) viewed mental illness or abnormal behavior as a normal response to a stressful situation. In fact, he even encouraged people to get in touch with their own psychosis as a means of letting go of these stressors in their lives. Laing developed hospitals in England where individuals could go to become schizophrenic, and he would periodically "allow" himself to "become" schizophrenic.

Today, there is growing evidence that biological and genetic factors affect personality development, and the belief that genes determine one's personality at birth has been dismissed, with the current thinking being that genetic influences "are dynamic over the life span" (Nigg & Goldsmith, 1994, p. 349). For instance, it is now pretty much taken for granted that alcoholism often runs in families and probably has genetic links. Growing evidence indicates that **schizophrenia,** and perhaps even **major depression,** have genetic links. Most developmental models that examine **psychopathology** and abnormal behavior have room for genetic and biological ties to such behaviors.

The various types of developmental models we examined in this chapter approach the understanding of abnormal behavior differently. For instance, psychoanalytic theorists state that psychopathology is a result of dysfunctional parenting in the first five years of life. Such early patterning of one's personality is represented through the development of the individual's id, ego, and superego. These theorists also believe that the earlier the dysfunction, the more serious the pathology and the more difficult it is to change.

On the other hand, although not dismissing possible biological and genetic determinants of behavior, the humanistic and learning theorists state that change can occur at any point in one's lifetime and that, although pathology may be a function of learning or parenting styles early in life, new ways of learning can occur throughout one's lifetime.

Finally, the life-span developmental theorists view behavior as being affected throughout the life span as a function of specific predictable developmental tasks. Not dismissing biological or genetic determinants of behavior, these theorists also believe that problems in any one of these stages can seriously affect healthy functioning.

As our understanding of development has become clearer, many individuals now believe that the psychoanalysts, humanists, learning theorists, and life-span development theorists all offer some bits of truth to our understanding of normal and abnormal behavior.

Diagnosis and Abnormal Behavior:
What Is the *DSM-IV-TR?*

The American Psychiatric Association in consultation with the other mental health associations has over the years developed a manual to help in the diagnosis of mental disorders. In its fourth edition, the manual describes a full range of descriptive behaviors that epitomize different types of mental illnesses and emotional problems. The *Diagnostic and Statistical Manual of Mental Disorders-IV-TR (DSM-IV-TR)* (APA, 2000) is a complex manual that can be of great assistance in our understanding, diagnosis, and treatment of individuals. This manual has also become extremely important for the payment of mental health benefits because most health insurance companies will not pay for mental health counseling unless there is an appropriate diagnosis from a duly licensed clinician.

The *DSM-IV-TR* also has its critics. Some say that it is too reductionistic—that is, it tries to reduce mental illness and emotional problems into very neat categories, categories that some believe do not really exist. Others say a diagnosis tends to be a self-fulfilling prophecy in that once a client is given a diagnosis, others tend to see the client in that light and will tend to reinforce those behaviors in the person.

Despite its critics, the *DSM-IV-TR* seems to offer us a means of understanding emotional problems and is an important step toward our treatment of various mental health concerns.

ETHICAL AND PROFESSIONAL ISSUES

Abnormal Behavior
and Mental Illness—Myth or Fact?

Over the years, I have seen individuals argue over whether there is such a thing as mental illness. I have seen some vehemently state that mental illness is a disease, genetically or biologically caused, and should be treated as such. Others have just as strongly expressed the view that mental illness is the result of societal or family pressures or irresponsible behavior. Where lies the truth? Despite making great strides in the fields of personality development and its effect on mental illness, as well as giant leaps in our understanding of the **psychobiology** of mental illness, there is still much to learn. It appears to me that to come to any conclusions at this date about the **etiology,** or origins, of various forms of mental illness would be a mistake. Most important, the human service professional needs to be well read concerning the most recent literature in this area. Current knowledge along with an open mind can help the human service professional make important decisions when working with those who have severe emotional problems. These decisions may very well affect our clients for the rest of their lives.

When working with the mentally ill, we must ask ourselves what are the wisest decisions we can make to protect the welfare of our clients. Because there still seems to be much for us to find out about the etiology of mental illness, it seems that the wisest decisions for us to make would be to gather the data and keep an open mind before assisting our clients in treatment planning. Whatever decisions are made, they should be made with the welfare of our clients in mind.

Human service professionals respect the integrity and welfare of the client at all times. Each client is treated with respect, acceptance and dignity. (See Appendix B, Statement 2)

THE DEVELOPMENTALLY MATURE HUMAN SERVICE PROFESSIONAL

Constantly Changing, Constantly Examining

What is it about my development that I have lived 42 years, never married, yet now so want a family? Why did I end up in the field of human services and teaching? Why do I sometimes feel an emptiness inside that seems insatiable and at other times feel so totally filled with joy and excitement that I wonder how I could ever feel empty?

This is what I wrote for the first edition of this book. My own personal development has changed dramatically since that time. Where I was single, I now am married. Where I was not a parent, I now am a father, twice. Where I was not a son-in-law, I now am one. Then I was in what Donald Super calls the establishment stage of career development, now I have moved into my maintenance stage (see Chapter 9). I have developed—moved on. We all are constantly changing. If we do it with relative ease, and a little support, we can cherish each moment and enjoy our aging process. In a sense, each new developmental milestone brings with it a new birth and new growth ahead.

We all have unique developmental stories related to how we transverse developmental stages. By reflecting on our developmental history, we can better understand ourselves and the underlying reasons why we have developed in our unique ways. As there are reasons why I waited until my 40s to get married, there are explanations for all aspects of your personality development. In fact, *not* attempting to understand our own developmental histories can negatively affect our work with our clients through countertransference. It is our responsibility to put ourselves in situations that help expand awareness of self. Vehicles such as counseling, self-help groups, meditation, and reading literature on personal development are just a few of the many ways in which we can better understand self.

SUMMARY

This chapter presented an overview of human growth and development from birth through old age. The chapter started by defining some themes common to most developmental schemes. Thus, we saw that most developmental models imply change, are painful yet growth producing, are hopeful, and are continual, orderly, sequential, and build upon themselves.

In this chapter, we briefly reviewed the importance of knowing about the physical development of a child, especially as compared with the child's peer group. We next presented the model of cognitive child development as presented by Piaget. We noted that Piaget found that children pass through specific identifiable stages of cognitive growth that are called sensorimotor, preoperational, concrete-operational, and formal-operational. We also noted that Piaget stated that children either assimilate new information or accommodate to it. We next examined the moral development models of Kohlberg and Gilligan. Kohlberg, we showed, identified three levels of moral development with six stages. These include the preconventional, conventional, and postconventional levels. Gilligan, who also studied moral development, challenged some of Kohlberg's ideas and noted that she believed women's moral development was different from men's. Gilligan stated that when making moral decisions women use a "standard of care."

We also highlighted personality development as presented by Freud; the learning theorists, such as Skinner; and the humanists as symbolized by Rogers. We noted that Freud identified five stages of psychosexual development: oral, anal, phallic, latency, and genital. Freud also stated that defense mechanisms are important to development through these stages and affect the formation of the id, ego, and superego. The learning theorists, on the other hand, stress the role that operant conditioning, classical conditioning, and modeling have on the development of the person. Some of the more important learning concepts that we reviewed included positive reinforcement, negative reinforcement, schedules of reinforcement, discrimination, generalization, extinction, and spontaneous recovery. From the humanistic perspective, we noted that Rogers believed that the development of the person has to do with the kinds of nurturing received from significant others in the form of empathy, congruence, and unconditional positive regard, and that conditions of worth can dramatically affect the development, or lack thereof, of the "real self." We noted that the humanistic approach is a departure from the deterministic views of Freud and the reductionistic ideas of the learning theorists in that the humanists stress the importance of significant relationships to our understanding of personality development.

Finally, viewing development as a life-span model, we presented the stage models of Erikson and Kegan. Erikson offered eight stages that all individuals pass through as we go through life: (1) trust versus mistrust, (2) autonomy versus shame and doubt, (3) initiative versus guilt, (4) industry versus inferiority, (5) identity versus role confusion, (6) intimacy versus isolation, (7) generativity versus stagnation, and (8) integrity versus despair. Each stage, Erikson noted, has its own unique tasks that all of us face. Kegan, on the other hand, believes that life-span development is a function of how we construct reality as a result of our interactions with others as we pass through life. Kegan's theory includes six stages and is similar to Erikson's in the sense that each individual can pass through them. However, contrary to Erikson, he notes that passage through the adult stages may occur at different rates, or not at all, as a function of environmental factors such as education and the kinds of nurturing received. His stages are called incorporative, impulsive, imperial, interpersonal, institutional, and interindividual.

We noted in this chapter that understanding the developmental level of the client is crucial to working effectively toward client goals. Key components to using a developmental perspective when working with clients includes assessing developmental level, devising developmental-based techniques, and supporting yet challenging the client toward growth.

As we neared the end of this chapter, we explored the differences between normal and abnormal development and the ways we have tried to understand psychopathology, especially as presented by Szaz, Glasser, and Laing. We then discussed major differences in understanding abnormal behavior, along with one attempt to classify mental illness and emotional maladjustment as presented in the *DSM-IV-TR*.

Finally, we concluded the chapter by noting the importance of understanding our own development and how it can affect our work with our clients and the significance of finding activities that can assist us in our own personal developmental history.

EXPERIENTIAL EXERCISES

1. Reflecting on Your Personality Development

Refer to the personality theories of Freud, Rogers, and the learning theorists and then reflect on your personality development as it might be described from each of those perspectives.

1. How does each perspective explain characteristics of your personality?
2. In explaining your personality development from the differing perspectives, what commonalities do you see between the varying theories?
3. In explaining your personality development from the differing perspectives, what differences do you see between the varying theories?

2. Examining the Development of an Adult with a Developmental Disability

The following is the story of Gloria. From a developmental perspective, describe Gloria from the following viewpoints:

1. Child development

2. Personality development

3. Life-span development

Gloria's life story: Gloria, a 53-year-old developmentally disabled adult, was born mildly mentally retarded and with cerebral palsy. Soon after her birth, her parents hospitalized her in an institution for the developmentally disabled. She lived in this institution until she was 31, at which time she was placed in a group home for the mentally retarded.

As a child, Gloria's language development was delayed. She could not speak in sentences until she was 4 years old. She was not toilet trained until age 7. Although her parents would visit her periodically, her main caretakers were the social service workers at the institution. Gloria was schooled at the institution where she acquired the equivalent of a second-grade education. Gloria had few friends in the institution and was considered a loner. Despite working on social-ization skills while in the institution, Gloria still prefers to be alone and spends much of her time painting. She has become a rather good artist, and many of her paintings are found in the institution and in the group home. Visitors often com-ment on the paintings and are usually surprised that a developmentally disabled person can paint so well. Gloria has a part-time job at a local art supply company where she generally does menial work.

Although Gloria does have some friends at the group home and at the art sup-ply store, usually, when she spends much time with someone, she ends up having a temper tantrum. When this happens she will usually withdraw—often to her painting. Gloria generally blames other people for her anger.

Gloria is a rules follower. She feels very strongly about the list of rules on the bulletin board at her group home. She methodically reports people who break the rules. She always feels extremely guilty after having a temper tantrum because she sees herself as breaking the rule "talk things out rather than get into a fight." In a similar vein, Gloria feels that laws in the country "are there for a purpose." For instance, at street crossings she always stops at red lights and waits for the light to change.

Gloria has no sense of her future. She lives from day to day and, despite peri-ods of depression, generally functions fairly adequately. She states she wants to get married, but her lack of socialization skills prevents her from having any meaning-ful relationships with men.

Overall, the human service professionals who have contact with Gloria describe her as a rigid, conscientious, talented person who has trouble maintain-ing relationships. They note that, despite being in individual counseling and in a socialization support group, she has made little progress in maintaining satisfying relationships. Their feeling is that she probably will maintain her current level of functioning, and they see little hope for change.

3. Examining the Development of a Gifted Child

The following is the story of Joe. From a developmental perspective, explain Joe's development from the following viewpoints:

1. Child development

2. Personality development

3. Life-span development

Joe's life story: Joe is 13 years old and is the only child, grandchild, and niece or nephew on his mother's side of the family. Joe's parents separated when his mother was five months' pregnant with him. His parents, both of whom are highly educated, went through a tumultuous separation and divorce but now have a cordial relationship. Following his birth, his mother was distraught over the breakup of her marriage but subsequently has maintained a strong sense of self and high self-esteem. Following Joe's birth, his mother, who works full-time, was fortunately able to afford a live-in nanny. This woman still lives with them and has been a significant help for the family and an additional source of comfort for Joe.

Joe's mother remarried when Joe was 10 years old, and his father has been involved in a long-term relationship. Joe lives with his mother but spends every other weekend, some weekdays, and extended periods during the summer and holidays with his father. Joe seems to have a good relationship with both parents, his stepfather, and his father's girlfriend.

Joe, who has always done well in school, currently attends a private school. He maintains very high grades and has a high IQ. Joe is at ease in relationships, as evidenced by his many friends and his ability to relate to people of all ages. He has many skills and is just beginning to examine those things that he is best at. He is just entering puberty, and girls are becoming more important to him. Overall, most people would describe Joe as a bright, personable, and thoughtful young man who is at ease with himself.

Although sometimes he may appear a little "spoiled," he generally is thoughtful and can recognize other people's feelings. He can think abstractly, and it would not be difficult to have a conversation with him concerning such philosophical matters as death and the existence of God.

4. Counseling Gloria

If you were to counsel Gloria, how would your knowledge of her development help you in the strategies you used?

5. Counseling Joe

If you were to counsel Joe, how would your knowledge of his development help you in the strategies you used?

6. Understanding Defense Mechanisms

Provide an example of each of the following defense mechanisms:

1. Repression

2. Denial

3. Projection

4. Rationalization

5. Regression

6. Other defense mechanisms?

7. Examining Defenses People Use

Can you think of other kinds of defenses people use to protect themselves from past pains and current hurts?

8. Developmental Differences Between Men and Women

Using the concepts as presented by Kohlberg and Gilligan, discuss your views on how men and women approach moral reasoning. What differences and similarities do you see between how men and women approach morality?

9. Examining Differing Perspectives on Abnormal Behavior

Respond to the following statements concerning abnormal behavior:

1. Using a situational point of view, make an argument for abnormal behavior being a function of one's surroundings.

2. Using a personality development perspective, make an argument for abnormal behavior being a function of early child rearing.

3. Using the perspective of Laing and Szaz, make an argument that abnormal behavior is a normal reaction to stressful life events.

4. Using a genetic and biological orientation, make an argument for abnormal behavior being determined.

10. Using the *DSM-IV-TR*

Go to your college library reserve desk and obtain a copy of the *DSM-IV-TR*. Pick one diagnostic category and review the behavioral characteristics of that disorder along with a possible etiology of that disorder. In class, discuss the varying diagnostic categories you found.

11. Ethical and Professional Vignettes

Reflect on the following ethical vignettes and discuss them in class:

1. A colleague with whom you work continually uses pathological language in describing her clients. You believe that this behavior is demeaning to her clients and wonder about her ability to work with them. Is the colleague acting ethically? Professionally? What, if anything, should you do?

2. A human service professional who does not believe in mental illness insists on treating clients with severe pathology in a proactive, humanistic manner and refuses to explore the possibility of medication as an adjunct to counseling. Is this ethical? Professional? Legal?

3. A human service professional who is working with a severely depressed client tells the client that she needs to seriously consider taking some

antidepressant medication. She then refers the client to a psychiatrist. Is this ethical? Professional? Legal?

4. A human service professional offers, for a fee, educational workshops to help individuals understand developmental tasks and unique developmental issues. Can the helper ethically and legally do this without being licensed?

5. A psychologist places an ad in the local newspaper that states, "Holistic, nonintrusive, nonpsychopathologically oriented counseling. See a helper who cares and can offer hope to all individuals." Is this type of ad ethical? Professional? Legal?

6. A human service professional who is a colleague and a friend has had little training in developmental stages and normal transitions in life. You notice that often the treatment planning for his clients is based on a medical model, and you believe that some of his clients are being served poorly because normal developmental struggles are being viewed as pathology. What is your responsibility to this professional? To his clients? What should you do if you explain your concerns and he does not do anything differently?

6

Systems: What Are They, and How Do We Work with Them?

The concept of system thus treats people and events in terms of their interactions rather than their intrinsic characteristics. The most basic principle underlying the systems viewpoint has been understood for some time. An ancient astronomer once said, "Heaven is more than the stars alone. It is the stars and their movements." (Baruth & Huber, 1984, p. 19)

My sister is 5 years older than I, my brother 5 years younger. My father, who died when I was 26 years old, was a hard-working, kind, thoughtful man, somewhat on the quiet side and not particularly expressive of his feelings. My mom was (and still is) a nurturing, sometimes opinionated, yet mostly supportive woman on whom we could always rely in time of need. Both my parents were college educated and first generation in this country. Dinner was a very special time for my family. My mother (and sometimes my sister) would prepare dinner while the rest of us would watch television in the den. During dinner, we would often have lively discussions about politics or other contemporary issues. As much as I loved these family interactions, I clearly remember being both overwhelmed by and particularly in awe of my sister's ability to argue her point of view.

Because I was sickly as a child and overweight, my self-esteem was not very high. Although I loved the family interactions, I had a sense that I could not hold my own in the nightly discussions; I would often find myself going inward to my feelings rather than relying on my intellectual ability. I remember arguing over issues such as capital punishment and the war in Vietnam. My arguments often became very passionate because I had become comfortable in the feeling world and less comfortable presenting a factual argument.

It seems as if we began to take on particular roles in the family—my father being the strong yet quiet debater; my sister, the verbally fluid family member; my mom, the mediator; me, the passionate member; and my brother, being the youngest and perhaps because the feeling and verbal roles were already taken, seemed on the quiet side. There was a kind of balance in the family. Things seemed a little off if we suddenly were out of our family roles. Perhaps it's not surprising that my sister became a lawyer; I, a mental health professional; and my brother, an engineer—professions that match the personality characteristics of the roles we chose.

My first therapeutic experience was in a counseling group in college. It is not accidental that I was the advocate for "expression of feelings," for invariably the roles we took on as children in our families are repeated in these groups. A woman of that same group, who had always taken on what might be considered male qualities, wanted to experiment with her feminine side. Therefore, she decided to try to act more feminine in the group. A third member of the group was always considered the outcast in school. He quickly took on this role in the group, and the group leader helped him examine why this continually happened to him.

My first job as a mental health professional was at a street-front crisis and drop-in center. There, we would often have homeless people seeking shelter. These people, most of whom had abusive or deprived childhoods, were often unkempt and uneducated, and many had emotional problems. Unfortunately, because of their inability to communicate effectively, which many times was a function of early roles played out in their families of origin, they would sabotage their attempts to receive aid from local social agencies. I remember how effective Vanessa, a woman who had been on welfare herself, was in helping these individuals work with the local social service systems.

When I accepted my current job at Old Dominion University, I discovered that a colleague of mine, Garrett, had grown up in an Irish-American neighborhood a few miles from my predominantly Jewish neighborhood in Queens. I had not even known that his neighborhood existed. Despite the fact that we grew up close to each other, our neighborhoods were so insulated that there was little shared between these cultures. These closely knit neighborhoods had somewhat rigid boundaries that prevented a sharing of cultural wealth.

What do all these vignettes have in common? They all are expressions of the complex interactions in systems. From the family systems in which we grew up, to the groups in which we now interact, to the community and organizational systems in which we live and work, systems play an important role in our lives. Thus, I don't find it surprising that, in a survey of graduates of human service programs, most respondents rated knowledge of organizations, families, and groups as particularly significant (Sweitzer & McKinney, 1991).

In this chapter, we will examine how human service professionals can use knowledge of systems to enhance their work with clients. We will begin by reviewing general systems theory and examining how this theory can help us understand all kinds of systems. Then, we will take a look at three systems in particular—families, groups, and communities—and examine how the human service professional can affect each of these systems to induce change. In addition, we will discuss ethical and professional issues related to working in systems. Finally, we will examine the importance of understanding the complex interactions of systems for the developmentally mature human service professional.

GENERAL SYSTEMS THEORY

Living systems are processes that maintain a persistent structure of relatively long periods despite rapid exchange of their component parts with the surrounding world. (Skynner, 1976, pp. 3–4)

Although knowledge of the amoeba may seem like a far cry from our understanding of systems, in actuality there is much we can learn from this one-celled animal. The amoeba has semipermeable boundaries that allow it to take in nutrition from the environment. This delicate animal could not survive if its boundaries were too rigid or too permeable. Boundaries that are too rigid would prevent it from ingesting food, and boundaries that are too loose would not allow the amoeba to maintain and digest the food it has found.

General systems theory was developed to explain the complex interactions of all types of systems including living systems, family systems, and community systems (Bertalanffy, 1934, 1968). Each system has a **boundary** that defines its **information flow** and allows it to maintain its structure while the system interacts with other systems around it. Thus, the action of the amoeba, a small living system, affects the surrounding environment. Similarly, the action of a family unit will affect other families with which it interacts, and the action of a community group will affect other aspects of the community.

Components in a system tend to maintain their typical ways of functioning, whether those actions within the system are functional or dysfunctional. A much-used analogy is that of the thermostat in the house. When the temperature drops in the house, the thermostat, based on the temperature setting, switches on. If the thermostat is set for 70 degrees and the temperature drops below that, the heater turns on. However, if the thermostat is set for 40 degrees, the heater will not turn on until the temperature drops below 40 degrees. This tendency toward equilibrium is called **homeostasis.**

In families and in groups, members take on typical ways of behaving, regardless of whether these typical patterns are dysfunctional. Because families and groups become comfortable with their typical ways of behaving, members in these systems will exert covert or overt pressure to have atypical behaviors suppressed. For instance, it was unusual for any member of my family to express anger. When I was a teenager, the few times I got very angry I distinctly remember my mother saying, "I don't understand why you're so angry; maybe we should take you to see a psychologist." My anger was atypical (rather than wrong), and the family system was attempting to deal with my unusual behavior.

General systems theory views a healthy system as one that has **semipermeable boundaries** that allow new information to enter the system and be processed and incorporated. When a system has **rigid boundaries,** information cannot flow easily into or out of the system, and the system has difficulty with the change process. Alternatively, a system that has **loose boundaries** allows information to flow too easily into and out of the system, resulting in the individual components of the system having difficulty maintaining a sense of identity.

Regardless of the types of boundaries within a system, its regulatory mechanism maintains its homeostasis through a series of rules that define how it will interact. Therefore, finding families and community groups (for example, religious organizations) with a fairly rigid set of rules that maintains their functioning in relatively healthy ways is not unusual. Alternatively, there are also families and community groups that allow a wide range of behaviors within the system (for example, encounter groups). Although American culture allows for much variation in the permeability of various systems, systems that have very rigid or very loose boundaries have a tendency toward dysfunction. Sometimes these systems have disastrous results when breakdown occurs (see Box 6.1).

FAMILY SYSTEMS

Divorce has ripple effects that touch not just the family involved, but our entire society. As the writer Pat Conroy observed when his own marriage broke up, "Each divorce is the death of a small civilization." When one family divorces, that divorce affects relatives, friends, neighbors, employers, teachers, clergy, and scores of strangers. (Wallerstein & Blakeslee, 1989, p. xxi)

BOX 6.1   Jim Jones and the Death of a Rigid System

In the 1950s and early 1960s, Jim Jones was a respected minister in Indiana. However, Jones became increasingly paranoid and grandiose, believing he was Jesus. He moved his family to Brazil and later relocated to California where approximately 100 of his church followers from Indiana joined him. In California, he headed the People's Church, and he began to set more rigid rules for church membership. Slowly, he became more dictatorial and continued to show evidence of paranoid delusions. He insisted that church members prove their love for him, demanding sexual intercourse with female church members, having members sign over their possessions, sometimes having them give their children to him, and having members inform on those who broke his rules. In 1975, a reporter uncovered some of the tactics Jones was using and was about to write a revealing article about the church. Jones learned about this and, just before publication of the article, moved to Guyana, taking a few hundred of his followers with him. As concerns about some of the church practices

reached the United States, California Congressman Leo Ryan and some of his aides went to Guyana to investigate the situation. Jones and his supporters killed the congressman and some of the aides. Jones then ordered his followers to commit suicide. Hundreds killed themselves. Those who did not were murdered.

Jones developed a church with a rigid set of rules. The publication of a revealing article and the congressman flying into Guyana were threats to the system. As in many rigid systems, attempts at change from the outside were seen as potentially lethal blows to the system. Jones dealt with the reporter's threat to the system by moving his congregation to Guyana. Then, rather than allow new information into the system, Jones killed off the system, first killing the congressman and then ordering church members to commit suicide. The members had become so mired in the rules of the system that nearly 900 of them committed suicide or were murdered. This is a tragic example of how dysfunctional a rigid system can be.

Today, nearly 50% of marriages end in divorce. So great is the impact of divorce on the family that Wallerstein and Blakeslee (1996) found that 10 to 15 years following a divorce, many of the children of divorce continued to have strong negative feelings about the divorce, and a large percentage of the parents who divorced felt as if life was unfair and disappointing. Divorce affects everyone in the family and many outside of it. Families are systems, and each unique family system affects other systems around it. In this section, we will explore the family system, how it functions and how it becomes dysfunctional, and the role of human service professionals in their encounters with families.

The Development of the Healthy Family

Healthy family systems have semipermeable boundaries that allow information to flow in, be evaluated, and through healthy communication channels, make change as needed. A healthy family has parents or guardians who are the main rule makers (a healthy family system can also have a single parent or guardian). Although rules differ from family to family, healthy families have a clear sense of **hierarchy.** This means that the parents are the main rule makers and that children, although possibly consulted in the rule making, are the recipients of those rules. **Virginia Satir** (1967) noted that when one member of the family feels pain, the whole

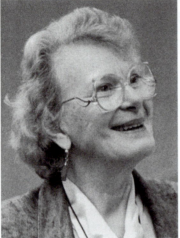

Virginia Satir, world-renowned family therapist (1916–1988), noted that the actions of one family member resonate throughout the family system.

family is affected. This is because the family is a system with a delicate homeostasis, and the actions of one member resonate throughout the whole system.

Salvadore Minuchin (1974) sees families as going through **situational crises** and **developmental cycles.** He states that families may face unexpected problems that are situationally specific and will encounter predictable struggles as the family ages and goes through the life stages. For example, when a husband and wife have their first child, the spousal dyad faces its first potential crisis. The husband and wife will face a disruption in their relationship because rules in their family change to deal with the new family member. As children age, families will continually face **developmental crises** (see Chapter 5) that necessitate changes in family rules. A healthy family has the mechanism to successfully pass through these developmental stages. Like Satir, Minuchin notes that when one member of the family is affected by a situational crisis or developmental milestone, the whole family is affected. If the family has healthy ways of communicating and if the family members can support one another as individual members go through changes, then the family will survive in a healthy manner (see Box 6.2).

Dysfunctional Families

All husbands and wives bring to their marriage **unfinished business** from their pasts. Invariably, this unfinished business will affect their relationship. The more serious the issue, the more likely it will affect their marriage and, from a systems point of view, affect the family. A family that has serious problems is often called a **dysfunctional family.** For instance, a wife who was sexually molested as a child and has not worked through her pain will undoubtedly bring this unfinished business into the relationship. She might have developed mistrust of men and therefore unconsciously have chosen a man who is distant (and safe). Perhaps he is a workaholic. Alternatively, a man who has difficulty with intimacy might unconsciously pick a wife who allows him to be distant (and safe). As the relationship

---

BOX 6.2   A Situational Family Crisis

When I was between the ages of 8 and 13, I had a heart disorder called pericarditis. This somewhat debilitating illness enlarged my heart, caused me much chest pain, and left me periodically bedridden with a resulting mild depression. Although not considered extremely serious, this illness certainly affected my life in a major way. However, it also affected my parents' lives and the lives of my siblings.

Although my illness potentially could have been a threat to the homeostasis in the family, it became clear that the family was strong enough to deal effectively with this situation. Because my parents' marriage was solid, the added stress did not dramatically affect their relationship. In addition, they were able to maintain the functioning of the family in a relatively normal way. This normalization of family patterns during a period of stress speaks highly of the strength of the family.

---

unravels, each spouse's issues are played out either on one another or on a child (or children). The husband may become stressed at work and take this out on his wife, children, or both. The wife may crave more intimacy, become discontent with the marriage, and take this out on her husband or children. Is it surprising that there are so many affairs and divorces?

When spouses are discontent with each other and when they unconsciously take out their anger on a child rather than work it through with each other, that child is said to be a **scapegoat.** When a member of the family is scapegoated, he or she often becomes the **identified patient** (IP) in the family, or the member that is identified as the "one with the problem." In actuality, the whole family has the problem. When a child acts out in the family, in school, or in the community, it is often the result of that child being the member carrying the pain for the family (see Box 6.3).

Family Guidance, Family Counseling, and the Role of the Human Service Professional

Therapists who do family counseling have in-depth knowledge of family systems and how to facilitate change in the family. Such counseling often involves the whole family being involved in intensive family sessions. Today, there are many models of family therapy, each of which has a slightly different twist on how to work with families. However, they all tend to adhere to the following broad guidelines borrowed from general systems theory:

1. Families (and other social groups) are systems having properties which are more than the sum of the properties of their parts.

2. The operation of such systems is governed by certain general rules.

3. Every system has a boundary, the properties of which are important in understanding how the system works.

BOX 6.3   An Example of a Dysfunctional Family

When I was in private practice as a psychologist, a school counselor referred a 12-year-old boy to me because the boy's grades had dropped considerably and he was acting out in school. I asked him and his parents to come in for family counseling. For the first two months, the parents insisted that everything was fine in their marriage. As I continued to explore the situation, I could not understand why this boy was doing so poorly in school and was demonstrating such a dramatic personality shift. Then, during one session, the father revealed to me that he was extremely depressed, in fact, suicidally depressed. His depression stemmed back to his childhood. Soon, the mother revealed that she was bulimic, and later I discovered she was having an affair. The secretness of the father's depression and the mother's bulimia and affair were symptoms of deep discontent in the marriage, and all stemmed back to issues in their childhoods.

Rather than dealing with these very painful issues with each other, the couple had taken out their discontent on their oldest child. They did this through the mother becoming overly protective, the father becoming overly distant, and, whenever they would get angry at each other, both focusing on their son's problems. When the school tried to involve them in assisting the boy, they sabotaged whatever they were asked to do, as if they had something at stake in keeping him the identified patient. In essence, as long as he was seen as the one with the problem, they did not have to deal with their problems. As soon as they became aware of what they were doing, the mother became less protective, the father became closer to his son, and the couple stopped scapegoating their son and began to deal with their own issues. The son's acting-out behaviors immediately stopped, and his grades improved dramatically.

---

4. The boundaries are semi-permeable; that is to say that some things can pass through them while others cannot. Moreover, it is sometimes found that certain material can pass one way but not the other.

5. Family systems tend to reach a relatively, but not totally, steady state. Growth and evolution are possible, indeed usual. Change can occur, or be stimulated in various ways.

6. Communication and feedback mechanisms between the parts of the system are important in the functioning of the system [cybernetics: positive and negative feedback loops].

7. Events such as the behavior of individuals in the family are better understood as examples of *circular causality*, rather than as being based on linear causality.

8. Family systems, like other open systems, appear to be purposeful.

9. Systems are made up of *subsystems* and themselves are parts of larger *suprasystems*. (Barker, 1998, p. 28)

Over the years, a number of approaches to family counseling have been developed (see Nichols & Schwartz, 2001). Some of these include **strategic family therapy** (Haley, 1973, 1976), family therapy from a **communication perspective** (Satir, 1972a, 1972b), **structural family therapy** (Minuchin, 1974, 1981), **multigenerational family therapy** (Bowen, 1976, 1978), **experiential family therapy** (Napier & Whitaker, 1978; Whitaker, 1976), psychodynamic family therapy (Skynner, 1981), and **behavioral family therapy** (see Foster & Gurman,

1985). Although each of these approaches has its unique take on the family counseling process, they all follow, to some degree, the tenets Barker noted.

Training in family counseling is rigorous and requires at least a master's degree. Although human service professionals do not have the training to do family counseling, knowledge of family systems can help them provide family guidance. Family guidance does not include intensive family counseling; however, human service professionals may refer to family counselors, suggest workshops to attend, offer reading materials regarding how families interact, and give basic advice on family matters. It is important that the human service professional make an assessment about the seriousness of the family dysfunction and act accordingly.

Individual Counseling Versus Family Counseling

When should a family member be referred to individual counseling rather than the whole family being referred for family counseling? Although some therapists might suggest it is always appropriate to refer the whole family for counseling rather than just one member (Napier & Whitaker, 1978; Satir, 1967), most therapists today agree that it is often a matter of making a decision based on an assessment of the situation. For instance, a child who comes from an extremely dysfunctional family may be better off seeing a therapist individually because working with the family may be an extremely long process, whereas individual counseling may give some immediate relief to the child. Or it may be prudent to refer a spouse for individual counseling to work on his or her unfinished business because this will facilitate change in the whole family. Also, individual members in a family will often seek out individual counseling while the family undergoes family treatment. If you are unsure what might be the best referral for a client, seek advice from a more experienced human service professional.

GROUP SYSTEMS

Groups, like families, can be viewed from a systemic perspective in which individuals in the group can be understood by examining the dynamic interaction of its members and how that interaction results in specific communication patterns, power dynamics, hierarchies, and the system's unique homeostasis (Durkin, 1972; Gazda, 1989; Lonergan, 1994). Like members of families, group members will bring in their unfinished business, which may cause problems in the healthy functioning of the group. Groups tend to create their own homeostasis, and members may be scapegoated in this process. Therefore, when a group member is scapegoated, he or she is reflecting problems within the whole system. Although community and social groups have always existed, groups whose intent is to explore human interactions are relatively new.

A Brief History

Gladding (2003) notes that before 1900, the purpose of group treatment was to assist individuals in ways that were functional and pragmatic. This often revolved around helping people with daily living skills and arose out of the social group work movement where individuals like **Jane Addams** organized group discussions that centered on such things as personal hygiene, nutrition, and self-determination (Pottick, 1988). Using groups as their vehicle, social reformers like Addams were particularly concerned with community organizing as an effort to assist the poor.

At the turn of the century, schools began to offer "Vocational and Moral Guidance" in group settings. These efforts were often "preachy" in their nature, and group members had little opportunity to discuss personal matters in reflective ways. However, with the spread of psychotherapeutic theory and with the beginnings of sociological concepts concerning group interactions, the first use of counseling and therapy groups that had more of an introspective nature arose in the 1920s and 1930s (Gladding, 2003).

During the 1940s, the modern group movement emerged. During this decade, Carl Rogers brought together therapists to discuss what problems they might encounter in working with returning war veterans. He soon found that within this group setting there was a deepening of expression of feeling and, in many instances, an uncovering of new awarenesses concerning themselves. Thus began the **encounter group** movement (Rogers, 1970). At about the same time, **Kurt Lewin** and other nationally known theorists developed the **National Training Laboratory (NTL)** to examine **group dynamics** or the ways in which groups tend to interact (Gladding, 2003; Shaffer & Galinsky, 1974). NTL still exists and continues to train individuals in understanding the special dynamics of groups. Over the years, many different types of groups with unique characteristics have arisen. For instance, we have seen the proliferation of self-help, psychoeducational, and counseling and therapy groups.

Defining Self-Help, Psychoeducational, and Counseling and Therapy Groups

Although systems dynamics occur in all groups, there are some differences in the functioning of **self-help groups, psychoeducational groups, and counseling and therapy groups** (Capuzzi & Gross, 2002; Trotzer, 1989). Regardless of the type of group, however, all groups have rules regarding membership behavior, leadership style, technical issues (for example, when and where to meet, number of group members, length of meeting times), and ground rules (for example, limits of confidentiality, socializing outside of the group, nature and purpose of the group).

Self-Help and Personal Growth Groups

The growth of **self-help groups,** sometimes called **support groups** or **personal growth groups,** in this country has been phenomenal during the past 25 years. From Alcoholics Anonymous (AA), to codependency groups, to eating disorder and diet groups, to men's and women's groups, to self-help groups for the chronically mentally ill, the kinds of self-help groups that have emerged seem endless. Their purpose is the education, affirmation, and enhancement of existing strengths of the group member (Andrews, 1995). Generally, a nonpaid volunteer leader focuses the discussion and assists in defining the rules of the group.

However, sometimes there may be no leader at all. Self-help groups are generally free or have a nominal fee and can be facilitated by a trained layperson or mental health professional.

Self-help groups are not in-depth counseling groups and hardly ever require a vast amount of self-disclosure by the group members. In fact, because self-help groups tend to be open groups, their composition is constantly changing, and this can hinder the building of group cohesion, a critical element for in-depth work. Usually individuals in self-help groups are encouraged to only share that amount that feels comfortable for that member. Some self-help groups even discourage intense self-disclosure as that would be seen as more appropriate for individual or group counseling. Although self-help groups have had limited evaluation and their effectiveness is unclear (Andrews, 1995; Yeaton, 1994), many people swear by them, and they have become an ever increasing referral source for mental health professionals.

With self-help groups, the number of group members, length of meeting times, and atmosphere of the group setting can vary considerably. Some groups have 200 members, but others are limited to just a few people. Some groups meet in the basement of a church, whereas others meet in the comforts of the office of a therapist who has lent the group space. Some self-help groups are ongoing, others are time limited, and some demand confidentiality, but others do not (see Box 6.4).

Psychoeducational Groups

Psychoeducational groups attempt to increase self-understanding, promote personal and interpersonal growth, and prevent future problems through the dissemination of mental health education in a group setting (ASGW, 2000; Capuzzi & Gross, 2002). A few examples of the many topics that psychoeducational groups have focused on include sex education, conflict resolution, AIDS awareness, career awareness, communication skills, diversity issues, chemical dependence, stress management, and lifestyle adjustment.

In recent years, the term *psychoeducational groups* has become more popular than the term *guidance* because guidance has been misconstrued as being too highly advice oriented, has held negative connotations for people, and has been particularly associated with the schools (Brown, 1998; Kottler, 1994).

Compared with self-help groups, psychoeducational groups always have a designated, well-trained group leader, and generally, their purpose is the education and support of the group members. Leaders will usually offer a didactic presentation, and although there is not much in-depth self-disclosure, there may be an opportunity for some sharing of personal information. With their purpose being more educational than psychotherapeutic, the result of this group is to increase members' knowledge. Such groups may be ongoing or can occur on a one-time basis. Psychoeducational groups can vary in their length, and other technical issues can also vary depending on the focus of the group. Like self-help groups, psychoeducational groups may be free of charge; however, some psychoeducational groups involve a fee (see Box 6.5).

BOX 6.4   A Men's Self-Help Group

For two years, I participated in a men's self-help group, which was started by 10 men who had an interest in discussing issues particularly relevant to our maleness. Although there was no defined leader, we all took a leadership role at various times. When we first started meeting, we defined some of the rules of our group. We decided not to have designated topics to discuss (although generally, the discussions revolved around male issues—for example, relationships with women, how men express feelings, our relationships with our fathers). We decided to meet every Sunday for two hours and used our homes as a meeting place on a rotating basis. We also decided that we would not share details of our talks with others outside the group, although we felt it was all right to talk in generalities about what we discussed in our group. Our group afforded each of us a place where we could feel supported, discuss issues about being male, and receive feedback about ourselves from other group members. Although, as in all groups, we had our ups and downs, generally we all agreed that the group was a positive experience.

Counseling and Therapy Groups

Like individual counseling and therapy, many people differentiate a counseling group from a therapy group by the depth of self-disclosure and the amount of personality reconstruction expected during the therapeutic process. However, counseling and therapy groups probably have more similarities than differences. For instance, both counseling and therapy groups have a designated, highly trained leader. Generally, there are between 4 and 12 group members. Such groups usually meet for a minimum of eight sessions, and some continue on an ongoing basis. Most counseling and therapy groups meet at least once a week for one to three hours. Confidentiality of the group is critical, and individual members are asked not to reveal information about other members outside the group. Although leadership styles may vary, members usually will have the opportunity to freely express their feelings and to eventually work on behavioral change. Many of the counseling and therapy approaches noted in Chapter 3 have been adapted for this group process (see Box 6.6).

Group Membership Behavior

We all have typical ways of behaving in life. These typical patterns are repeated in groups as they are in our daily interactions with friends and acquaintances. Therefore, groups are often called minilabs of our world, and they give us the opportunity to look at how we present ourselves to others. In addition, they allow us to obtain feedback about our typical ways of interacting. In counseling, therapy, and self-help groups, we will often be given the opportunity to examine these behaviors and work on changing those that we might identify as maladaptive. As members pass through the stages of group development, their typical patterns of behavior will emerge. Some group specialists have identified certain characteristics or roles taken on by members (Gladding, 2003; Vander Kolk, 1990). For

---

BOX 6.5   An AIDS Psychoeducational Group

Jonathan is a human service professional who works for the local AIDS awareness center. His main job is to visit local schools, businesses, and community centers, and present workshops on how one contracts HIV, current diagnostic procedures for HIV, and treatment of AIDS. His two-hour workshop is information based, and he allows time for questions and self-disclosure when appropriate. When requested, he will extend his presentation for one to four additional meetings. He also provides referrals to AIDS self-help groups and to therapists who work with HIV-positive individuals, their families, and their friends.

---

instance, some members may be dominators, mediators, manipulators, caretakers, nurturers, or facilitators, whereas other members may be withdrawn, hostile, blockers, or opinionated. These are just a few of the types of roles members assume. Can you think of others?

As the group process continues, **group membership behaviors** (the roles that members take on) may vary. For example, whereas some members might be withdrawn near the beginning stages of the group, others might become withdrawn at later stages. Whether a member is withdrawn, manipulating, or nurturing, I prefer to not place a value judgment on the behavior. Instead, I view group membership roles as a statement about the individual, a statement about the needs of the group, and a role that can be beneficial or harmful to the group process. For instance, consider the individual who is a great nurturer near the beginning of the group. Such a role may come easily to a particular member of the group and thus be a statement about the member's way of being in the world. Also, the group may need a member to be the nurturer, so the group allows this behavior to emerge so all the members can build a sense of trust. Finally, although such a role can be beneficial as it helps to build group cohesion, it can also be harmful if it is used by group members to avoid focusing on other issues or if the nurturer uses this behavior as a means of avoiding other behaviors (for example, anger, deep hurts, and so on).

Group Leadership Styles

Although **group leadership styles** will vary depending on the leader's theoretical orientation (Corey, 2000; Gladding, 2003), all leaders need to be aware of basic group theory and process to facilitate groups appropriately (Brown, 1992). Therefore, knowledge of systems, familiarity with membership roles, awareness of group stages of development, and adeptness at basic as well as advanced counseling techniques are crucial. Good leaders are aware of the composition of their groups and have adjusted their styles to the needs of the groups. A good leader will be strong without being authoritarian, knowledgeable about the rules and technical issues, yet flexible in the ways they are implemented. He or she can facilitate the interactions of the group members as they pass through the stages of group development. Such a leader feels comfortable working with a vast array of member behaviors and can set the stage for the group to unfold in a natural way.

BOX 6.6   William's Therapy Group

William has been struggling his whole life with mild depression. When he married two years ago, he thought he would feel better. However, after an initial period of being pretty mellow, his depressive feelings again began to emerge. He entered individual counseling and began to work on some of his issues, discovering that he often had expectations that women in his life would bring him happiness. He found that he often relies on them for comfort and nurturing and becomes upset when they do not meet his needs. After some initial gain in self-awareness during individual counseling, his therapist suggested that he might want to enter a mixed (male and female) counseling group to experiment with new ways of relating to women. Although he has found this to be difficult, as he continues to build trust in the group, he is beginning to examine his behaviors more closely and explore new ways of relating.

Stages of Group Development

Over the years, many authors have identified typical stages of group development (Gladding, 2003; Tuckman & Jensen, 1977; Ward, 1982; Yalom, 1995). Although the terms for these stages vary from author to author, general characteristics of membership behavior are exhibited as group members pass through these stages.

Pregroup Stage Before forming a group, the leader has to decide a method to prescreen potential group members. This **pregroup stage** can be accomplished in many ways. Some group leaders will have a pregroup group meeting with all potential members. Other leaders will provide potential members with thorough written or even videotaped knowledge of the expectations of the group in an effort to have potential members screen themselves out. However, probably the most effective and common method is the individual interview. Couch (1995) notes that the interview can accomplish many things, including (1) identifying needs, expectations, and commitment of the potential group member; (2) challenging myths and misconceptions of the potential member; (3) conveying information to and procuring information from the potential member; and (4) screening out (or in) potential members.

The Initial Stage This beginning of a group is often highlighted by anxiety and apprehension by group members (and to a lesser degree, by the group leader). Members are learning about the rules and goals of their group and are wondering whether they can trust the other members.

During this **initial stage,** group members are often self-conscious and worried about how others might view them. Because of this initial apprehension and lack of trust, group members will often avoid talking about in-depth feelings, and discussions are relatively "safe." Therefore, it is common for conversations to be superficial, for members to talk about things not related to their lives, and for discussions to revolve around past feelings rather than current feelings. Corey and Corey (2002) call this a "self focus" as compared with an "other focus."

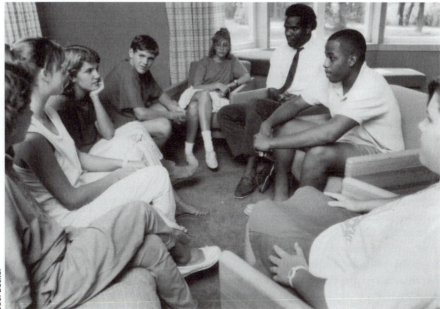

Joel Becker

Groups can offer a safe environment in which one can share feelings and gain feedback about oneself.

The major task for the group leader in this stage is to define the ground rules and to build trust. In building trust, the ability to set limits, to use empathy, and to show unconditional positive regard is crucial. As members become comfortable with the ground rules and as they begin to feel comfortable with one another, they move on to the next stage of group development.

The Transition Stage During the early **transition stage**, group members understand the goals and rules of the group but continue to remain anxious concerning the group process. Issues of control, power, and authority become increasingly important in this stage as members position themselves within the system (Corey & Corey, 2002; Vander Kolk, 1990; Yalom, 1995). Hostility during this stage can be viewed as a type of resistance that gives members a way to avoid dealing with their issues. The leader needs to be aware of any scapegoating that could occur as one manifestation of this hostility. Although empathy is still crucial, the leader must actively prevent a member from being scapegoated or attacked. Therefore, the leader will often take an active role in preventing coalitions from forming and in preventing verbal attacks on members.

As this stage continues, group members begin to settle in and can focus more on themselves (Higgs, 1992). This is highlighted by a sense of self-acceptance of the member's life predicaments. Members now demonstrate the ability to take ownership of their feelings, to talk in the here and now, and to not blame others for their problems. This is an important step toward actually making change that occurs in the next stage. As members move into this part of the transition stage and begin to take more responsibility for their feelings and actions, the leader's role becomes much easier. No longer is it necessary for the leader to "protect" members, and during this part of the transition stage the leader can usually relax and let the group develop on its own.

The Work Stage As group members gain the capacity to take ownership for their feelings and life predicaments, a deepening of trust and a sense of cohesion emerge within the group (Corey, 2000). Now, group members experience a sense of readiness to work on their identified problem areas. During this **work stage**, the group has developed its own homeostasis. Now it is important that the group leader prohibit members from becoming too comfortable in their styles of relating because this can prevent change and growth. Members readily give feedback to other members, and as they identify problem areas, they begin to take an active role in the change process. At this point, members might attempt new ways of communicating, acting, or expressing feelings. The leader can best facilitate movement by asking questions, using problem-solving skills, giving advice, offering alternatives, encouraging feedback by members, and affirming members' attempts at change.

As members accomplish their goals, they begin to gain a sense of high self-esteem. This is a product of receiving positive feedback from other members as well as a personal sense of accomplishment for the work that they have done. As members meet their goals, they are near the completion of the group process.

The Closure Stage As group members reach their identified goals, there is an increased sense of accomplishment and the beginning awareness that the group process is near completion (Corey, 2000; Gladding, 2003). During this **closure stage**, the leader will often summarize the learning that has taken place and begin to focus on the separation process. Because members typically have shared deep aspects of themselves, a sense of togetherness, cohesion, and warmth has developed. Therefore, saying good-bye can be a difficult process for many, and it is important that the leader facilitate this process in a direct yet gentle fashion. Often this is done by members sharing what they have learned about themselves and one another, through expression of feeling toward one another, and by defining future goals for themselves. This important final stage in the group process allows members to feel a sense of completion and wholeness about what they have experienced.

In this stage, the leader might actively encourage members to express their feelings concerning the group process as well as their feelings about ending the group. Asking questions and encouraging members to express their feelings might accomplish this. Of course, using empathy to listen to members' feelings regarding the closure of the group is extremely important.

Conclusion Whereas all types of groups should pass through these stages to be effective, the depth of work and intensity of feeling expressed will vary dramatically depending on the nature of the group. For instance, clients of psychoeducational and self-help groups will work on more superficial levels as they pass through these stages, whereas clients of counseling and therapy groups will deal with deeper levels of experience; in these groups, the work accomplished will be at the level of personality reconstruction. Therefore, when conducting groups, expectations of group behavior should be partially based on the type of group being offered.

Individual Counseling Versus Group Counseling

When does one refer a client to group counseling as an alternative or adjunct to individual counseling? First, the most current research indicates that group counseling is as effective as individual counseling (Faith, Wong, & Carpenter, 1995; Tillitski, 1990; Toseland & Siporin, 1986), which suggests that group work should always be considered an alternative to individual treatment. Although there is no easy method of determining when to use group or individual counseling, a few guidelines might help. Refer clients to group counseling in the following situations:

1. For a client who cannot afford the cost of individual counseling.
2. When the benefits of individual counseling have gotten so meager that an alternative treatment might offer a new perspective for the client.
3. When a client's issues are related to interpersonal functioning and a group might facilitate working through these issues in a "real to life" manner.
4. When a client needs the extra social support that a group might offer.
5. When a client wants to test new behaviors in a system that will support him or her while receiving realistic feedback about the new behaviors.
6. When the experiences of others who are working through similar issues as the client's can dramatically improve the client's functioning (for example, alcoholism, bipolar disorder).

COMMUNITY SYSTEMS
AND SOCIAL CHANGE

One way that American culture has attempted to equalize the inequities found throughout various communities in our society is to provide social service agencies that offer services to the poor, disabled, and deprived. Many of these agencies offer free or low-cost aid to individuals in need. In almost any community today, we find state and federally supported programs such as mental health centers, shelters for the homeless, vocational rehabilitation, child protective services, Medicare and Medicaid programs, food stamp programs, Aid to Families with Dependent Children (AFDC), and so forth. In addition, it is becoming increasingly common to find agency staff focusing on making broader systemic changes in the community. To work effectively with clients, the human service professional must work in a healthy agency, and, to make wider systemic changes, the professional must have a deep respect for the community and work closely with community members (Close, 2001; McMillen, 2001).

Working with Clients in Agencies

In most social service agencies, we can find human service professionals providing direct services to those in need. Their ability to effectively serve client needs is central to American society's attempt to change the face of American culture (McMillen, 2001). For human service professionals to work effectively with clients, they must have effective client skills (see Chapter 4) and have a clear understanding of the boundaries, rules, hierarchy, and information flow within the system.

Boundaries We hope that the system in which a human service professional works is healthy in that it has semipermeable boundaries that allow for open communication, flexibility, and change. Boundaries that are too rigid are indicative of an agency struggling with issues of power and control. Boundaries that are too loose are often a sign that the agency has not yet gotten its act together and needs to formulate rules to help govern itself effectively.

Rules Every agency has both overt rules and covert rules. Human services professionals need to understand the unique rules of the agency in which they work and at times make difficult ethical and moral decisions about whether or not they will follow the rules. In fact, sometimes, the system's rules may be contrary to your ethical guidelines. For instance, a system may have a rule that any use of illegal substances by a client should be reported to the police. Because this rule is contrary to the ethical guidelines of confidentiality, the human service professional will need to struggle with ways of dealing with this conflict. An example of a covert rule might be an agency that verbally states there is no dress code, yet looks askance at those professionals who come in dressed in blue jeans.

Hierarchies Knowing who's in charge, and when, is critical if one is to be a "team player" at an agency. For instance, knowing when to consult with one's supervisor is important for ensuring the proper treatment of clients, lowering one's liability risk, and maintaining the relationship balance at an agency. However, sometimes you might be willing to avoid seeking or to not listen to advice from a person in authority, such as when you believe the authority's feedback will harm the client. Although rebuking a person in authority can result in the loss of one's job, it is a decision that some professionals will periodically make if they believe there is a moral reason for doing so. Usually, however, such conflicts can and should be worked out:

> When a conflict arises between fulfilling the responsibility to the employer and the responsibility to the client, human service professionals advise both the employer and client of the conflict, and work conjointly with all involved to manage the conflict. (See Appendix B, Statement 34)

Information Flow Healthy information flow in agencies is a result of a clear understanding of the rules, semipermeable boundaries that allow open communication, and respect of the hierarchy because the hierarchy deserves that respect (e.g., a supervisor who is a strong, knowledgeable, ethical, and flexible leader). When these ingredients are in place, one has a healthy functioning agency. If there are, however, problems in the agency, the human service professional has an ethical obligation to work on improving conditions:

> Human service professionals participate in efforts to establish and maintain employment conditions which are conducive to higher quality client services. They assist in evaluating the effectiveness of the agency through reliable and valid assessment measures. (See Appendix B, Statement 33)

Working with the Community to Effect Client Change

> We also know that the social environment has a significant impact on individual behavior and development. Therefore, we must create programs that attend to the development and enhancement of the community and its climate. This will require that substantial attention be given to addressing systemic and environmental issues . . . (McMillen, 2001, p. 234)

Change tends to occur from the larger system to the smaller system, and often in very complex ways. Thus, if we are to affect the individual, we must make inroads in the community. A number of strategies for changing the community have been suggested over the years; however, today, it is clear that whatever intervention one makes, it should be undertaken with an attitude of respect and collaboration with community members (Close, 2001; McMillen, 2001). Six steps for implementing community change include the following:

1. Accurately Define Your Problem A clear understanding of the problem is necessary before one attempts to make change. If a community has a widespread drug problem, one needs to make sure the problem is indeed drugs and not a high unemployment rate.

2. Collaborate with Community Members Before developing strategies for change, it is critical that the agency staff is not seen as a group of "outsiders" pushing their ideas for change on the community. Individuals in the community will have vital ideas about how to develop change strategies that can be incorporated into a broader plan.

> Human service professionals keep informed about current social issues as they affect the client and the community. They share that information with clients, groups, and community as part of their work. (See Appendix B, Statement 11)

3. Respect Community Members Human service professionals must not have a "better than" attitude if change is to occur. Only when the professional is seen as respectful of the community, and even a part of the community, can effective change take place.

> Human service professionals are knowledgeable about the cultures and communities within which they practice. They are aware of multiculturalism in society and its impact on the community as well as individuals with the community. They respect individuals and groups, their cultures and beliefs. (See Appendix B, Statement 18)

4. Collaboratively Develop Strategies for Change In consultation with the community, develop strategies for change. Make them attainable and publicize them.

5. Implement Change Strategies Develop a timeline for implementing the change strategies, and with the help of community members, apply the strategies.

6. Assess Effectiveness In consultation with community members, evaluate whether or not your change strategies have had a positive impact on the community. If not, why not? And if not, start over.

Conclusion

To effect change in a person we can work directly with that person at an agency, or we can induce change in the community with hopes that such change will positively affect the lives of many community members. Regardless of whether you're working with the individual client at an agency or the community at large, understanding the complexity of systems will help you work effectively toward creating positive change.

ETHICAL AND PROFESSIONAL ISSUES

The System and Confidentiality

Human service professionals have a responsibility to protect the confidentiality of the client, whether it be in individual, group, or family counseling.

> Human service professionals protect the client's right to privacy and confidentiality except when such confidentiality would cause harm to the client or others, when agency guidelines state otherwise, or under other stated conditions. (See Appendix B, Statement 3)

At the same time, human service professionals have a responsibility to the broader system, as noted in the *Ethical Standards of Human Service Professionals:*

> Human service professionals understand the complex interaction between individuals, their families, the communities in which they live, and society. (See Appendix B, Statement 12)

Therefore, the ethical guidelines recognize the complexity of the system and acknowledge that a person is not an island unto himself or herself. Human service professionals are responsible for being aware of any agency regulations and of laws that could affect their work with clients relative to confidentiality and for making wise decisions when dealing with complex issues related to confidentiality.

When working with groups or families, human service professionals can ensure clients that they will not break confidentiality except in the situations noted earlier; however, human service professionals cannot ensure that group or family members will uphold such standards. Therefore, when working with groups or families, stressing that confidentiality be maintained is important. When the human service professional becomes aware that a group or family member has broken confidentiality, appropriate action must be taken. Such action may be simply to discuss the breaking of confidentiality; however, with more extreme cases in a group, a specific member may be asked to leave the group. Any such action should be taken after careful reflection and with sensitivity to the client and the group.

In social service systems, client confidentiality also must be maintained. This means that your work with clients should not be discussed with your colleagues unless it is for consultative or supervisory reasons, and in those cases, your consultation must be kept in confidence:

> All consultations between human service professionals are kept confidential unless to do so would result in harm to clients or communities. (See Appendix B, Statement 25)

Finally, if human service professionals are sharing information concerning their clients with other mental health professionals, a signed release-of-information form should be obtained from the client before the sharing of such information. In addition, all client records should be secured so that only employers and supervisors have access to such records.

> Human service professionals protect the integrity, safety, and security of client records. All written client information that is shared with other professionals, except in the course of professional supervision, must have the client's prior written consent. (See Appendix B, Statement 5)

Rules of Group Behavior

Depending on the type of group you are leading, rules may vary. Rules are often determined by the leader but can be altered after consultation with the group members. In determining the rules of the group, the following questions should be considered:

1. What are the limits of confidentiality?
2. Can members socialize outside the group?
3. Can members date outside the group?
4. What expectations do you have concerning attendance in group sessions?
5. What expectations do you have concerning self-disclosure of members?

6. What are the repercussions and limits of physical acting out during group sessions?

7. Are there expectations concerning the types of things to be discussed during group sessions?

8. What expectations do you have concerning members being punctual and staying for the group meeting?

9. What expectations do you have concerning how members communicate during group sessions?

10. What is your responsibility to a member and to the group should you suspect that a specific member might cause harm to himself, herself, or others?

11. What other agency rules might determine specific conduct within the group?

Any group rules that are determined by the leader should be clearly defined to the group members. Members can then give their informed consent to these rules or decide that they do not want to participate under such conditions.

Training and Competence

The *Ethical Standards of Human Service Professionals* states,

> Human service professionals know the limit and scope of their professional knowledge and offer services only within their knowledge and skill base. (See Appendix B, Statement 26)

Therefore, when working with families or conducting groups, or when working with community members, human service professionals need to know the limits of their professional competence.

For instance, although many human service professionals have the training to lead psychoeducational and self-help groups, generally, counseling and therapy groups should be left to more highly trained professionals. Similarly, human service professionals are not trained to do family counseling and family therapy but may offer family guidance as an aspect of the human service professional's job function. In either case, when human service professionals believe that their training is not at the level to work effectively with specific clients, they need to either refer those clients to other mental health professionals, seek out supervision and consultation, or gain additional training (Cogan, 1989; Corey et al., 2003).

Finally, it should be remembered that training does not just take place in school. Depending on the circumstances, additional training can be gained through workshops or other continuing education activities. Ultimately, human service professionals need to carefully review the helping relationships in which they are working and decide whether their training is adequate for each specific situation.

THE DEVELOPMENTALLY MATURE
HUMAN SERVICE PROFESSIONAL

Using a Systems Approach toward Understanding
the Complexity of Interrelationships

Developmentally mature human service professionals do not view clients in isolation, unaffected by the systems in which they interact but, instead, understand the complexity of the interactions in the clients' world. Mature human service professionals understand that families, groups, and social systems have a large impact on the client. Therefore, they view depression, anxiety, economic deprivation, acting out behavior, and so forth as symptoms of client problems *and* as issues related to the systems in which clients interact. Many times, I have seen human service professionals make statements such as, "That client just has no motivation to change; he will do nothing for himself." If one were to take an individualistic view of this client, then such statements may seem to be true. However, human service professionals who view clients as being affected by the systems around them understand the power that such systems may have on the behavior of clients. When working with clients, viewing them from both an individual and a systems perspective is important.

SUMMARY

In this chapter, we examined the complex interactions of systems. I noted that general systems theory states that all systems have regulatory mechanisms that maintain their unique homeostasis. In addition, we learned that all systems have semipermeable boundaries that can become rigid or loose. In an effort to maintain a system's unique homeostasis, members of it will act covertly or overtly to maintain the homeostasis of the system. We highlighted the fact that healthy systems change by permitting information to flow into the system and allowing this information to be evaluated by the system. We noted that family counseling applies the knowledge of systems in a variety of ways. Some of the more prevalent family counseling approaches we listed included Haley's strategic family therapy, Satir's communication perspective, Minuchin's structural approach, the multigenerational approach of Bowen, the experiential approach of Whitaker, the psychodynamic approach of Skynner, and the behavioral family therapy approach.

In this chapter, we also noted that families are affected by situational factors and developmental milestones and that healthy families have clear hierarchies and semipermeable boundaries that allow for open communication. Such families can adapt in times of stress, and although all spouses bring their unfinished business to the family, healthy families can work through these issues, whereas dysfunctional families allow their issues to have a deleterious effect on them. This is often seen by scapegoating one or more family members, often the children. Often the individual who is scapegoated becomes what is called the Identified Patient (IP). With some background in understanding systems, human service professionals can provide family guidance; however, family counseling and family therapy are usually reserved for more highly trained therapists.

In addition to the family system, in this chapter we examined a second system—the group—and noted that as in all systems, groups develop a homeostasis with rules that govern their behavior. We then presented a brief history of the development of group treatment and suggested that crude types of groups started during the 1800s as "moral guidance" but have evolved over the years. Today, we noted the three major categories of groups include self-help groups, psychoeducational groups, and counseling and therapy groups. Today, a group leader's role often is to gently challenge the homeostatic regulatory mechanism to induce change. We noted that groups can be viewed as minilabs of the world; that is, typical styles of behavior will be repeated during the group process. These behaviors can then be examined and changed, if desired.

Although all groups can be expected to pass through stages of development, the intensity of change during the process will be partially based on the type of group. Five typical stages of development we highlighted were the pregroup stage, the initial stage, the transition stage, the work stage, and the closure stage. We noted typical behaviors that occur within each stage and pointed out that leadership styles will vary as a function of stage. In addition, we stated that style of leadership will vary from professional to professional and will be based on the type of group being offered. We also noted that membership roles in groups will vary as a function of the stage of the group and the personality of the members, and leaders need to be aware of how to work effectively with different types of member roles.

Next, we noted that human service professionals could have a positive impact on clients through their work in social service agencies or their effect on the community. In social service agencies, the human service professional must have effective client skills and have a clear understanding of the boundaries, rules, hierarchy, and information flow within the system. We then suggested six steps for effecting change in the community, including accurately defining your problem, collaborating with community members, respecting community members, collaboratively developing strategies for change, implementing change strategies, and assessing effectiveness.

As we neared the end of the chapter, we examined the ethical and professional issues of the rules of group behavior, confidentiality, and training and competence as they relate to systems. We highlighted the importance of confidentiality in systems, exceptions to confidentiality, and the difficulty of ensuring confidentiality when working with systems. Finally, we noted that the developmentally mature human service professionals can use a systems approach in understanding the complexity of the interrelationships of clients' lives.

EXPERIENTIAL EXERCISES

1. Reflecting on Your Family of Origin

After reflecting on your family of origin, write responses to the following questions:

1. What roles did your family members take as you were growing up?
2. Do you think your family had rigid boundaries, loose boundaries, or boundaries that allowed for healthy communication?
3. Were there predictable patterns of behavior that you could identify in the various members of your family?
4. What would happen if a member in your family acted differently than expected?
5. Was there a family member who was scapegoated or an identified patient?
6. How did your family handle conflict?
7. When your family experienced periods of stress, how were they handled?
8. What situational crises did you or members of your family experience? How were they handled?
9. Reflect on the developmental cycles of your family. How were they handled?

2. Developing a Psychoeducational Group Program

Develop an outline of a psychoeducational program on a topic of your choice. Discuss the following issues in the development of your program:

1. The title of the program
2. A brief outline of your program
3. Technical issues related to your program
   a. Number of sessions
   b. Number of clients
   c. Ground rules
   d. Type of meeting place
4. Expected responses of clients as they pass through the group stages of development
5. How you would handle closure of the program
6. Any follow-up you might do

3. Developing a Self-Help Group Program

Using the outline in Exercise 2, develop a self-help group program on a topic of your choice.

4. Working with a Family in Need

Read the following description of a family that sought aid from your agency. Then respond to the questions that follow.

The Family: David, Jan, and their three children have just moved to the area. They made the move because David thought he would have an easier time finding a job. Having left family and friends, they no longer have the support that they had at their prior residence. They noted that, when they first moved, they were living out of their car and then at the "hotel from hell," but they recently moved into a low-income subsidized housing project.

David is an unemployed construction worker, and Jan works part-time at the local convenience store. David is age 28 and Jan is age 29. They have been married 10 years. Jan states that David "sometimes drinks too much"; David denies this. David states that Jan has "gotten too fat"; Jan admits having gained some weight but states, "David should love me anyway." During your meeting with them, you find that they often argue with each other about work, the children, and Jan's weight.

Mark, the oldest child, is 11 and has been autistic and unable to form relationships since birth. Jan and David have received disability for him in the past and previously placed him in a residential treatment center. They are unsure about how to care for him now that they have moved. Jordan, who is 9 years old, has had behavioral problems in school and has been involved in some vandalism in his neighborhood. Jan thinks he may be "drug running" for some of the older kids in the neighborhood. Jordan is entering the third grade (he was held back 1 year at his previous school). David and Jan are unclear on how to register Jordan in his new school. In fact, they're not sure where his new school is located. They describe their youngest child, Jessica, as "their gem." She is 6 years old and entering the first grade. They state that she is the only one who has not caused them problems.

As you work with this family, respond to the following questions:

1. Do you think this family's boundaries are healthy (not too rigid or too loose)?
2. Do you think any member(s) of this family is (are) being scapegoated?
3. Is there an identified patient in this family?
4. What helping skills would you need to work effectively with this family?
5. How would you diagnose the problem areas in this family?
6. What needs does this family have?
7. What goals would you help the family set for itself?
8. What referrals would be appropriate for this family?
9. What type of follow-up would you want to do?

5. Working with an Individual in Need

Read the following description of an individual who sought aid from your agency. Then respond to the questions that follow.

Alice: Alice is a 16-year-old single female who is 3 months pregnant. She seeks your advice concerning her pregnancy. She lives with her parents and her 15-year-old sister. She has not told her parents about the pregnancy and is concerned that they will find out before long. Her family has little money, and she is concerned about paying for the pregnancy and birth. Her parents do not have medical insurance.

Alice has come to your agency because she is depressed and feels at the "end of her rope." She is looking for help. When you meet with her, she sobs throughout the interview and at times seems to whine. Alice's father Arnold, who is 34 years old, is a part-time truck driver. Alice states that he has rigid views and tends to be rather "authoritarian." She also thinks that he will "lose it" if he learns she is pregnant and will want to "take care of the situation" to make it go away. Although he has not abused her in the past 2 years, when she was younger he would often "take a belt to me." At times, he drinks too much, and there seem to be conflicts between him and his wife. He was married at age 18.

Alice states that her mother "cares a lot about me"; however, Alice also notes that her mother would never go against her father's wishes. Alice's mother, Linda, who is 35 years old, works part-time at a fast food restaurant and is very concerned about her daughter's well-being. Because she got married when she was pregnant with Alice, Alice thinks that her mother will probably understand her situation.

Joan is Alice's 15-year-old sister. Alice states that Joan is a good student but at times acts like a "wise-ass." She feels as if Joan has always received all the attention in the family; now that Alice is pregnant, she is concerned that she will be even more of an outcast. Alice notes that Joan has many friends and is often out of the house doing things rather than staying home with her "drunk dad" and her mom.

As you work with Alice, respond to the following questions:

1. What helping skills would you need to work effectively with Alice?
2. How would you diagnose Alice's problems?
3. What needs does Alice have?
4. What goals would you help Alice set for herself?
5. What referrals would be appropriate for Alice?
6. Would you consider a referral for family counseling or family guidance for Alice and her family?
7. Do you think this family's boundaries are healthy (not too rigid or too loose)?
8. Do you think any member(s) of this family is (are) being scapegoated?
9. Is there an identified patient in this family?
10. Would you consider a referral to a group for Alice?

11. If you were to consider a referral to a group for Alice, what type of group might you consider? Why?

12. What type of follow-up would you want to do?

6. Wearing Labels

Using the following phrases or other terms your instructor lists, do the following exercise in class. Have the instructor cut out the phrases and tape one on each student's forehead (students should not know which phrase they have on their foreheads). Then find an open space and "mill around," responding to one another based on the phrase an individual has on his or her forehead. After a few minutes, sit in a large circle and, without removing the phrase, discuss your response to how people interacted with you.

Look at me intensely.	Walk away from me.
Tell me you like what I'm wearing.	Look at my shoes.
Frown at me.	Act as if I don't exist.
Be loving toward me.	Yell at me when I speak.
Speak softly to me.	Be angry at me.
Look at my stomach.	Treat me humanely.
Touch me when you talk to me.	Act disgusted toward me.
Be nice to me.	Disagree with anything I say.
Be rude to me.	Reflect back anything I say.
Talk to me but don't listen to me.	Act as if you like me even though you don't talk to me.
Treat me like an object when talking.	

After you have finished the exercise, discuss the following questions:

1. What's it like being labeled?

2. Do we all wear labels as we go through life? (Are there certain personality characteristics that we tend to exhibit?)

3. If we do exhibit certain personality characteristics, is it possible that we create other people's responses to us by the personality characteristics that we exhibit?

4. How can the group process help us understand the labels (personality characteristics) that we tend to exhibit?

7. A Detailed Examination of an Agency

To fully understand the nature of an agency system, a thorough review of its policies and practices is needed. Using the following guidelines, you and a partner pick a social service agency and interview someone who can respond to the items. Write down the individual's responses and compare agencies in class.

1. What is the name of the agency?

2. What is the agency's address?

3. How many total staff members does the agency have?

4. How many administrative staff are there and what are their roles?

5. What are the approximate salaries of administrative staff?

6. How many direct-service personnel (mental health professionals who work with clients) are there?

7. What are the types of direct-service personnel (for example, mental health aides, therapists, supervisors, program coordinators, group leaders, family counselors)?

8. What degrees are held by direct-service personnel?

9. What are the approximate salaries of direct-service personnel?

10. What are the number and type of support staff (for example, secretaries, clerical staff)?

11. Is this a private or a public agency?

12. Where does the agency get its funding?

13. Does the agency have a policy and practices statement (a written statement that explains the functions of the agency and the roles of the staff)?

14. Who are the clients of this agency?

15. How does the agency obtain its clients?

16. What happens when a client initially contacts this agency?

17. Is there a process where client problems are diagnosed, client needs are assessed, goals are established, referrals are made, and follow-up is accomplished?

18. How do clients pay?

19. What types of counseling or assistance take place at this agency (for example, individual, group, family)?

20. How long are typical counseling/interviewing sessions?

21. What kind of paperwork do the direct-service personnel have to fill out?

22. How many hours, days, weeks, months, or years would a typical client spend at this agency?

23. How are services for the typical client terminated?

24. How does the agency evaluate itself?

25. Does a staff development effort take place at the agency (for example, in-house workshops, guest speakers, monetary support for conferences)?

26. How does the agency deal with ethical concerns related to confidentiality, counselor training, and competence?

27. Does the policy and practices statement of the agency match what is actually going on within the agency?

8. Ethical and Professional Vignettes

Reflect on the following vignettes and then share your thoughts in class. You may want to refer to the NOHSE Ethical Standards in Appendix B.

1. Before meeting with a family for a family guidance session, a human service professional gives a written document explaining to the parents the limitations of confidentiality and the general direction the session will take. After reading this informed consent document, the parents sign it and bring the family in. The informed consent document is not given to or described to the children. Has the helper acted ethically? Professionally?

2. You are seeing a family in family guidance when you realize the father is extremely depressed, perhaps suicidally so. You decide to refer him for individual counseling. Is this ethical? Is this the professional thing to do? Is this the wise thing to do?

3. In deciding on how to act on an ethical concern with a family, a human service professional notices that the code of ethics of the American Association for Marriage and Family Therapy (AAMFT) has a different response to a situation than does the Ethical Standards of Human Service Professionals. The human service professional decides to go with the code of ethics that best matches her view of the situation. Is this ethical? Is this the professional thing to do?

4. A human service professional you know is practicing family counseling even though she doesn't have advanced training in this area. Is this ethical? Professional? Legal? What, if anything, should you do?

5. A few months after working with a family on some parenting issues, you are subpoenaed to testify against one of the spouses. You believe she has major issues that are unfinished from her family of origin. Is it ethical to testify? Is this professional? Legal?

6. While running a psychoeducational group for substance abusers, you realize that a couple of the members of the group are using illegal substances. What should you do?

7. After setting a ground rule that group members cannot date, a group leader finds that two members of a group are seeing one another. He immediately throws them out of the group. Is this ethical? Is this professional?

8. Despite the fact that a group leader stresses the importance of confidentiality, the leader discovers that some intimate information about a group member has been "leaked" by another member. The group member asks who in the group broke confidentiality and no one answers. Therefore, the leader decides to meet individually with each member in an attempt to find out who broke confidentiality. Is this ethical? Professional? Do you have other ideas about what the leader should do?

9. A group member shares that he has committed a robbery. Subsequently, the police arrest him, and the group leader is subpoenaed to court to testify to what she heard in the group. Can she be forced to testify?

10. When you are running a psychoeducational group on safe sex, a 16-year-old member of the group reveals that he committed a date rape when out with a "friend." The human service professional does not act on this knowledge because he wants to protect the confidentiality of the student. Is this ethical? Professional? Legal?

11. A human service professional decides to run a short-term group for students at risk. While running the group, some of the girls ask him where they can get information on birth control. He gives them the phone number and address of the local Planned Parenthood agency. Is this ethical? Legal?

12. After learning that a girl in a teen responsibility group is pregnant and wants to have an abortion, a group leader encourages the girl to consider keeping the child or adopting it out. Most of the group members concur and the group leader gets them to promise that they will support her. Is this ethical? Professional? Legal?

13. The director of the agency in which you work tells all employees to report any client who is using illegal substances to the police. Can the director do this? Is this ethical? Professional? What, if anything, should you do?

14. After working at an agency for a few months, you realize that there are many breaches of confidentiality. What, if anything, should you do?

15. After working at an agency for a few months, you realize that many of your co-workers tend to make fun of their clients during break. What, if anything, should you do?

16. Your agency is meeting with individuals from the community to discuss a proposal to offer an HIV prevention program at a number of after-school programs. An irate member of the community accuses you of promoting sexual promiscuity and endorsing the use of condoms even though you didn't mention any specifics of the program. You then ask the rest of the individuals at the meeting to raise their hands if they had heard you promoting these values. Is this ethical? Is this professional? Was this the best way to respond? If not, what are some other ways you could have responded?

7

Human Service Professionals in a Pluralistic Society

You scorn us, you imitate us, you blame us, you indulge us, you throw up your hands, you tell us you have all the answers now shut up and listen. (Lamar, 1992, p. 90)

Growing up in New York was a world unto its own—the ethnic foods, the multicultured music, the people; oh, how I loved to watch the people. Walk down a Manhattan street and you could watch a sea of endless people, a sea that seemed to change color as it flowed by you. A sea whose shape transformed constantly, and if you flowed with it long enough, you could visit every part of the world. Unquestionably, New York gave me a multicultural perspective that many people don't have an opportunity to obtain. However, despite this exposure to a variety of cultures and ethnic groups, I really never got "below the surface." I could taste the foods, I could see the people, and I could listen to the music, but that experience alone was still from a detached perspective. Even though I might see the brightly colored clothes of the Nigerian, I still didn't know that person. Even though I could taste the sushi, I didn't understand the world of the Japanese. And even though I could listen to the Latino music, I didn't really understand the people.

When I lived in New Hampshire, I learned to adapt. No longer would I be this brash New Yorker. I mellowed. New Hampshire's population has a very large percentage of Catholics. My friend John, a priest at the Catholic college at which I worked, would often tell me that some of the nuns thought I was on the verge of a conversion. They saw me as searching. Maybe I was . . . a little, but not enough to convert to another religion. These nuns could not understand how a person with my values could not be more religious. They didn't really know me. Perhaps, if they had taken the time to find out who I am, they could understand me.

From New Hampshire, I moved to Norfolk, Virginia, from an area that was mostly Catholic to a part of the country that had many fundamentalist Christians. I found that a small minority of these fundamentalist Christians would confront me on my religious orientation. For instance, one day I was eating lunch with a friend and a friend of hers. As my friend momentarily got up from the table, her friend slowly reached into her purse, pulled out some flyers, and placed them in front of me without saying a word. I looked down and was aghast to see that they were "Jews for Jesus" flyers. I said to her, "Are you trying to tell me something?" She responded that perhaps I would be interested in this. I felt intruded upon. I felt disrespected. Not unlike the nuns in New Hampshire, here was another person trying to place her values on me. If she had tried to talk with me, tried to understand me, tried to have a conversation regarding different approaches to religion, I would have talked with her.

This chapter is about differentness. It is about understanding people. It is about cultural and ethnic diversity. In this chapter, we will examine the cultural mosaic that makes up the United States. From the different cultural and ethnic groups, to the varying religious orientations, to understanding sexual orientation and gender sex role issues, we will try to make sense out of the varying lifestyles that make up the United States.

Besides gaining knowledge about diversity in the United States and throughout the world, in this chapter we will examine ways in which the human service professional can be effective with clients from diverse backgrounds. Finally, we

Table 7.1 Number and Percentage of Individuals from Select Racial, Ethnic, Cultural, Religious, and Sexual Identity Backgrounds in the United States

Ethnicity/Race*	Number (millions)	Percentage	Religion**	Number (millions)	Percentage
White	211.5	75.1	Protestant	169	64
Black or African American	34.7	12.3	Baptist	56	21.1
Hispanic	35.3	12.5	Methodist	32	12.1
Asian	10.2	3.6	Lutherans	20	7.7
American Indian and Alaska Native	2.5	0.9	Presbyterian	12	4.5
			Episcopalians	6	2.6
Native Hawaiian and Other Pacific Island	0.4	0.1	Roman Catholic	66	25
Some Other Race	15.4	5.5	Muslim	?	?***
Two or More Races	6.8	2.4	Jewish	5	2.3
			Eastern Orthodox	4	1.5
Sexual Orientation****			Other religions	5	2.0
Gay		1–10	No preference	18	16.7
Lesbian		2–6			
Heterosexual		90–95			

*Figures from U.S. Census Bureau (2002)

The majority of Asians have the following ancestry: Chinese, Filipino, Indian, Vietnamese, Korean, and Japanese. The majority of Hispanics have the following ancestry: Mexican, Puerto Rican, Cuban, and Dominican. The majority of whites have the following ancestry: German, English, Irish, Slavic, French, Italian, Scottish, Scandinavian, and Dutch (Allen & Turner, 1988).

**Percentage of religions from *Compton's Encyclopedia* (1996).

***Muslims probably range in the millions, but most have not officially registered as a religious sect.

****Studies on percent of homosexuality range from 1% to 10%, with most from 3% to 6%. Number of bisexuals vary considerably based on study (see Singer & Deschamps, 1994).

will examine the professional issue of individual rights and personal dignity of our clients and how the developmentally mature cross-cultural helper can gain increased sensitivity toward working with diverse clients.

CULTURAL DIVERSITY
IN THE UNITED STATES AND THE WORLD

America is the most diverse country in the world—a country that is truly a conglomerate of ethnic groups, races, cultures, and religions (see Table 7.1).

In addition to the data in Table 7.1, some additional select groups include 53 million individuals who have a disability (U.S. Census Bureau, 2001a), almost 37 million people who are over 65 (U.S. Department of Commerce, 1991; U.S. Census Bureau, 2000a), more than 32 million individuals who are poor (U.S. Census Bureau, 2000b), 8 million individuals who are mentally ill (NIMH, 1998), and between 600,000 and 800,000 individuals who are HIV-positive (Centers for Disease Control, 2002). We are truly a diverse nation and thus are called to offer services to individuals from many diverse backgrounds.

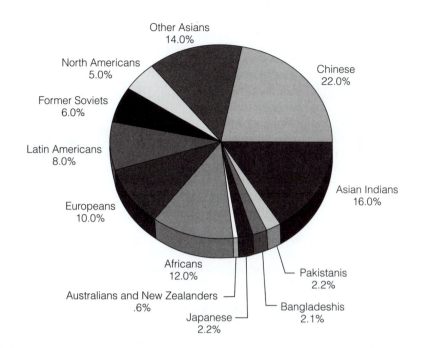

FIGURE 7.1 People of the world

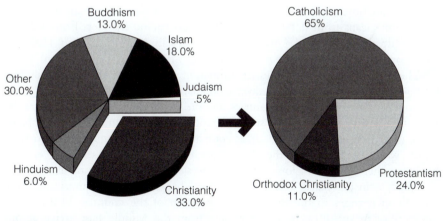

FIGURE 7.2 Religions of the world

As can be seen in Figures 7.1 and 7.2, the world, too, is a diverse place. Sometimes, when we become sheltered within our communities, or become focused on our own country, we lose sight of the great diversity that exists on this planet. As we become increasingly more worldly, not only will we have to know diversity within our country, but we will also have to understand the diversity that exists on this place we call earth.

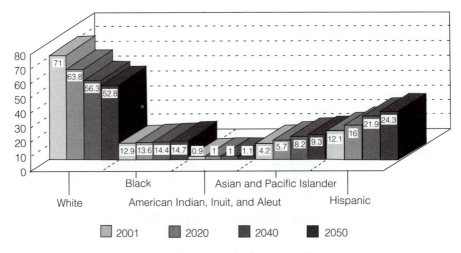

FIGURE 7.3 Percent of population by race and culture over time

THE CHANGING FACE OF AMERICA

America is becoming increasingly diverse. In fact, today, almost 30% of Americans are racial and ethnic minorities (U.S. Census Bureau, 2001b), and midway through this century minorities will constitute almost 50% of the American population (U.S. Census Bureau, 2001c). Some of these changes will include an increase in Native Americans from 0.9% to 1.1%, Asian and Pacific Islanders from 4.2% to 9.3%, Hispanics from 12.1% to 24.3%, and African Americans from 12.9% to 14.7%, and a decrease in white Americans from 71% to 52.8% (Figure 7.3).

These changing demographics are a function of a number of factors, including the higher birth rates of culturally diverse populations, the fact that most immigrants no longer come from western countries, and the fact that immigration rates are the highest in American history. Most immigrants are now Asian (39%) or Hispanic (43%) (U.S. Census Bureau, 2001d), as compared with past immigrants who were mostly white European, and they have a greater tendency to assert their cultural heritage rather than be swallowed up by the western-based American culture.

Changes in the racial, ethnic, and cultural backgrounds of Americans bring with them changes in the religious composition of the country. As increasing numbers of Asians, Hispanics, and people from the Middle East arrive at our shores, we will find religions that were previously rare in America. But diversity in religion is not only brought to us by our immigrants. Although America is a country that is largely Christian, diversity in Christianity in America is now greater than ever. From a multitude of Protestant faiths, to Roman Catholics who are increasingly varied in their beliefs, to Eastern Orthodox, Mormons, Christian Scientists, Seventh Day Adventists, Amish, Mennonites, and on and on, Christian religion in America is a religious mosaic in and of itself.

The age of our population is also changing. In 1900, 3% of the population of the United States was over 65 years of age. By 1960, this figure rose to 9.2%, and

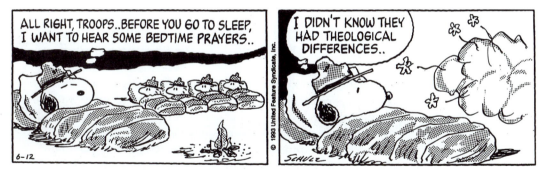

SOURCE: Reprinted by permission of United Feature Syndicate, Inc.

in 2000, 12.7% of the population was over 65 (U.S. Department of Commerce, 1991; U.S. Census Bureau, 2000a). It is estimated that by the year 2030, fully 20% of the population will be over 65 years old (U.S. Census Bureau, 2000c).

In addition to the changing ethnic, cultural, and religious diversity in America, today there are changes in sex-role identity. The macho male is no longer considered a model for maleness, and expectations concerning the woman's role in the workplace and as a child-care provider have changed dramatically. Also, in America today we see increased awareness of the gay and lesbian subculture. Whereas in the past many homosexuals felt a need to hide their sexual preference for fear of discrimination, today we find an increasing number of gays and lesbians coming out. In addition, changes in federal, state, and local laws as well as a gradual move toward more tolerance of difference in our culture has given us an increased sensitivity and awareness of a number of special groups, including the physically challenged, older persons, the homeless and the poor, individuals who are HIV positive, the mentally ill, and others. With the diversity that currently exists in the United States, and with every indication that America will become more diverse, the human service professional must be effective when counseling and working with clients from diverse backgrounds.

DEFINING MULTICULTURAL COUNSELING

I believe that all helping relationships are multicultural helping relationships, even when clients are seemingly from the same cultural background. However, if we were to define multicultural counseling in such a broad context, we would be faced with a monumental task and would detract from examining the important issues that face those clients that have already been greatly damaged by the helper's lack of awareness of multicultural issues. Consider the analogy of the emergency room. A number of individuals come in at once, some with minor wounds, some with major. Whom do we treat first? Clearly, we treat the ones who most need immediate attention. And thus it is with multicultural counseling. Even though it would be important to attend to the needs of all groups, the needs of those who have been most harmed by prejudice and discrimination in society are most pressing. Consequently, I think we need to limit ourselves to those who have been clearly discriminated against. Therefore, borrowing from Axelson (1999), but keeping in mind that some groups have more pressing needs than others, we will view multicultural counseling within the following context:

> [Multicultural counseling] encompasses all the components of the many different cultural environments in a democratic society, together with the pertinent theories, techniques, and practices of counseling. In this regard, the approach takes into specific consideration the traditional and contemporary backgrounds and environmental experiences of diverse clients and how special needs might be identified and met through the resources of the helping professions. (p. 22)

In examining differences within American society, many have differentiated between such terms as culture, race, minority, ethnicity, social class, and power while highlighting how stereotyping, prejudice, racism, and discrimination have affected our clients and our work with them (Atkinson, Morten, & Sue, 1998; Baruth & Manning, 1998). Understanding terms gives all of us a common ground with which to communicate. The following are brief definitions of some of these terms.

Culture

Shared values, symbols, language, and *ways of being in the world* are some of the words and terms I think of when reflecting on the word *culture.* **Culture** represents the common values, norms of behavior, symbols, language, and common life patterns that people learn and share with one another. For instance, despite great diversity in the United States, most Americans do have a similar cultural heritage because within this society there is a shared language, symbols that most of us recognize, and patterns of behavior with which most are familiar. Traveling throughout this country, we find many symbols of a common culture (e.g., fast-food restaurants, music, laws, basic values, shared language). Yet, even as I acknowledge this common culture, I am acutely aware of the unique patterns of behaviors and values that distinguish many **subcultures** within our country. Examples of some subcultures include urban gays and lesbians; various racial, ethnic, and religious groups; subcultures based on gender; and subcultures based on the region of the country in which one lives (e.g., "the South") (Samovar & Porter, 2001). In attempting to delineate cultural identity, Whitfield, McGrath, and Coleman (1992) have identified 11 elements that can be used in helping to understand specific cultural patterns. They include how each culture does the following:

1. Defines its sense of self
2. Dresses and values appearances
3. Embraces specific beliefs and attitudes
4. Relates to family and significant others
5. Plays and makes use of leisure time
6. Learns and uses knowledge
7. Communicates and uses language

8. Embraces certain values and mores

9. Uses time and space

10. Eats and uses food in its customs

11. Works and applies itself

Race

Genetic heritage, skin color, and *ambiguity* are some of the words and terms I think of when reflecting on the word *race.* Whereas the concept of culture has been based on such characteristics as shared learned traits, race has traditionally been defined biologically, with people of the same race being said to share similar genetic heritage (Krogman, 1945). However, recently, this definition has been challenged. For instance, research on the human genome shows that humans share much more genetically than was at one time thought. In fact, genetic differences between humans are far less than those found between chimpanzees (NOVA, 2000). Behaviorally, there seem to be more differences within racial groups than between them (Atkinson et al., 1998). In addition, gene pools throughout the world, and especially in the United States, have become increasingly mixed because of migration, exploration, invasions, systematic rape as a result of wars and oppression of minorities, and intermarriage (see Box 7.1). With some sociologists saying there are no races, others saying there are three, and still others concluding that there are as many as 200, the issue of race is cloudy and perhaps doesn't matter. Because of the confusion concerning this term, some now advocate for discontinuing its use (Cameron & Wycoff, 1998). Generally, I agree with this stand, and for the most part I have instead used the words *culture, ethnic background,* or *minority.*

Ethnicity

Heritage, ancestry, and *tradition* are some of the words that come to mind when I reflect on the word *ethnicity.* More specifically, when a group of people share a common ancestry, which may include specific cultural and social patterns, they are sometimes said to be of the same ethnic group (Davis, 1978; Rose, 1964). **Ethnicity,** as opposed to race, is not based on genetic heritage but on long-term patterns of behavior that have some historical significance and may include similar religious, ancestral, language, or cultural characteristics. Therefore, Jews, who share religious and perhaps similar ancestral characteristics, may be considered an ethnic group but may not share the same culture (Jews live in many different cultures throughout the world). Similarly, people of Asian heritage, although considered a race by some, may not share the same culture or the same ethnic background.

Social Class

Money, power, status, hierarchy—these are the words that come to mind when I think of the term *social class.* Calling it the "missing dimension" in understanding diversity, Hannon, Ritchie, and Rye (1992) note that social class has been largely overlooked when examining issues of diversity. One's social class represents the

BOX 7.1 Dr. Cheryl Evans

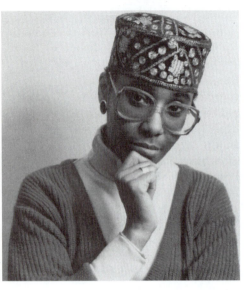

Cheryl Evans

Dr. Cheryl Evans was born outside of Boston in the oldest continuous African American community in the Northeast. From a very young age, she remembers being aware of her color because she was treated in a prejudicial manner or was made aware that she was "different" from others. Cheryl's family history is as diverse as that of most African Americans. Some of this history includes a great-grandmother who was Native American, a great-grandmother who was born a slave, a great-grandfather who was a "traveling preacher," a Lithuanian Jewish grandmother who was illiterate and immigrated to this country when she was 12 years old, a grandmother who was disabled at an early age from a stroke, an African American grandfather who worked for the railroad, and a grandfather who was an Ethiopian "Falasha"—a Jewish rabbi who immigrated to this country via Europe and Jamaica. Because Cheryl's mother was a child of a mixed marriage, her mother and her mother's siblings were taken away from their natural parents and brought up in foster homes. Although Cheryl's parents were married in the Catholic Church, she describes her mother as always being a "seeker"; therefore, Cheryl was exposed to a number of religions, including Jehovah's Witnesses, Islam, Mormonism, and Judaism.

Cheryl's parents, particularly her mother, strongly encouraged education, and Cheryl always found herself in the honors classes in school. Cheryl's mother stressed to her that others could take away her material things, but they could not take away her education. Being one of the few African Americans in her classes, Cheryl tended to feel highly visible and responsible for the whole race. By the age of 10, Cheryl became more aware of the civil rights movement; as she grew older, it was not uncommon to find her at a civil rights protest march or listening to Malcolm X or Martin Luther King, Jr. Cheryl speaks emotionally about the impact that Malcolm X, Martin Luther King, Jr., and other leaders of the times had on her.

In her adult life, Cheryl has been a teacher of human development at a college, worked for a major radio station in Boston; helped run the diversity-sensitive human resource support company called Manpower for the Dukakis governorship; recruited African American students for Rutgers University; administered a business for women; and ran for political office. After completing her master's and doctoral degrees, Cheryl obtained a job as a faculty member at Bloomfield College, teaching human services. With all of this, Cheryl has also found time for one of the major driving forces in her life—building bridges between diverse groups.

perceived ranking of an individual within a society and is based on a number of dimensions, including the amount of money an individual has, the kind of status one holds (e.g., one's occupation, one's position in the community), and the amount of power an individual wields (see "power differentials," later) (Macionis, 2001). An individual's social class may cut across a person's ethnicity, cultural identification, or race (Ihle, Sodowsky, & Kwan, 1996). Therefore, even though individuals share a similar culture, ethnicity, or race, they might have little in common with one another because of differences in social class. For instance, it is not unusual to find a poor African American who may have little in common with a wealthy African American.

Power Differentials

Potential abuse, force, control, and *superior/underling* are some of the words and terms that come to my mind when I think of the term power differential. **Power differentials** may represent greater disparities between people than culture, ethnic group, race, or social class. Power can be a function of race, class, gender, occupation, and a host of other factors and can easily be misunderstood. Whether perceived or real, power can be abused. For instance, the professor may abuse his or her power by sexually harassing the student. The upper-management Mexican-American female who does not abuse her power could still be disliked because the workers believe that Hispanic females should not hold positions of power. And the white male could be given a leadership position in a management group, not because of his expertise, but because the other group members unconsciously believe that white males have power.

Minority

A **minority** is any group of people who are being singled out because of their cultural or physical characteristics and are being systematically oppressed by those individuals who are in a position of power. Using this definition, a minority could conceivably be the numerical majority of a population, as was the case for many years in South Africa and as is the situation with women in the United States (Atkinson et al., 1998; Macionis, 2001).

Stereotypes, Prejudice, and Racism

Stereotypes are rigidly held beliefs about a group of people that assume that most or all of the group has certain characteristics, behaviors, or beliefs (e.g., Asians are intelligent people, American Indians are alcoholics) (Lum, 2000). Whereas the word *stereotype* refers to *specific* behaviors or beliefs of a group, **prejudice** is a positive or negative bias about a group as a whole (e.g., "I hate gays"). Whereas prejudice can be toward any group, **racism** is a specific belief that one race is superior to another (e.g., whites are better than blacks). Some authors have taken the position that racism is a disease, noting that, like other mental disorders, racism is based on a distortion of reality (Skillings & Dobbins, 1991).

Discrimination

Whereas the words *stereotypes, prejudice,* and *racism* refer to attitudes held by people, **discrimination** is an active behavior, such as gay bashing or unfair hiring practices, that negatively affects individuals within ethnic or cultural groups (Lum, 2000).

What is the extent of prejudice and discrimination in America? A study by the Anti-Defamation League (ADL, 1992) found that in surveying American households, many people felt that prejudice and discrimination were experienced by a wide variety of subcultures in this country. In particular, Americans felt that a considerable amount of discrimination was experienced by blacks (76%) and homosexuals (74%), and more than 50% of Americans felt that Jews, Asians, Hispanics, and women experienced some discrimination. Unfortunately, the most recent hate crime statistics from the FBI (1999) indicate that we still have much work to do in this country:

> Of the 7,876 incidents, nearly 55 percent were motivated by racial bias; 18 percent by religious bias; 17 percent by sexual orientation bias; 11 percent by ethnicity/national origin bias; and less than one-half of one percent by disability and multiple biases. (p. 5)

POLITICAL CORRECTNESS, OR, OH MY GOD, WHAT DO I CALL HIM OR HER?

Hispanic, Latino, Latina, Chicano, Chicana, black, Negro, African American, Afro American, Oriental, Asian American, Chinese American, Japanese American, Native American, Indian, Eskimo, Inuit, Aleut, native, American Indian, Asian Indian, Jew, Hebrew, Jewish American, Protestant, WASP, Muslim, Moslem, Islamic, Born Again, Fundamental Christian, Christian, Catholic (are Catholics Christians?), white, Caucasian, European American, American, gay, homosexual, straight, heterosexual, bisexual, lesbian, transgendered, transsexual, transvestite, disabled person, individual with disability, handicapped person, physically challenged, and on and on.

Did I offend anybody? I hope not, but in these days of political correctness, finding the correct term is often difficult. And, once you find the correct term, you will still offend somebody. Although there is a great amount of variety concerning how individuals should be addressed, usually the following terms have been used. For Americans with African heritage, the term *African American* is generally used, although black is still acceptable in some circles and even preferred by a few. *Asian American* refers to any of a number of individuals with heritage from Asia and the Pacific Islands, including approximately 40 distinct subgroups that differ in language and cultural identity (Sandhu, 1997). *Hispanic* refers to Mexican Americans, Puerto Ricans, Cuban Americans, individuals with Central and South American heritage, and individuals with roots from Spanish-speaking countries in the Caribbean. However, not all individuals from these countries are comfortable with the term *Hispanic,* especially many Cuban Americans. Islam is a religion whose followers are called *Muslim* (less commonly called Moslem). Homosexuals today generally use the terms *gay,* for men; and *lesbian,* for women. The term *straight* is generally not used to describe heterosexuals because of the implication that it is better than another type of orientation (e.g., "on the straight and narrow"). Individuals who have been born in this country and identify with their cultural or ethnic background often place the word "American" following their heritage. Therefore, it is not unusual for us to find individuals referring to themselves as Irish American, Italian American, Arab American, and so forth. Individuals who are naturalized citizens generally do not use the term "American" following their country of origin (see Box 7.2). Finally, rather than saying "handicapped," or "disabled person," generally people now say "individual with a disability," although some prefer the term "physically challenged."

Although I cannot describe the politically correct term for individuals from every culture, ethnic, or minority group, I have attempted to use politically correct terms throughout this text. Of course, people vary in how they wish to be addressed. However, I believe that making an effort to use terms correctly shows our sensitivity to individuals from diverse cultures.

BOX 7.2   Dr. Martha Muguira: A Woman of Mexican Heritage

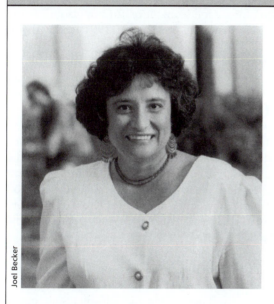

Joel Becker

Dr. Martha Muguira was raised in Mexico City in a family that included her parents and three younger siblings. Marty, who is a naturalized citizen, considers herself Mexican, rather than Mexican American, because she was raised in Mexico.

Marty's paternal and maternal great-grandparents were of Spanish and Mexican-Indian descent. Marty notes that the population of Mexico is mostly Catholic, and the rituals include many Indian customs that are not ordinarily found in the United States. She comments that, until recently, light-skinned Mexicans (usually Mexicans of Spanish heritage) were treated preferentially in the country. She mentions that Mexico has tended to be a male-oriented society with preferential treatment toward men, particularly concerning careers.

As a female, Marty remembers that she received mixed messages from her parents. On the one hand, they valued education, particularly bilingual education, and sent her to an American school in Mexico City. In fact, when Marty was 17 years old, she received a scholarship to live in North Carolina with a banker's family and go to a private school. On the other hand, even though Marty received this scholarship, her father encouraged her to stay in Mexico, pursue a more traditional education, and have a family. Despite these mixed messages, Marty went on to finish her doctorate, raise a family, and now works at a counseling center at a university in Virginia.

Although Marty states that she has not experienced overt discrimination, she notes that throughout her life people would have expectations of her because of her Mexican heritage. For instance, while living in North Carolina, she was asked to fit in better by wearing American rather than Mexican-style clothes. Also, when she worked at a Veterans Administration hospital, she was chosen to run a special program for Spanish-speaking employees, mostly because she was Mexican. Dr. Muguira is proud of her Mexican heritage, values her bilingual education, and is another prime example of the diversity in the United States.

THE NEED FOR
MULTICULTURAL AWARENESS

Counseling is not working for many clients from diverse backgrounds. A large body of evidence shows that minority clients are frequently misunderstood, often misdiagnosed, find therapy less helpful than their majority counterparts do, attend therapy at lower rates than majority clients do, and tend to terminate therapy more quickly than do majority clients (Garretson, 1993; Gonzales et al., 1997; Good, 1997; Lee & Mixson, 1995; McKenzie, 1999; Morrow & Deidan, 1992; Poston, Craine, & Atkinson, 1991; Solomon, 1992; Wilson & Stith, 1991). In addition, clients from cultural backgrounds different from that of their helper may experience the helping relationship more negatively than if the helper is of the same culture (Atkinson, 1985; Atkinson, Poston, Furlong, & Mercado, 1989; Phelps, Taylor, & Gerard, 2001). Thus, it is understandable that today we find minority clients underrepresented at mental health centers (Sue & Sue, 1999).

Why is counseling not working for a good segment of our population? Some have suggested the following reasons (Midgette & Meggert, 1991; Sodowsky & Taffe, 1991; Solomon, 1992; Yutrzenka, 1995):

1. *The melting pot myth.* Some believe this country is a **melting pot** of cultural diversity. However, this is not the experience of many minority clients, who find themselves on the fringe of American culture, view themselves as different from the mainstream, and cannot relate to many of the values and beliefs held by the majority. In truth, people from most cultures want to maintain their uniqueness and are resistant to giving up their special traditions. In fact, identifying with one's own culture instead of the broader culture can affect one's understanding of the world (see Box 7.3). Thus, the human service professional who assumes the client should fit into and conform to the values of the majority culture could turn off some clients. Probably, viewing American society as a **cultural mosaic,** a society with a myriad of diverse values and customs, more accurately represents the essence of diversity that we find today.

2. *Incongruent expectations about the helping relationship.* The western, particularly American, approach to counseling has a number of assumptions concerning the helping process. For instance, it assumes that the helping process should emphasize the individual; stress the expression of feelings; encourage self-disclosure, open-mindedness, and insight; and show cause and effect. However, many cultures do not place high value on these attributes, and clients from those cultures will therefore enter such a relationship with much trepidation, face disappointment when a helping relationship does not meet their expectations, and could even be harmed by the helping relationship (Sodowsky & Taffe, 1991; Yutrzenka, 1995). For example, the Asian client who is proud of her ability to restrict her emotions might leave the helping relationship feeling as if she disappointed her helper who has been pushing her to express feelings.

3. *Lack of understanding of social forces.* Although helpers may be effective at attending to clients' feelings concerning how they have been discriminated against, abused, or affected by other "external" factors, the same human service

---

BOX 7.3   Blackbirds Sitting in a Tree

A white female elementary school teacher in the United States posed a math problem to her class one day. Suppose there are four blackbirds sitting in a tree. You take a slingshot and shoot one of them. How many are left? A white student answered quickly, That's easy. One subtracted from four is three. An African immigrant youth then answered with equal confidence, Zero. The teacher chuckled at the latter response and stated that the first student was right and that, perhaps, the second student should study more math. From that day forth, the African student seemed to withdraw from class activities and seldom spoke to other students or the teacher.

If the teacher had pursued the African student's reasons for arriving at the answer zero, she might have heard the following: If you shoot one bird, the others will fly away. Nigerian educators often use this story to illustrate differences in worldviews between United States and African cultures. The Nigerians contend that the group is more important than the individual, that survival of all depends on interrelationships among the parts. (Sue, 1992, pp. 7, 8)

---

professionals will often de-emphasize the actual influence these social forces have on clients. Human service professionals often assume that most if not all negative feelings are created by the individual, and they often have difficulty understanding the power of social influences. By de-emphasizing social forces, human service professionals are likely to have a difficult time building a relationship with a client who has been considerably harmed by external factors. For instance, the client who has been illegally denied jobs because of his disability or his sexual orientation might be discouraged when a helper says, "What have you done to prevent yourself from obtaining the job?" (see Box 7.4)

4. *Ethnocentric worldview.* Human service professionals who are not cross-culturally aware tend to view the world through the lens of their own culture. These individuals have an **ethnocentric worldview** in that they tend to falsely assume that their clients view the world in a similar manner or believe that when one presents a differing view of the world he or she is emotionally disturbed, culturally brainwashed, or just simply wrong. Although the importance of understanding a client's unique worldview is always crucial to an effective helping relationship, this is particularly significant when working with minority clients whose experience of the world could be particularly foreign to our own. For instance, a helper may inadvertently turn off a Muslim or Jew when she says to her client, "Have a wonderful Christmas" (see Box 7.5).

5. *Ignorance of one's own racist attitudes and prejudices.* Of course, the helper who is not in touch with his or her prejudices and racist attitudes cannot work effectively with minority clients and could indeed be harmful to those clients. Understanding our own stereotypes and prejudices takes a particularly vigilant effort because our biases are often unconscious. For instance, the heterosexual helper who unconsciously believes that being gay is a disease but consciously states he is accepting of all sexual orientations could subtly treat a gay client as if there is something wrong with him.

6. *Inability to understand cultural differences in the expression of symptomatology.* What may be seen as "abnormal" in the United States may be considered quite

---

BOX 7.4   Scott King

Forty-five-year-old Scott was born the eldest of four children in a small town in Maine. He remembers his early years as being almost a stereotype of the early 1960s American family: his father worked and his mother stayed at home and raised the children. Scott remembers having the expectation to grow up, get married, and have children. He was not aware of any individuals who were gay or lesbian when he grew up.

After graduating from high school, Scott attended Bates College, a liberal arts school where the world outside Maine made its first impact. Although for years he had realized that he found men much more attractive than women, he dated the opposite gender mainly because that was the only option that he felt was possible. Soon after college, he began graduate school and for the first time started to realize there was a gay community out there. During a summer job in Texas, he began to come to terms with his own homosexuality and in the process left graduate school and decided to start living what he saw as a more truthful life. Shortly after his coming out, Scott met and moved in with the man who would become his partner of 15 years, Lee. Scott subsequently began working in international student services and has remained in this profession for almost 20 years.

Being in an openly gay relationship caused difficulties and was a significant factor in Scott's departure from jobs at three universities. Although no supervisor ever directly raised the issue of sexual orientation, some supervisors created an uncomfortable atmosphere that made work unpleasant. In 1991, Scott accepted a university job in Virginia, a decision that was to some extent made because of the school's inclusion of sexual orientation in its antidiscrimination statement. During the first year at the university, he was, for the first time, fully open about his sexual orientation and took leadership positions in gay/lesbian/bisexual issues on campus. In 1992, Lee died of AIDS, and the support provided by the campus community cemented Scott's desire to work toward equality for gay, lesbian, and bisexual people.

Recognized as a leader within the Association of International Educators, Scott founded a gay/lesbian/bisexual caucus and led that for the first two years of its existence. In addition, Scott advises the campus gay/lesbian/bisexual student organization, has taken leadership within the local gay/lesbian/bisexual community through such activities as cochairing the annual Pride festival and chairing the area chapter of the gay/lesbian/bisexual ministry of the Episcopal Church. Scott King is a true leader who happens to be gay.

---

usual and customary in another culture. The human service professional's lack of knowledge about cultural differences as they relate to the expression of symptoms can seriously damage a helping relationship and result in misdiagnosis, mistreatment, and early termination of culturally different clients from the helping relationship. For instance, whereas many individuals from European cultures would show grief through depression, agitation, and feelings of helplessness, a Hispanic might present with somatic complaints.

7. *The unreliability of assessment and research instruments.* Over the years, assessment and research instruments have notoriously been culturally biased. Although advances have been made, one can still readily find tests that have cultural bias, and research that does not control adequately for cultural differences. One common problem in the use of assessment instruments is that individuals from other cultures may inadvertently be answering questions in a manner that would be considered "abnormal" by American standards when indeed they do not have an

---

BOX 7.5   A Jewish-American Woman

Eleanor is a 75-year-old widowed Jewish woman. Both her parents immigrated to the United States from Eastern Europe and Russia when they were children. They came looking for a better life and to escape anti-Semitism in their countries of origin. Like many Jews who came to the United States around the turn of the century, they came with little and had to work hard to survive in their new homeland. Because of the turmoil when leaving their countries of origin, Eleanor notes, there is little history of her family genealogy.

Eleanor grew up in a mostly Jewish section of New York and states that this resulted in her maintaining her sense of Jewish heritage. For instance, because her community was exclusively Jewish and because she would only meet Jewish men, it was unlikely that she would marry outside her faith, even though she might have entertained that idea. Although Eleanor was brought up speaking English, Yiddish was commonly spoken among her parents and grandparents. (Yiddish is a mixture of German and Baltic languages. Some Yiddish words have entered into English—for example, nosh, schmooz, chutzpah, and oy-vey.)

Even though Eleanor does not view herself as being highly religious, she identifies herself strongly as a Jew, noting that for her, being Jewish today is mostly cultural and brings to her "a sense of belonging and an association with people who are more or less like me." Although Eleanor states that she has encountered little overt anti-Semitism in the United States, she feels this is partly a result of living mostly around other Jews. She notes that rather than encountering overt prejudice, she often runs into people who are ignorant about Judaism and ask questions such as, Do Jews believe in God? One example of anti-Semitism that she did encounter was when she applied for a bookkeeping position in the Navy a number of years ago. Having passed the interview, she was about to be hired when the officer asked her what her religious affiliation was. When she told him she was Jewish, he threw her application in the trash.

Eleanor is proud of her Jewish heritage and maintains a sense of her ethnicity through affiliation with friends, membership in a synagogue, and attendance at Jewish cultural events.

---

emotional disorder. For example, when an item on a test asks if a person "hears voices," a religious Hispanic client might answer "yes," thinking that she "talks to God"—a normal response in her culture. Although Americans might also "talk to God," they have learned to deny that they "hear voices" because that implies psychopathology in this culture.

8. *Institutional racism.* Because **institutional racism** is embedded in society and even within the professional organizations (D'Andrea & Daniels, 1991, 1999), materials used by human service professionals will likely be biased, and helpers will unknowingly have gained a skewed understanding of culturally different clients. Examples are plentiful. For instance, some diagnoses that have been listed in the DSM-IV-TR have been shown to be culturally biased; some counseling approaches endorsed by professional associations have been shown to be practically useless when working with clients from some cultures; and some human services programs have, until recently, not stressed multicultural issues. No doubt there are culturally biased statements in this text of which I am not aware.

In summary, the eight reasons that the helping relationship does not always work for the minority client are (1) the melting pot myth, (2) incongruent expectations about counseling, (3) lack of understanding of social forces,

(4) ethnocentric worldview, (5) ignorance of one's own racist attitudes and prejudices, (6) inability to understand cultural differences in the expression of symptomatology, (7) unreliability of assessment and research instruments, and (8) institutional racism. Human service professionals who are not familiar with these reasons and who have not examined their own biases will assume that some culturally different clients resist treatment because they are not embracing the values consistent with the goals of the traditional helping relationship (Sodowsky & Taffe, 1991; Yutrzenka, 1995).

What happens when a helper is not attuned to cultural differentness? Robertiello and Schoenewolf (1992) note "101 common therapeutic blunders" that were made by helpers because of their own naivety. In brief, a few examples include the following:

1. The liberal white therapist who refuses to deal with an African American client's mistrustful and suspicious dreams of him because of the helper's denial of the tension in the relationship.

2. The feminist helper who blindly encourages her client to leave her husband because he is a batterer. The client leaves her husband but ends up in another battering situation because the helper did not examine what part the woman was playing in picking abusive men.

3. The helper who reassures her client that the client's homosexual feelings do not mean she is a lesbian. The helper does this out of fear of dealing with the client's sexuality and instead tries to ignore the subject. The client may or may not be homosexual, but reassuring her that she is not does not allow the client to explore her sexuality.

4. The helper who refuses to hear his client's atheistic views because they are contrary to the helper's religious beliefs. This had the effect of cutting off meaningful conversations in other areas because the client lost trust in the helper.

The human service professional must have knowledge of the many cultures that exist within this diverse country if he or she is to be effective when working with the culturally different client.

THE HELPING RELATIONSHIP
AND CULTURAL DIVERSITY

Every person is like all persons, like some persons, and like no other person. (Paraphrased from Kluckhorn & Murray, in Speight, Myers, Cox, & Highlen, 1991, p. 32)

Existentialists have noted that in trying to understand individuals, we need to be aware of their uniqueness **(Eigenwelt),** the common experiences held in groups and cultures **(Mitwelt),** and shared universal experiences **(Umwelt)** (Binswanger, 1962, 1963). Keeping this in mind, we need to ask ourselves, "How

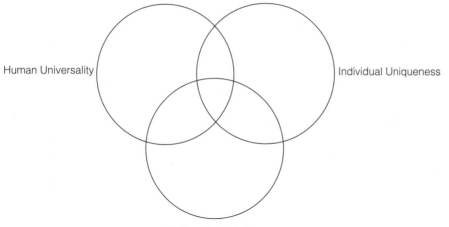

Human Universality   Individual Uniqueness

Cultural Specificity

FIGURE 7.4 Each sphere represents a unique aspect of the individual. The overlapping of the spheres suggests that we can only understand the totality of our clients' situation if we can understand the uniqueness of these three components.

SOURCE: From "A Redefinition of Multicultural Counseling," by S. L. Speight, J. Myers, C. F. Fox, and P. S. Highlen, 1991, *Journal of Counseling and Development, 70*, 29–36. Copyright 1991. American Counseling Association. Reprinted by permission.

can the helper be effective with culturally different clients?" Using this existential framework, one model of working with all clients assumes that each client has specific issues related to his or her culture, is unique unto himself or herself, and shares universal issues common to all people (Speight et al., 1991, p. 32) (see Figure 7.4). Each of these spheres represents a unique aspect of the individual. The overlapping of the spheres suggests that we can only understand the totality of our clients' situation if we can understand the uniqueness of these three components.

The Culturally Skilled Human Service Professional:
Beliefs and Attitudes, Knowledge, and Skills

A number of authors have stated that to work effectively with clients, culturally skilled mental health professionals must be aware of their attitudes and beliefs toward culturally diverse populations, have a knowledge base that supports their work with diverse clients, and have the necessary skills to apply to clients with diverse backgrounds (Pedersen et al., 1996; Sue et al., 1982; Sue et al., 1992).

Beliefs and Attitudes Culturally skilled human service professionals have an awareness of their own cultural backgrounds, biases, stereotypes, and values, and such helpers should have the ability to respect differences. Although culturally skilled human service professionals might not hold the same beliefs as their clients do, they can accept differing worldviews as presented by the helpee. Being sensitive to differences and one's own cultural biases allows culturally skilled human service professionals to refer a minority client to a human service professional of the client's own race or culture when such a referral will benefit the helpee.

Knowledge Culturally skilled human service professionals have an awareness of sociopolitical issues in the United States, have knowledge of the barriers that hinder culturally diverse clients from using social service agencies, and possess specific knowledge about clients' cultural or ethnic groups. Such skilled human service professionals have or are willing to gain knowledge of characteristics of specific cultural, racial, and ethnic groups (for example, personality styles, customs, traditions). (See Box 7.6.) At the same time, such human service professionals do not assume that clients necessarily have these characteristics just because they come from a specific cultural background. In other words, human service professionals have knowledge of the group from which clients come, yet do not "jump to conclusions" about clients' ways of being.

Skills Human service professionals who are effective with culturally diverse populations are able to apply generic interviewing and helping skills with culturally diverse populations while being aware of and able to apply specialized interventions that might be effective with specific populations. Also, culturally sensitive human service professionals understand the verbal and nonverbal language of clients and can communicate effectively with them.

PRACTICAL SUGGESTIONS FOR WORKING WITH A CULTURALLY DIFFERENT CLIENT

The following are suggestions for working with a select group of clients. These clients are often discriminated against and the manner in which we work with them may be unique (see Neukrug, 2001, for a more involved discussion). In addition, the human service professional will likely find these client groups prominent in the 21st century (see Chapter 10).

Counseling Individuals from Different Ethnic and Racial Groups

Although cultural differences are great among African Americans, Asian Americans, Hispanics, and Native Americans, there are some broad suggestions one can make for working with individuals from these and other cultures (Westwood & Ishiyama, 1990; Neukrug, 2001):

1. *Encourage clients to speak their own languages.* Although you are not necessarily expected to be bilingual, you can make an effort to know meaningful expressions of your client's language.

2. *Learn about the culture of your clients.* Make sure you have taken courses, read, or have asked your clients about their cultural heritage.

BOX 7.6   Counseling a Retired Polish-American Mine Worker

As a young therapist at a mental health center, I had the opportunity to work with a Polish-American client who had recently retired from working most of his life in the coal mines in northeastern Pennsylvania. I quickly realized there were a number of cross-cultural issues at work. I knew little of what it was like to be Polish American, had not worked with older clients, and had no idea what it was like being a blue-collar worker, working in the mines. Because of this, I wondered how I would connect with this man who was depressed. My choices seemed clear: I could either ignore these cultural differences or find out more about his heritage, what it meant to be retired, and his lifetime occupation. I therefore started counseling with him by spending a number of sessions asking him what it was like working in the mines and growing up Polish-American. At the same time, I reflected on developmental theory related to retirement age. It was clear that this client wanted to share his background with me. I could see he was proud of his heritage and loved telling me about the mines. I could see that my ability to not feel defensive about my lack of knowledge and my desire to learn about his social and cultural heritage made him feel close to me. This created an atmosphere of trust, and I soon understood his depression, which was partly a result of his belief that he was no longer a productive member of his community.

Using the model presented in Figure 7.4, you can see that in working with this client I tried to understand his unique situation and tried to gain knowledge of the culture from which he came. My ability to gain an understanding of this client's uniqueness and cultural specificity made it easier for me to gain a deep understanding of some of the universal concerns with which he was dealing. These included lack of meaning in life (which he had obtained partially through his work) as well as the sense of emptiness and loss he was currently experiencing.

---

3. *Assess the cultural identity of your clients.* Try to understand how your clients view their cultural identity. For example, an acculturated client may have little identification with his or her culture whereas a new immigrant will likely be embedded in his or her culture.

4. *Check the accuracy of the nonverbals of your clients.* Don't assume that nonverbal communication is consistent across cultures. Ask about nonverbals when in doubt.

5. *Use alternative modes of communication.* Because of cross-cultural differences, some clients will be reluctant to talk and for others, English may be a second language. When reasonable, use other modes of communication such as acting, drawing, music, story telling, collage making, and so forth, which might draw out clients.

6. *Encourage clients to bring in culturally and personally relevant items.* Encourage clients to bring in items that will assist you in understanding them and their culture (e.g., books, photographs, articles of significance, culturally meaningful items, and so forth).

7. *Vary the helping environment.* The helping relationship may be unfamiliar territory for some clients and sitting in a small private room might create intense anxiety. Consider using alternative helping environments (e.g., take a walk, have a cup of coffee at a quiet restaurant, initially meet clients at their homes, and so forth).

8. *Don't jump to conclusions.* Don't assume clients will act in stereotypic ways. Many clients won't match a stereotype.

9. *Know yourself.* Assess your own biases and prejudices to ensure that they will not negatively affect the helping relationship.

10. *Know appropriate skills.* Take courses and workshops and keep informed about the most recent professional literature to ensure you know the most appropriate helping skills to use.

Counseling Individuals
from Diverse Religious Backgrounds

In working with any individual, it is important to understand his or her religious background because it could hold the key to understanding underlying values. Some pointers to keep in mind concerning religion and the helping relationship include the following:

1. *Determine the religious background of your clients.* Know the religious affiliation of your clients to assist in treatment planning. This can be acquired at the initial interview; however, be sensitive to any client who may initially resist such a discussion.

2. *Ask how important religion is.* Many clients have only a rudimentary understanding of their religious tradition, even if they present themselves as deeply religious. Assess the part religion plays in the lives of clients to assist you in goal setting and treatment planning.

3. *Assess the level of faith development of your clients.* Low-stage faith development clients are dualistic, concrete, and work better with structure. High-stage clients are complex thinkers, value many faith experiences, and are comfortable with abstractions and self-reflection. Assessing the faith development of your clients will assist you in treatment planning (see Fowler, 1981).

4. *Don't make false assumptions.* False assumptions can lead to misunderstanding and a lack of trust. For instance, some helpers might falsely believe that all Jews keep a kosher home. Or, some Christian helpers might assume that all faiths believe people are born with original sin (this is solely a Christian belief) (personal communication, Dr. John Lanci, June 15, 2002).

5. *Educate yourself.* Know about the religious affiliation of clients. Take a course or workshop, read, attend a client's place of worship, and, if appropriate, ask the client.

6. *Be familiar with holidays and traditions.* To not accidentally embarrass or offend your clients, take time to familiarize yourself with the more important religious traditions of your clients (e.g., a Muslim would not want to be offered food during the month of Ramadan).

7. *Understand that religion can affect clients on many levels.* Some clients who deny any religious affiliation could still be unconsciously driven by the values they

were originally taught. Look at a client's actions; don't only listen to his or her words (e.g., a "lapsed Catholic" may continue to feel guilty over certain issues).

8. *Know yourself.* Assess your biases and prejudices to ensure they will not affect the helping relationship.

9. *Know appropriate skills.* Take courses and workshops and keep informed with the most recent professional publications to ensure you know the most appropriate helping skills to use.

Counseling Women

Several authors have made suggestions about how to assist women through a counseling relationship (Downing & Roush, 1985; Fitzgerald & Nutt, 1995; Gladding, 1967; McNamara & Rickard, 1989). They suggest that women have special issues to address and that the helping relationship offers women an opportunity to develop their female identity:

1. *Understand issues unique to women.* Be knowledgeable about how social, political, biological, and psychological issues affect women.

2. *Establish a relationship.* Using skills that women might find particularly helpful (e.g., empathy, self-disclosure), form a close relationship with the client, and encourage women to trust themselves.

3. *Model positive behaviors.* Use nonsexist language. Female helpers in particular should model empowerment, and male helpers should model sensitivity. Female clients should view new, positive ways of living in the world from the helper.

4. *Validate and legitimize women's feelings.* As female clients begin to talk more freely about their lives, validate their feelings about how women's issues have affected them.

5. *Combat feelings of powerlessness and low self-esteem.* As female clients increasingly understand the sociopolitical issues that have negatively affected them, encourage them to combat these feelings and to actively make positive changes.

6. *Help clients with conflicts between traditional and newly found values.* Insight might bring conflicting feelings between former and newly found values (e.g., wanting to stay home to raise children and wanting to work). Validate these contradictory feelings, acknowledge the confusion, and assist clients to explore their belief systems fully.

7. *Explore behavioral change.* As women gain new insights into self, they may wish to practice new behaviors. Help clients identify and try out new potential behaviors.

8. *Encourage new female relationships.* As female clients grow, encourage them to find new female friendships. For instance, women's groups can help clients express new feelings, develop more intimate relationships with women, feel supported, and be challenged to change.

9. *Encourage integration of new feelings, new ways of thinking, and new behaviors.* The expression of new feelings and new ways of thinking and acting will slowly take on a life of their own and be integrated into the client's way of living. Actively reinforce these new ways of being.

10. *Say goodbye.* Although many women may want to continue in counseling, it's important to encourage newfound independence. Be able to say goodbye and end the relationship. This will allow the client to test out new behaviors and come back to counseling later, if necessary.

Counseling Men

Helpers must be aware that there are men's issues and understand how they affect men and the helping relationship (Kelly & Hall, 1992; Osherson, 1986). Some ideas that can be used when working with male clients include the following (Osherson, 1986; Scher, 1981):

1. *Accept men where they are.* Men are particularly on guard when initially entering the helping relationship. Accept men as they are in an effort to build trust. Once men feel safe, they work hard on their issues (Moore & Haverkamp, 1989; Scher, 1979).

2. *Don't push men to express "softer feelings."* Men tend to be uncomfortable expressing certain feelings (e.g., deep sadness, feelings of incompetence, intimacy) and more at ease with "thinking things through," and problem solving. Don't push a man to express "softer feelings" too quickly or you'll push him out of the helping relationship.

3. *Early in therapy, validate men's feelings.* To protect their egos, men tend often to blame others and society for their problems. Initially validate these feelings that men express.

4. *Validate the view of many men that they have been constrained by sex-role stereotypes.* Initially validate men's beliefs that they have been constrained by sex-role stereotypes and pressure in society (e.g., the father must work particularly hard for his family). Validation of these views helps to build trust and establish the relationship.

5. *Have a plan for therapy.* Men like structure and a sense of goal directedness. Be clear with men that you want to collaborate with them on a plan for the helping relationship.

6. *Begin to discuss developmental issues.* Although each man has his own unique issues, he will likely also be struggling with common male developmental issues. Be aware of and willing to discuss these issues (e.g., mid-life crises) (see Levinson, 1986).

7. *Slowly encourage the expression of new feelings.* As trust is formed, men will begin to express what are typically considered to be more feminine feelings (e.g., tears, caring, feelings of intimacy). Reinforce the expression of these newly found feelings.

8. *Explore underlying issues and reinforce new ways of understanding the world.* As new feelings are expressed, underlying issues will emerge (e.g., childhood issues, feelings of inadequacy). One critical issue for men is their relationship with their fathers. How fathers modeled, distanced, and showed love becomes a template for men's relationships. Help the male client *"heal his wounded father"* (Osherson, 1986).

9. *Explore behavioral change.* As men gain insight, they may wish to try new behaviors. Help men identify new potential behaviors and "try them out."

10. *Encourage the integration of new feelings, ways of thinking, and new behaviors.* The expression of new feelings and new ways of thinking and acting will slowly take on a life of its own and be integrated into men's way of living. Actively reinforce these new ways of being.

11. *Encourage new male relationships.* As male clients change, new male friendships allow them to freely express feelings while maintaining their "maleness." Men's groups can allow men to develop more intimate relationships, feel supported, and be challenged to change (Moore & Haverkamp, 1989; Williams & Myer, 1992).

12. *Say goodbye.* Although some men may want to continue in the helping relationship, many will see it as time limited, a means to a goal. Be able to say goodbye and end the relationship. Doing this sets the seeds for him to come back, if he so desires.

Counseling Gay Men and Lesbians

Because of gender differences, there are actually many differences in counseling gays and lesbians, and human service professionals must remember that gender issues are powerful, regardless if you are gay or lesbian. Keeping this in mind, there are some common concerns that should be acknowledged when counseling gays and lesbians (Browning, Reynolds, & Dworkin, 1995; Pope, 1995; Shannon & Woods, 1995):

1. *Adopt a nonhomophobic attitude.* Make sure your biases do not interfere with the helping relationship.

2. *Make few assumptions about lifestyle.* Don't make assumptions about the gay and lesbian "lifestyle," often portrayed in movies and on TV. This lifestyle is usually only found in larger metropolitan areas. Most lesbians and gays have a wide variety of "lifestyles."

3. *Know the unique issues of lesbians and gays.* By reading professional literature, gay and lesbian literature, and by becoming involved with local lesbian and gay community groups, gain an understanding of some of the unique issues of gays and lesbians.

4. *Know community resources.* Have available community resources that might be useful to gays and lesbians.

5. *Know identity issues.* Be familiar with the identity development of gays and lesbians, especially as it relates to the coming out process (e.g., see Cass, 1979).

6. *Understand the idiosyncrasies of religion toward homosexuality.* Be familiar with particular religions and spiritual concerns unique to lesbians and gays (e.g., some religions view homosexuality as abnormal).

7. *Be tuned into domestic violence issues.* Be aware that domestic violence can occur in gay and lesbian relationships just as it occurs in heterosexual relationships.

8. *Know about substance abuse.* Have a firm foundation in substance abuse treatment as gays and lesbians may have a greater tendency toward the use of substances as a method of dealing with the coming out process and the inherent prejudices in society (Dyne, 1990).

In addition, when counseling gays, it is important to be knowledgeable about AIDS. AIDS is not a gay disease, but there are a disproportionate number of gays who are HIV positive. And, when counseling lesbians, be particularly cognizant that a large percentage of lesbian women have been sexually abused before the age of 18 (38% according to Loulan, 1987).

Counseling Individuals Who Are HIV Positive

A number of challenges face the helper who works with a person who is HIV positive or who has AIDS. Shannon and Woods (1995) and others have highlighted some points to consider when counseling the individual with HIV:

1. *Know the cultural background of the client.* Be prepared to work on cross-cultural issues if the client is from a diverse background because HIV positive individuals are found in all cultures.

2. *Know about the disease, and combat myths.* Be knowledgeable about the disease so you will feel comfortable working with an HIV positive individual and so the client will feel comfortable working with you.

3. *Be prepared to take on uncommon helper roles.* Be prepared to be an advocate, caretaker, and resource person, roles with which helpers have not always been comfortable.

4. *Be prepared to deal with unique treatment issues.* Become familiar with a number of treatment issues unique to HIV positive individuals, including (a) loss of income as a result of inability to work and the high cost of medical treatment, (b) depression and feelings of hopelessness, (c) loss of friends who may have died from AIDS, and (d) prejudice from society.

5. *Deal with your own feelings about mortality.* Be able to deal effectively with your feelings about the client's possible death and how those feelings may bring to the surface issues concerning your own immortality.

Counseling the Homeless and the Poor

A number of unique points should be considered when counseling the homeless and the poor (Axelson & Dail, 1988; Blasi, 1990; Rossi, 1990), including the following:

1. *Focus on social issues.* Be prepared to focus on social issues, such as helping a person obtain food and housing, rather than working on intrapsychic issues.

2. *Know your client's heritage.* A disproportionate number of homeless and poor persons come from diverse cultural groups, so know about the cultural heritage of your client.

3. *Be prepared to deal with multiple issues.* Be prepared to deal with multiple issues such as homelessness, poverty, mental illness, substance abuse, and medical problems. The homeless are at great risk for all of these.

4. *Know about developmental delays.* Homeless and poor children are more likely to have retarded language and social skills, be abused, and have delayed motor development, so know how to identify developmental delays and know referral sources.

5. *Know psychological effects.* Know how to respond to the psychological and emotional response to homelessness and poverty, which can include despair, depression, and a sense of hopelessness (Blasi, 1990).

6. *Know resources.* Helpers should be aware of the vast number of resources available in the community and make referrals when appropriate.

Counseling Older Persons

Older persons have a number of concerns that need to be addressed when they are counseled (Gibson & Mitchell, 1995; Schlossberg, 1995). The following are some issues that you should be aware of when counseling an older person:

1. *Adapt one's counseling style.* Be prepared to adapt the helping relationship to fit the older client's needs. For instance, use journal writing or art therapy for older persons who have difficulty hearing. For non-ambulatory clients, have a session in the client's home.

2. *Build a trusting relationship.* Older persons seek counseling at lower rates than do others (Hashimim, 1991), and those who do may be less trustful, having been raised when counseling was less common. Thus, be prepared to spend additional time building a trusting relationship.

3. *Know potential sources of depression.* Depression can come from many sources for the older person, including the loss of loved ones, lifestyle changes, health issues, and thoughts about dying and if one's life has been meaningful. Thus, helpers should be capable of identifying and discussing the many potential sources of depression.

4. *Know about identity issues.* Many older persons had based their identities on their careers, families, or roles in the community. Identity changes and loss of status can lead to despair, anxiety, and depression. Be prepared to help older persons define themselves in new ways.

5. *Know about possible and probable health changes.* Predictable health changes (e.g., loss of vigor) can lead to depression and concern for the future. Unpredictable changes (e.g., heart attack) can lead to loss of income and emotional problems. Know potential health problems and their emotional counterparts that are common to the elderly.

6. *Have empathy for changes in interpersonal relationships.* Aging brings changes in significant relationships as a result of such things as the death of a spouse, partner, and friends; changes in health status; and relocation. Know about and have empathy toward your clients concerning these changes.

7. *Know about physical and psychological causes of sexual dysfunction.* Be aware of the possible physical and psychological causes of sexual dysfunction in the elderly, and remember that regardless of age, people are always sexual beings.

Counseling the Mentally Ill

Helpers who work with the chronically mentally ill need to understand psychiatric disorders, psychotropic medications, and the unique needs of the chronically mentally ill. Specific treatment issues when working with this population include the following:

1. *Help clients understand their illnesses.* Many clients do not have an understanding of their illnesses, the courses of the illness, and the best treatment methods. You should fully inform your client with up-to-date knowledge about their mental illnesses.

2. *Help clients work through feelings concerning their illnesses.* Mental illness continues to be stigmatized in this society, and many clients are embarrassed about their disorders. Support groups and a nonjudgmental attitude can help to normalize the client's view of self.

3. *Help ensure attendance in counseling.* Clients miss appointments because of denial about their illnesses, embarrassment, or simply not caring. Call clients before appointments, have relatives or friends assist clients, or work on strategies to help clients remember appointments.

4. *Ensure compliance with medication.* Clients discontinue medication because of forgetfulness, denial about the illness, a belief that they won't relapse, or a belief that the medication is not helpful. Find strategies that ensure medication compliance.

5. *Ensure accurate diagnosis.* A diagnosis is crucial for treatment planning, and its accuracy can be greatly increased if you use a combination of diagnostic procedures including testing, clinical interviews, interviewing others, and the appropriate use of supervision.

6. *Reevaluate treatment plans, and do not give up.* The mentally ill are some of the most difficult clients, and it is easy to become discouraged. Helpers need to continue to be vigilant about their work with the mentally ill and continually reevaluate treatment plans.

7. *Involve the client's family.* Families can offer great support, and they can be a window into the client's psyche. Ensuring adequate family involvement helps you better understand a client and helps families better understand the client's diagnosis and prognosis.

8. *Know resources.* The mentally ill are often involved with many community resources (e.g., social security disability, housing authority, support groups). Have a working knowledge of these resources.

Counseling Individuals with Disabilities

As federal laws have increasingly supported the rights to services for individuals with disabilities, helpers have taken increasingly active roles in their treatment and rehabilitation (Lombana, 1989). Some treatment issues include the following:

1. *Have knowledge of the many disabling conditions.* Know the emotional and physical consequences of disabilities so you can work effectively with clients.

2. *Help the client know his or her disability.* Ensure that clients are fully informed of their disabilities, the probable courses of treatment, and their prognoses. Knowledge of their disabilities will allow them to be fully involved in any emotional healing that needs to take place.

3. *Assist the client through the grieving process.* Clients who become disabled go through stages similar to Kubler-Ross's (1997) stages of bereavement. You should expect denial, anger, negotiation, resignation, and acceptance. Facilitate passage through these stages.

4. *Know referral resources.* Be aware of community resources (e.g., physicians, social services, physical therapists, experts on pain management, vocational rehabilitation, and so forth).

5. *Know the law and inform clients of the law.* Know the law so you can ensure that clients receive all necessary services, are not discriminated against, and can empower themselves.

6. *Expect career counseling.* Often, one result of a disability will be a career transition. Be prepared to do career/vocational counseling or refer a client to a career/vocational counselor.

7. *Include the family.* Families can offer support, assist in long-term treatment planning, and help with the emotional needs of the client. Whenever reasonable, include the family.

8. *Be an advocate.* Individuals with disabilities are faced with prejudice and discrimination. Advocate for clients and help them learn how to advocate for themselves. Clients who know their rights and who advocate for themselves will feel empowered.

COUNSELING THE CULTURALLY DIFFERENT

An Ongoing Process

Not ours, not theirs; no one way of counseling surpasses another in the international arena. As cultures differ, so must counseling. (Romano, 1992, p. 1)

Throughout this text we have stressed specific methods of working effectively with clients, but it should be noted that counseling is not fixed, and, indeed, many international counseling theories may approach the helping relationship in ways foreign to the American helper (Locke, 1992b). Usher (1989) notes, "it is widely acknowledged that current counseling theories are products of Western

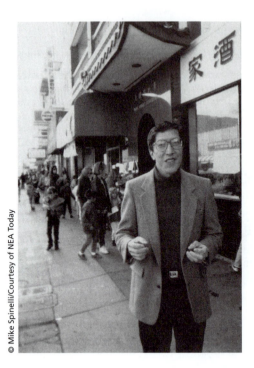

Dr. Derald Sue, one of the leaders in the field of multicultural counseling, has developed models for working with clients of diverse backgrounds and for incorporating cultural diversity in business, education, and mental health organizations.

culture and, as such, are not universally applicable to cross-cultural counseling situations" (p. 62).

Sue and Sue (1999) note that working with culturally different clients should be viewed as a constantly changing process. In this context, they note that the helping relationship "is an active process, that it is ongoing, and that it is a process that never reaches an end point. Implicit is the recognition of the complexity and diversity of the client and of client populations, and acknowledgment of our own personal limitations and the need to always improve" (p. 227).

Acknowledging the importance of ongoing training in cross-cultural counseling, a number of models have been suggested (see Landis & Bhagat, 1996). For instance, some authors have advocated weaving multicultural perspectives throughout human service programs (Garcia, Wright, & Corey, 1991), whereas others have spoken of the importance of having a separate course in multicultural awareness. Still others have suggested establishing peer counseling programs for students of diverse backgrounds (Stokes et al., 1987).

The **triad model** of cross-cultural training (Pedersen, 1981, 1983, 1987) suggests the counselor, an anticounselor, and a procounselor all meet together during an interview. The function of the anticounselor is to highlight the differences in values and expectations between the client and counselor, whereas the procounselor highlights similarities in values and expectations. In this model, the procounselor and anticounselor give continual and immediate feedback to the helper in an effort to increase the helper's ability to understand the client's perspective, recognize client resistance, recognize the helper's defensiveness, and learn how to recover from mistakes that the helper might make during the interview.

Finally, the **Association for Multicultural Counseling and Development (AMCD),** a division of the American Counseling Association (ACA), has developed **31 multicultural counseling competencies** that are considered essential in the training of mental health professionals (see www.counseling.org/resources/competencies.htm). You may want to review these competencies in class and decide if your program adheres to them.

Regardless of the model used, it is crucial that human service programs adapt a process that can offer ongoing training in cross-cultural counseling in an effort to meet the needs of an increasingly diverse America.

ETHICAL AND PROFESSIONAL ISSUES

The Culturally Diverse Client's Right to Dignity, Respect, and Understanding

The culturally diverse client deserves a human service professional who has left his or her biases behind. Such a human service professional is knowledgeable about cultural and ethnic differences and is sensitive to the needs of the culturally different client. The importance of these attributes should not be underestimated. Examples of how mental health professionals have negatively affected culturally different clients because of their own biases and prejudices abound in the literature (Cayleff, 1986; Quintana & Bernal, 1995). All clients deserve the respect and understanding of the professionals with whom they are working.

Our prejudices are often beyond our awareness. In other words, even though you may think you are not biased, unconscious prejudicial attitudes could seep out during interviews with clients. Because of this, ethical guidelines often speak to the importance of sensitivity to clients from diverse populations. For instance, the *Ethical Standards of Human Service Professionals* states that professionals should be knowledgeable about different cultures, aware of their own cultural heritage and how that affects others, understand sociopolitical issues, and seek ongoing training and supervision to work effectively with the culturally different client (see Appendix B, Statements 18, 19, 20, and 21).

THE DEVELOPMENTALLY MATURE HUMAN SERVICE PROFESSIONAL

Being Open to the Continual Development of a Multicultural Perspective

Developmentally mature human service professionals are able to work with clients of diverse backgrounds. They attempt not to be prejudiced or to hold stereotypic views and instead approach each client as a unique person. Such human service professionals understand their limitations and are eager to learn about the culture or ethnic background of clients with whom they are working.

The effective human service professional who is cross-culturally astute is willing to examine his or her own cultural background. This individual understands that cultural awareness is developmental; that is, each of us can learn more about ourselves and others in predictable stages. D'Andrea (1996) and D'Andrea and Daniels (1991, 1992) suggest that these stages range from an affective/impulsive stage of racism, where an individual could respond impulsively and in a hostile fashion to individuals from diverse backgrounds, to the principled activist stage where one can understand and accept that culturally different people may hold varying values and beliefs and may behave in ways different from the helper. In addition, students in this final stage actively work for systemic change in society.

SUMMARY

We began this chapter by offering some statistics on cultural diversity in the United States and throughout the world and then we highlighted the fact that the United States is becoming increasingly diverse as we move into the 21st century.

Next, we defined multicultural counseling and noted that although all helping relationships are cross-cultural, when working with clients who are particularly different from ourselves we are faced with some unique challenges. We then offered a number of basic definitions related to cross-cultural counseling, including definitions of culture, race, ethnicity, social class, power differentials, minority, stereotypes, and prejudice, racism, and discrimination, and we also presented terms to use in an effort to be "politically correct."

We next examined several reasons for the importance of multicultural awareness, including (1) the melting pot myth, (2) incongruent expectations about the helping relationship, (3) lack of understanding of social forces, (4) ethnocentric worldview, (5) ignorance of one's own racist attitudes and prejudices, (6) inability to understand cultural differences in the expression of symptomatology, (7) the unreliability of assessment and research instruments, (8) institutional racism, and (9) the idea that the counseling process has not been developed for clients from diverse backgrounds.

Focusing on the helping relationship and cultural diversity, we discussed the need for culturally skilled human service professionals to embrace certain beliefs and attitudes and have the knowledge and skills to be effective in the cross-cultural relationship. We next offered a list of practical suggestions for the following client groups that tend to be discriminated against or have special concerns: (1) individuals from different ethnic and racial groups, (2) individuals from diverse religious backgrounds, (3) women, (4) men, (5) gays and lesbians, (5) individuals who are HIV positive, (6) the homeless and poor, (7) older persons, (8) the mentally ill, and (9) individuals with disabilities.

As we ended this chapter, we talked about the need for ongoing training in multicultural counseling and we highlighted the importance of human service programs infusing multicultural counseling into their curriculum and examining the multicultural competencies of AMCD. We also discussed one method of supervision of cross-cultural counseling, the triad model. Finally, we noted that the *Ethical Standards of Human Service Professionals* highlights the importance of multicultural counseling and that the developmentally mature human service professional is willing to examine his or her developmental maturity, prejudices, attitudes, and knowledge base in an effort to be effective with culturally different clients.

EXPERIENTIAL EXERCISES

1. The Alligator River.* Read "A Loving Story," and then fill in the grid as instructed.

A Loving Story:

Lovey is in a committed relationship with Fine who lives on the other side of the Alligator River. Lovey wants to see Fine, but the bridge is out due to a recent flood. Lovey could swim across the river, but would get eaten by the alligators. Therefore, Lovey goes to Popeye, who is the only person with a boat on the river, and asks Popeye for a ride to the other side of the river.

Popeye has always been infatuated with Lovey from a distance. Popeye has a severe speech impediment, low self-esteem, and has rarely dated. Popeye earns a meager living taking people across the river. When Lovey asks Popeye for a ride across the river Popeye states, "Lovey, I've always been infatuated with you, and I'll take you across the river if you'll make love with me." Lovey is initially disgusted and goes to a close confidant named Friend for advice. Friend states, "This is your problem, and you're going to need to work it out on your own." Lovey ponders the situation and thinks, "What the hell, I've slept with lots of people, one more won't make a difference." After they have sex, Popeye, as promised, takes Lovey across the river.

When Lovey gets to the other side of the river, out of a sense of honesty, Lovey tells Fine the whole story. Becoming enraged, Fine states, "Get out of my life, I never want to see you again." Lovey becomes distraught and seeks advice from a friend named Slug. Slug becomes infuriated and punches out Fine.

A. Examining Values as a Function of Gender and Ethnicity *Scoring your results:* Using the grid at the end of this exercise, rate each of the five characters in the story. Place an X under number 1 and across from the name of the person you like most; then place an X under number 2 and across from the name you like second most; and so forth. Your instructor will then count all the 1s, 2s, 3s, 4s, 5s, and

---

*This exercise is adapted from the book by Simon, Howe, and Kirschenbaum (1995), *Values clarification: A handbook of practical strategies for teachers and students* (revised edition). Sunderland, MA: Values Press. For a list of other books on values, phone Values Press at (413) 665–4800.

6s in the class and place them on a master grid on the board. Then, as a class, respond to the following questions:

1. What does the distribution tell you about how students in your class view individuals with differing values?

2. Based on the characters' roles, did you assume that certain characters in the story were male and others were female?

3. Consider how you might rate the characters if you changed their genders.

4. If the characters in the story were of differing ethnic, cultural, or religious backgrounds, would you have responded differently to them?

5. If you were in a helping relationship with any of the characters in the story, how would your positive and negative stereotypes affect your work with them?

B. Alternative to the Previous Exercise Instead of having the class complete Exercise A, the instructor will break the class into six groups and have each group make assumptions about the characters as noted.

Then, using the scoring instructions in Exercise A, collect the aggregate data in each of the six groups and compare the responses of the six different groups. (Feel free to create other groups of different gender and ethnic mixes.)

1. Group 1 (all characters are white): Lovey is female, Fine is male, Popeye is male, Friend is female, Slug is male.

2. Group 2 (all characters are African American): Lovey is female, Fine is male, Popeye is male, Friend is female, Slug is male.

3. Group 3 (female characters are white, male characters are African American): Lovey is female, Fine is male, Popeye is male, Friend is female, Slug is male.

4. Group 4 (male characters are white, female characters are African American): Lovey is female, Fine is male, Popeye is male, Friend is female, Slug is male.

5. Group 5 (all characters are female).

6. Group 6 (all characters are male).

	1	2	3	4	5	6
Lovey						
Fine						
Popeye						
Friend						
Slug						

2. Examining Our Heritage

In class, form small groups of four or five. Then state your full name (if you're married and use your husband's last name, include your maiden name). Then discuss the origins of your name. Note such things as the origins of your last name, why you were given your first name, and any other information about your family history of which you may be aware. If you are not familiar with the history of your family name, ask a parent, guardian, or relative and see what he or she knows.

3. Acknowledging Our Cultural/Ethnic/Religious Affiliation

In class, the instructor will ask each student to anonymously write on a piece of paper all ethnic, cultural, and religious groups to which each belongs (for example, Irish-American, Catholic, homosexual, individual with a disability). Then, have the instructor gather all papers and write on the board all the diverse groups found in your class. (Note to instructor: It is important to maintain anonymity.)

4. Finding Out About Other Cultural Groups (Follow-Up to Exercise 3)

After the various cultural, ethnic, and religious groups are written on the board, have each student anonymously write any question he or she would like to ask about any of the diverse groups on the board. Have the instructor collect the questions, and, as a class, all help answer the questions as best you can.

5. Interviewing a Person from Another Cultural Group

Using the following questions, interview a person from a different cultural, ethnic, or religious group. In class, share what you learned about that person.

1. What benefits does he or she attribute to being a member of that group?
2. What drawbacks does he or she attribute to being a member of that group?
3. What history does he or she know about his or her group?
4. What are the individual's feelings concerning stereotypes of the group?
5. What prejudice has he or she experienced?
6. How would he or she feel about seeing a helper of a differing ethnic, cultural, or religious background? Of the same background?

6. Experiencing Prejudice

Have the class divide into groups based on some physical attribute (for example, hair color, eye color, height). In addition, have the instructor randomly pick some of the groups to be of below-average, average, and above-average intelligence. Within your group, come up with stereotypes of the other groups. During class, respond to one another based on your stereotypes and on the chosen intelligence level. At the end of class, process how the experience felt to one another.

7. Counseling Myths Questionnaire*

Using the following scale, rate each of the statements listed on the Counseling Myths Questionnaire. When you are finished, discuss your responses in class. Before discussing your answers, your instructor might wish to gather all of your answers and give the breakdown of the responses to each item. Your answer choices are

SA	A	NO	D	SD
strongly agree	agree	no opinion	disagree	strongly disagree

_____ 1. Certain clients should be avoided because of their past experiences.

_____ 2. Cultural myths and stereotypes cannot be avoided when working with culturally different clients.

_____ 3. Cultural myths and cultural stereotypes are often a reality.

_____ 4. Large behavioral differences exist between clients as a function of their culture.

_____ 5. Helpers have fewer problems when they understand their clients' backgrounds.

_____ 6. Helpers should work only within their own cultural group.

_____ 7. Clients from the same ethnic background, religion, or culture have similar issues to work on.

_____ 8. Culturally different clients are usually referred to helpers from the same cultural group.

_____ 9. Cultural differentness of client and helper is a significant factor in the helping relationship.

_____ 10. Cultural variations exist regarding verbal and nonverbal communication across cultures.

_____ 11. Everyone is culturally different; therefore, helpers need a model that will serve all clients.

_____ 12. All types of social services are available for all persons who desire them.

_____ 13. All cultures receive fair treatment in the helping relationship.

_____ 14. Culturally different clients use profanity more often than nonculturally different clients do.

_____ 15. White clients are more likely to respond to helping interventions than are culturally different clients.

_____ 16. Generally, clients from low-income backgrounds are very difficult to help.

---

*Adapted with permission from Dr. Richmond Calvin, Indiana University–South Bend.

_____ 17. Many culturally different persons have shown they do not trust helpers.

_____ 18. Family ties are extremely weak with many culturally different clients.

_____ 19. Value systems for many culturally different clients are inferior.

_____ 20. Poor minority clients do not trust nonminority middle-class helpers.

_____ 21. Sociocultural history represents the most important ingredient in the helping relationship.

_____ 22. Culturally different clients do not possess qualities such as boldness, initiative, and assertiveness.

_____ 23. Culturally different clients are not logical thinkers, problem solvers, or good decision makers.

_____ 24. All helping relationships have a cross-cultural component.

_____ 25. Religious differences are not important in the helping relationship.

_____ 26. Age differences are not important in the helping relationship.

_____ 27. Gender differences are not important in the helping relationship.

_____ 28. Sexual-orientation differences are not important in the helping relationship.

8. Ethical and Professional Vignettes

After reflecting on the following vignettes, discuss your thoughts with other students in your class.

1. You realize when working with a client from Peru that the cross-cultural differences are making it difficult for you to be effective. Rather than referring the client, you decide to read more about your client's culture so you will gain a better understanding of him. Is this ethical? Is this professional?

2. You discover some fellow students making sexist jokes. What should you do? Have you encountered such behavior? Have you acted?

3. You find some family members making ethnic/cultural slurs. What should you do? Have you encountered such behavior? Have you acted?

4. A colleague of yours identifies herself as a feminist. You know that when she works with some women, she actively encourages them to leave their husbands when she discovers the husband is verbally or physically abusive. Is she acting ethically? Should you do anything?

5. You discover that a colleague of yours is telling a homosexual client that he is acting immorally. Is this ethical? Professional? Legal? What should you do?

6. A friend of yours advertises that she is a Christian counselor. You discover that when clients come to see her, she encourages reading parts of the Bible

during sessions and tells clients they need to ask for repentance for their sins. Is this ethical? Is this professional? Is this legal?

7. An African American human service professional who has expertise in running parenting workshops decides he should only work with African American clients. A white client has heard about his workshops and calls to sign up for one. The human service professional refers him to someone else and tells the client he works only with African Americans. Does this human service professional have a responsibility to see this client? Is he acting ethically? Professionally? Legally?

8. When offering a parenting workshop to individuals who are poor, you are challenged when you tell them that "hitting a child is never okay." They tell you that you are crazy and that sometimes a good spanking is the only thing that will get the child's attention. Do they have a point? What should you do?

9. A human service professional who is seeing a client who is HIV-positive discovers that his client is having sex with others without revealing his HIV status. You tell him that you have a responsibility to report him to the police. Would this be ethical? Professional? Legal?

10. You discover that a colleague of yours has a patronizing attitude about his clients who have a disability. He often can be heard saying things like "Poor Joe, he's blind," or "It's a pity that a pretty girl like Joan is missing a leg." What, if any, responsibility do you have to confront your colleague?

8

Research,
Program Evaluation,
and Testing

> The inquiry of truth, which is the love-making, or wooing of it, the
> knowledge of truth, which is the presence of it, and the belief of truth, which
> is the enjoying of it, is the sovereign good of human nature.
>
> SIR FRANCIS BACON

While I was living in Cincinnati and working on my doctorate, I was walking down the street one day and a person came up to me and said, "Do you want to take a personality test?" I said, "Sure!" I was brought into a storefront office and spent about 30 minutes completing an inventory. When I finished, I was asked to wait a few minutes while they scored the instrument. Then, a person came into the room and said, "Well, you have a pretty good personality and you're fairly bright, but if you complete L. Ron Hubbard's course on Dianetics, you will have a better personality and be even brighter." Having taken some course work in testing, I knew a number of things. First, I questioned whether the test truly measured personality and intelligence; second, I questioned the way in which the instrument was interpreted.

Ten years later, I'm walking down a street in Minneapolis and another person comes up to me and says, "Do you want to take a personality test?" Well, now I realize that this person is trying to get me to be involved with Dianetics. I say to him, "What proof do you have that this test is statistically valid and reliable?" He assures me that it is. I say, "I want some proof," at which point he tells me that at the headquarters in New York, they have that information. I say to him, "I'll buy the book Dianetics and read it after the information is sent to me." He agrees. I never hear from him again. The book is still sitting in my library.

After finishing my doctorate and while teaching at a small New England college, I was supervising a graduate student's thesis. Her hypothesis was that there would be a relationship between the number of years of yoga meditation and self-actualizing values; that is, the more you meditated, the more self-actualized you would be. She went to an ashram (a yoga retreat center) and had a number of individuals fill out an instrument to measure how self-actualized they were; she then collected information from the individuals concerning how long they had been meditating. After collecting her data and performing a statistical analysis, she found no relationship. Because she herself had meditated for years, she strongly felt that she would find such a relationship. Upon finding no relationship, she said to me, "There must be something wrong with this instrument or this research because people who have meditated for years are clearly more self-actualized than those who have just started meditating." I suggested there was nothing wrong with the research or the instrument, but that perhaps she had a bias because of her own experiences with meditation. I explained that this does not mean that meditation does not affect people, but that in this one area, using this instrument, the evidence showed that no relationship existed. I told her that research is not how you feel something is but what you find something is. When she was able to see her own biases, she realized that perhaps I was right.

I once received a federal grant to train school counselors how to be aware of and intervene in cases of chemical abuse. To receive the grant, I had to explain the need for and purpose of the training, how the training was to take place, and how we would evaluate the effectiveness of the training. Explaining how I would determine the effectiveness of this training, through evaluation, was considered a crucial factor in deciding whether I would get this grant. In this case, evaluation was used as a check to ensure that what we were presenting to the counselors was effective. In addition, evaluation was also viewed as a measure of whether it would be worthwhile to do similar training in the future and to examine which areas to revise if future training were to occur.

Unfortunately, many human service professionals have little knowledge of research, program evaluation, and testing, even though these three areas have permeated every part of our society and many aspects of our clients' lives (Mehrens, 1992).

> There is much ignorance about very basic measurement, evaluation, and research topics among the practitioners . . . and among those who are ignorant, there is, on occasion, a fair amount of hostility toward some useful data. (Mehrens, 1991, p. 439)

This chapter will help us become knowledgeable about research, program evaluation, and testing and show us how they are important in helping us understand our clients and in determining whether what we are doing benefits them. Because human service professionals will encounter research concerning client outcomes, evaluation of social service programs, and tests that clients take, they must understand each of these areas. Thus, this chapter will explore some of the major kinds of qualitative and quantitative research designs, examine types of program evaluation, and offer an overview of testing. Near the end of the chapter, we will review issues related to informed consent in research, program evaluation, and testing; the use of deception in research; and the proper use of testing data. The chapter will conclude with a discussion about how the information that we gain from research, program evaluation, and testing is an evolving process that allows us to continually add new knowledge to the field.

RESEARCH

Conducting Research

Research answers the questions "Are our hunches about the world correct?" and "How might what we are doing affect the future?" Best and Kahn (1997) define research as "the systematic and objective analysis and recording of controlled observations that may lead to the development of generalizations, principles, or theories, resulting in prediction and possibly ultimate control of events" (p. 18). In other words, researchers methodically analyze information so they can make predictions about the future. Research can be anything from counting the number of times a child acts out during the day, to surveying opinions of human service professionals, to performing a complex analysis of a specific counseling approach when working with clients. Before conducting research, however, one must develop a hypothesis or research question.

The Hypothesis, the Research Question,
and Literature Review

Kuhn (1962) said that all new knowledge is built on former knowledge and that, at times, shifts in our understanding of the world take place when former knowledge no longer explains current phenomena. In a sense, as Sir Francis Bacon said so eloquently, we are forever seeking the truth. In performing research, one of our first steps is to develop a **hypothesis** or **research question** in an effort to test propositions that are derived from theories and prior research (Leary, 2001; Sommer & Sommer, 2002). For us to come up with our hypothesis or question, we need to do a thorough **review of the literature.**

A review of the literature involves examining all major research done in the area we are exploring. This is accomplished by conducting a search of professional publications, usually articles and books. Three particularly popular electronic searches include **Educational Resources Information Center (ERIC), PsychINFO,** and **InfoTrac College Edition.** (Computer searches, such as ERIC and PsychINFO, are also valuable in helping the student identify sources for papers.) For instance, if I were interested in examining some aspect of the human services work environment, I might go to the computer and type in key descriptors; that is, major terms that the computer will search. In this case, such key descriptors might include *jobs, human services, social services, careers, occupations.* The computer would generate a list of abstracts that contained articles with one or more of these descriptors. Then, I would tell the computer to cross-reference all these descriptors so that I could remove duplications and focus only on those publications that are relevant to my topic. After cross-referencing, I would print out the abstracts of all the articles it found. After reading the abstracts, I would identify which articles I want to examine in more detail and obtain a copy of them. Next, I would begin to identify the variables I specifically want to examine in my research. A **variable** is "any characteristic or quality [for example, height, intelligence, self-esteem, job satisfaction] that differs in degree or kind and can be measured" (Sommer & Sommer, 2002, p. 85). For instance, in my computer search I might have found a number of articles on job satisfaction (Variable 1) of human service professionals who work at varying social service agencies (Variable 2). I could then begin to formulate a research question or a hypothesis around these variables.

In guiding research, when variables are measured and used to distinguish differences between groups, hypotheses are generally developed; when variables are measured and used to examine relationships between groups, hypotheses or research questions are generated; and when variables are measured and used to describe current events or conditions, research questions are generated. In the preceding example, one hypothesis might be the following:

> Human service professionals who work at mental health centers will be more satisfied than will those who work at child protective services (note the comparison of groups, thus a hypothesis).

On the other hand, a research question might be the following:

What roles and functions performed by human service professionals provide job satisfaction?

Defining the Research Design

Research designs can broadly be categorized as quantitative or qualitative in nature. **Quantitative research** relies on controlled research designs and can be applied in a laboratory setting or in the field. Quantitative research tests hypotheses or clarifies research questions. **Qualitative research** is generally field research that relies on the researcher to carefully observe and describe phenomena and to interpret the phenomena within a social context. Qualitative research attempts to clarify research questions.

Quantitative research assumes that there is an objective reality within which research questions can be formulated and scientific methods used to measure the probability that identified behaviors, values, or beliefs either cause or are related to other behaviors, values, or beliefs. Qualitative research, on the other hand, holds that there are multiple ways of viewing knowledge and that one can attempt to make sense of the world by immersing oneself in the research situation in an attempt to provide possible explanations for the problem being examined (Heppner, Kivlighan, & Wampold, 1992). Qualitative research allows one to examine phenomena that quantitative research cannot explore, like our understanding of abstract concepts such as empathy and the meaning we ascribe to God (Hanna & Shank, 1995).

Although quantitative and qualitative research designs vary dramatically, they both offer us unique and valuable ways of expanding our knowledge base (Borders & Larrabee, 1993; McMillan & Schumacher, 2001). What follows is a brief overview of some of the major kinds of quantitative and qualitative research. In the area of quantitative research, we will touch on **true experimental research, causal-comparative (ex post facto) research, correlational research,** and **survey research.** For qualitative research, we will examine **ethnographic** and **historical research.**

Quantitative Research

Although there are many forms of quantitative research, the following is a brief description of four of the more popular types, including true experimental designs, causal-comparative (ex post facto) designs, correlational research, and survey research.

True Experimental Research In true experimental research, you will be manipulating variables to see what effect they have on the outcome that you are examining. This type of research tests hypotheses and allows you to look at the causes of behavior. Usually, the variable that is being manipulated is called the **independent variable**, and the variable that you are measuring is called the **dependent variable**. For instance, if I wanted to examine the effect of different kinds of multicultural counseling training, I could randomly assign students to three groups, one where no training took place, and two other groups that provided different kinds of training in multicultural counseling. After the training was complete, I could measure how effectively they learned multicultural counseling skills. However, in some cases random assignment is difficult, if not impossible (see Box 8.1). In these cases, we might decide to conduct a causal-comparative study.

Causal-Comparative (Ex Post Facto) Research Because experimental research involves random assignment and the manipulation of variables, it is often impractical or impossible to implement even though hypothetically it might be more sound. Therefore, causal-comparative research, sometimes called ex post facto research, which allows us to examine variables of intact groups, is often employed. For instance, let's say I wanted to measure how satisfied 100 human service majors were at four different kinds of jobs (for example, mental health, social services, unemployment, rehabilitation), one year after graduation. If this were a true experimental design, I would have to randomly assign 100 graduates to these four jobs, and then compare how satisfied they were at their various jobs one year later. Clearly, this would be an impossible task. However, I could compare job satisfaction of human service professionals one year after they have been hired at these four kinds of jobs. First, I would give a satisfaction scale to each intact group, and then I would examine statistical differences among the four groups. In other words, I would score the satisfaction scales and statistically analyze whether some groups are more satisfied than other groups. Because random assignment is not used, any differences found cannot be attributed solely to the type of job (for example, perhaps people who have a tendency to be more satisfied pick certain jobs). Therefore, in this type of research, we cannot be assured that one variable causes another. However, this research can often give us a good sense of the relationship between variables.

Correlational Research Generally, correlational research is of two kinds, **simple correlational studies**, which explore the relationship between two variables, or **predictive correlational studies**, which are used to predict scores on a variable from scores obtained from other variables.

Correlational research uses **correlation coefficients** to show the strength of the relationship between two or more sets of scores. A correlation coefficient ranges from −1.0 to +1.0 and generally is reported in decimals of one-hundredths (see Figure 8.1). A positive correlation shows a tendency for two sets of scores to be related in the same direction. A negative correlation shows an inverse relationship between two sets of scores. For instance, if I was interested in the relationship between the ability to be empathic and dogmatism, I could obtain scores from one group of individuals on these two variables and correlate them. In this case, you would see a negative correlation, which would indicate that individuals who were more empathic tended to be less dogmatic and vice versa.

Generally, "r" is used to describe the strength of the relationship. For instance, if I found a correlation coefficient of .89 between height and weight I would say r = .89. Or, if I found that grades in college had a mild negative correlation of −.24 with the number of hours per week spent in pursuing leisure activities, I

BOX 8.1   A Failed Attempt at True Experimental Research

When I was living in New Hampshire, a colleague and I decided to do some research on the effects of aerobics on personality variables. After exploring the literature, we found some possible links between aerobics and the personality variables of self-actualization, depression, and anxiety. We approached our local YMCA, which was running a rather extensive aerobics program, and the staff agreed to let us talk with individuals who were about to start aerobics for the first time. They also agreed to let these people have 8 weeks of free membership at the Y if half of them (randomly chosen) would not start aerobics for 8 weeks. We found three instruments to measure our personality measures, with the intent of comparing, at the end of 8 weeks, the group that started aerobics with the group that

waited. We excitedly met with approximately 50 new aerobians. We told them our plans, and they looked at us and said, Are you kidding? We want to start now!

Our good intentions obviously were not going to sway these individuals who were ready to start exercising. Unfortunately for us, we could not implement our study. Instead, we moved to a causal-comparative study in which we compared individuals who had just finished 8 weeks of aerobics with those just starting. Because random assignment could not be used in this type of research study, it was not as solid a study as our original plan. I guess our desire to do research was not as powerful as the individuals' desire to exercise.

---

would present the correlation as r = −.24. It should be stressed, however, that correlational studies do not show cause and effect because other, often unknown variables may be responsible for the relationship between the two variables. For instance, in a study examining academic achievement, researchers found a high correlation between the number of bathrooms in the home and how children did in school. Certainly, having more bathrooms does not cause higher academic achievement. Other factors are undoubtedly the cause. For instance, those individuals who have more bathrooms likely have more money and are probably more highly educated. Thus, other variables are the cause for this unlikely correlation.

Survey Research   In survey research, a questionnaire is designed to gather specific information from a target population. For instance, we might send a questionnaire to human service professionals in an effort to understand what variables might be related to level of job satisfaction at various types of human service jobs. In this case, we could examine many variables such as salary, number of years at the job, and educational level and perhaps ask those surveyed to rate their job satisfaction. We could then use charts and graphs to illustrate the differences between the various jobs on these variables.

To illustrate the type of information one can obtain from surveys, Neukrug, Milliken, and Shoemaker (2001) completed a survey to determine if human service practitioners, educators, and students had had counseling for themselves, and for those who had, the kinds of characteristics they sought in a counselor. It was found that 75% had been in counseling, with women seeking counseling at higher rates than men, and practitioners attending at higher rates than educators or students. The researchers also found that the qualities most sought in choosing a counselor were competence, trustworthiness, warmth and caring, openness, and

−1, −.99,... −.80............. ....−.51...... −.25... −.10... −.02, −.01, 0, +.01, +.02... +10...+.25......+.51,............. .80... +.99, +1

     strong   moderate   low   none   low   moderate   strong

FIGURE 8.1 The range and strength of correlation coefficients

empathy, whereas research productivity, a reputation for being a therapist's thera-pist, and spiritual orientation were the least rated qualities deemed important for choosing a counselor.

Although survey research can be interesting, it cannot tell us the underlying reasons for our results. For instance, in our research on counseling attendance, we were not able to determine why individuals attended counseling and if certain types of counseling were more beneficial than others. Therefore, survey research can be limiting, although sometimes intriguing.

Qualitative Research

As noted earlier, the approach to qualitative research varies dramatically from quantitative research. Two of the most popular types of qualitative research are **ethnographic research** and **historical research.**

Ethnographic Research Ethnography refers to the description (*graphy*) of human cultures (*ethno*). Sometimes called **cultural anthropology**, ethnographic research was made popular by **Margaret Mead**, who studied aboriginal youth in Samoa by immersing herself in the people and their culture as she attempted to understand their lifestyle (Mead, 1961). Ethnographic research assumes that phe-nomena or events can best be understood within their cultural context. Take an event out of its context and its meaning is likely to be interpreted from the con-text of the researcher rather than from its original social context. Reality, there-fore, is a social construction that, to be understood, needs to be examined within the phenomenological perspective in which it occurred. Ethnographers, there-fore, seek to understand events by understanding the meanings that people place on them from within their natural contexts.

The first step in conducting ethnographic research is to identify the group to be studied and to identify a general problem to be researched. Conducting a liter-ature review can help the researcher gain a better understanding of the culture or group being studied and assists the researcher in defining the purpose of the research and in developing research questions. Next, the researcher decides on what method he or she wants to use to immerse himself or herself in the culture of the population. Before entering the culture, the researcher should develop a plan for implementing his or her data collection methods. Three common meth-ods used in ethnographic research include observation, ethnographic interviews, and collection of documents and artifacts.

Observation Ethnographers will often observe a situation or phenomenon and describe, using extensive notes, what they view. Although sometimes qualitative researchers take nonengaged roles when observing, more often they become

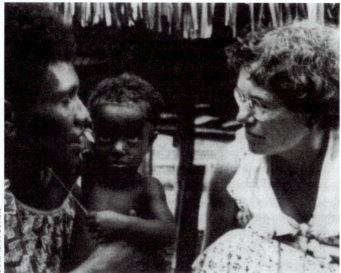

Bettmann/CORBIS

As a participant observer, Margaret Mead (1901–1978) gained a deep understanding of the culture she was observing by living with the people.

participant observers. In this kind of **observation**, the researcher immerses himself or herself into the group and interacts with the group being observed. He or she may actually live with the group and take notes about its interactions (Burgess, 1995; Cole, 1975); however, it is important that the observer does not interfere with the natural process of the group. During observation, the observer takes scrupulous notes and listens intensely to the individuals being observed in an effort to understand the unique perspective of the group. Only in this manner can the observer obtain a rich appreciation for the ways in which the group constructs reality. It is particularly important that the observer record what role he or she has taken while observing and what effect, if any, observation may have had on the group being observed (see Box 8.2).

Ethnographic Interviews **Ethnographic interviews** are a second popular qualitative method of collecting data from a culture or group. Such interviews involve open-ended questions in an effort to understand how the interviewees construct meaning. Interviews may be informal; guided, where questions are outlined in advance; or standardized, where the exact questions are determined before the interview, but the responses remain open-ended. As with participant observation, the interviewer must take scrupulous notes or record the interviews to obtain verbatim accounts of the conversation.

Collection of Documents and Artifacts **Artifacts** are the symbols of a culture or group and can provide multiple meanings to an understanding of the beliefs, values, and behaviors of the group. In understanding the meaning an artifact holds,

---

BOX 8.2   Disruptive Observation of a Third Grade Class

While working in New Hampshire, I was once asked to debrief a third-grade class that had just finished a trial period in which a young boy, who was paraplegic and severely mentally retarded, was mainstreamed into their classroom. During this trial period, these third graders had a stream of observers from a local university come into their classroom to assess their progress. Because this was not participant observation, the observers would sit in the back of the classroom and take notes about the interactions between the students. This information was supposed to be used later to decide whether it was beneficial to all involved to have the disabled student mainstreamed.

When I met with the students, they clearly had adapted well to this young boy who was disabled. Although the students seemed to have difficulty forming deep relationships with him, his presence seemed in no way to detract from their studies or from their other relationships in the classroom. However, almost without exception, the students noted that the constant stream of observers interfering with their daily schedule was quite annoying. Perhaps if participant observation was employed, where an observer interacted and was seen as part of the classroom, the students would have responded differently.

---

researchers need to know how the artifact was produced, where the artifact came from, the age of the artifact, how the artifact was used, and who used it. Interpretation of the meaning of artifacts should be corroborated from observations and through interviews. McMillan and Schumacher (2001) suggest the following major categories of artifacts: (1) personal documents such as diaries, personal letters, and anecdotal records; (2) official documents such as internal and external papers, records and personnel files, and statistical data; (3) objects that hold symbolic meaning of the culture (for example, Native American headdresses); and (4) erosion (for example, worn grass on college campuses indicating the quickest path that students use to get from one place to another).

Historical Research   The purpose of historical research is to describe and analyze conditions and events from the past in an effort to answer a research question. Historical research relies on the systematic collection of information in an effort to examine and understand past events from a contextual framework. When doing historical research, the researcher generally has a viewpoint in mind and needs to go to the literature to support this viewpoint. Then, the researcher will begin to collect data to show that his or her viewpoint has validity. At any point in this process, the researcher's point of view might change as he or she is influenced by the literature or by the sources of data obtained.

In collecting data for historical research, researchers can use a number of sources. Whenever possible, researchers attempt to use **primary sources,** or the original record, rather than **secondary sources,** which are documents or verbal information from sources that did not actually experience the event. Examples of primary sources include **oral histories, documents,** and **relics** (Gay & Airasian, 2003).

Oral Histories Oral histories are created when researchers directly interview an individual who had participated in the event or observed the event in question.

Documents Documents are records of events—such as letters, diaries, autobiographies, journals and magazines, films, recordings, paintings, and institutional records—that are generally housed in libraries or archival centers.

Relics Relics are any of a variety of objects that can provide evidence about the past event in question. Such things as books, maps, buildings, artifacts, and other objects are some examples of relics.

In conducting historical research, the researcher must attempt to interpret the information obtained from within the historical frame that is being examined. This is a long and tedious process but can result in obtaining more accurate information about the event being examined. For instance, examine the historical research in Box 8.3, written by a friend of mine when examining the letters of St. Paul from the New Testament (see Lanci, 1997, 1999).

Examining the Results Once you have completed your literature review, set up your design, and performed your study, you are ready to analyze your results. Many statistical analyses can be used in examining your research. Separate courses in both research and statistics, however, would be needed to comprehend the complexity of analyses that can be performed in good research.

Briefly, in quantitative research, when you are examining differences between groups or the relationship between groups, you can perform a number of analyses. Terms that you might see in the literature that examine group differences and relationships between groups include **t-tests, analysis of variance (ANOVA),** and **correlations.** To decide if there is statistical significance between groups, you will see a **probability level** set. Such levels tell you the probability that the results you have found could be found by chance alone. For instance, much research will set its probability at the .05 level. This means that there is less than a 5 out of 100 chance that the results you find happened by chance. Or, put another way, your results are probably caused by the factors you are examining. In the literature, this is reported as $p < .05$ (p = probability, < = less than).

In the reporting of survey research, **descriptive statistics** are usually used. Descriptive statistics include **measures of central tendency (mean, median,** and **mode), measures of variability** (for example, **range, standard deviation**), percentages, and frequencies (see the section "Measures of Central Tendency and Measures of Variability," pp. 245–246). These statistics are often presented in charts, graphs, and tables. This allows you to examine the overall results of the data you have collected. Table 8.1, based on a survey by Neukrug, Milliken, and Shoemaker (2001), is an example of a table using descriptive statistics with percentages.

Qualitative data collection, particularly ethnographic research, relies on a process called **inductive analysis,** which means that patterns and categories emerge from data (McMillan & Schumacher, 2001). Thus, the researcher who is

---

BOX 8.3   Historical Research: A New Temple for Corinth*

My project began because I thought it might be interesting to take a new look at the letters of St. Paul. They have been extremely influential in the formation of Christianity, and yet they are rarely examined as artifacts of a world that existed 2,000 years ago, a world very different from our own. Today, Christians look at them as theological treatises, but Paul wrote them as letters of guidance to specific Christian communities with specific challenges and problems.

I took one letter (1 Corinthians) and one image he uses (the community as a temple) in one passage (chapter 3, verses 16–17), and tried to see if traditional interpretations could be challenged by looking more closely at the actual historical and cultural context of the Corinthian people to whom Paul wrote. Traditionally, interpreters have assumed that Paul was spurning the Jewish temple in Jerusalem, the temple of his youth (since he was Jewish), and telling the Corinthian Christians that they were themselves THE new temple of God. I knew this to be historically uncertain, since there was no external evidence that Paul ever turned his back on the Jerusalem temple. I wondered how else this text might be interpreted.

I began by studying the conventional ways that people interpret the target passage and discovered some basic flaws in their views. To do this, I studied other primary texts to discover what functions temples played in cities like

Corinth. Some of these texts were inscriptions found at archaeological sites, including Corinth. Others were literary texts by Roman authors. In addition, I studied the archaeological remains of the temples of Corinth, visiting the site three times, talking with archaeologists and biblical scholars who were also studying Corinth.

What I found was that it is likely Paul was NOT referring to the Jerusalem temple, since his audience was Gentiles and there were plenty of other temples to which Paul could refer. And, I discovered that Paul was probably using the temple/community image to help the Corinthians understand who they were as a community, as opposed to attempting to get them to turn away from Jerusalem.

Past interpretations have unfortunately been used to support anti-Semitic attitudes because some interpretations are that Paul rejected his Jewish faith in favor of a new Christian one. This new, and I believe more historically accurate, interpretation supports the notion that Paul never stopped being a Jew; he just changed from being a traditional observer of Judaism to a Jew who believed that Jesus was the Messiah and was expressive of the fullness of Judaism. This sort of Jewishness was not rejected by other Jews until about 30 years after Paul died.

---

*By John Lanci, Ph.D.

---

examining the data collected through the various methods mentioned looks through the information for patterns, ways of categorizing information, and ways of selecting important pieces of information. As this process continues, the researcher begins to see particular points emerge.

Ethnographic researchers classify their data by a process called **coding.** This process breaks down large pieces of data into smaller parts that seem to hold some meaning to the research question. For instance, if I was involved in a study to determine what problems at-risk high school students might have in a specific school, I might observe the youths; interview them; interview their teachers, school counselors, parents, and peers; and collect school records. I would then go through all these pieces of information and try to select patterns and themes that seem to emerge from the data. I would carefully review all the data and look for words, phrases, and ways of acting that seem to be pointing in similar directions.

Table 8.1 Percentage of Attendance in Counseling by Type of Member and by Sex of Members of the National Organization of Human Service Education.

	Total in Counseling*	Individual (101)	Group (59)	Family (55)	Couple (30)	Other (18)
Educator (n = 102)	77 (75.5%)	73 (71.6%)	28 (27.5%)	18 (17.6%)	30 (29.4%)	2 (2.0%)
Practitioner (n = 59)	49 (83.1%)	47 (79.7%)	16 (27.1%)	7 (11.9%)	17 (28.8%)	1 (1.7%)
Undergrad (n = 56)	38 (67.9%)	35 (62.5%)	16 (28.6%)	11 (19.6%)	17 (30.3%)	1 (1.8%)
Grad (n = 31)	23 (74.2%)	21 (67.8%)	9 (29.0%)	7 (22.6%)	9 (29.9%)	0 (0%)
Other (n = 18)	16 (88.9%)	16 (88.9%)	8 (44.4%)	5 (27.8%)	5 (27.8%)	0 (0%)
Males (n = 43)	28 (65.1%)	27 (96.4%)	12 (27.9%)	5 (11.6%)	11 (25.6%)	1 (2.3%)
Females (n = 163)	126 (70.3%)	118 (72.4%)	47 (28.8%)	35 (21.5%)	34 (20.8%)	3 (1.8%)
Total (n = 206)	154 (74.8%)	145 (70.4%)	59 (28.6%)	40 (19.4%)	45 (21.8%)	4 (1.9%)

* Individuals may have identified themselves as more than one category (e.g., educator and practitioner). "Total" results eliminate duplications.

In both ethnographic and historical research, the researcher must go through a rigorous process of reviewing the data, synthesizing results, and drawing conclusions and generalizations. The researcher's original research question(s) may have been changed by this point as he or she has gone through the involved process of reviewing the literature and analyzing the sources. The results of the research are a product of a **logical analysis** of the materials obtained rather than a statistical analysis as we find in quantitative research. Finally, the researcher needs to be careful to not get caught up in his or her point of view and should be open to offering opinions that both support and contradict the ultimate findings.

The ability to provide reliable and valid results in qualitative research is based on how well the researcher is able to record information accurately and to use multiple methods in recording (Gall, Gall, & Borg, 1999; McMillan & Schumacher, 2001). For instance, this could involve taking verbatim accounts when interviewing people, using precise and concrete descriptions, using multiple researchers to get many perspectives and to look for similar themes among researchers, mechanically recording data, using primary data whenever possible, asking participants to make their own records and to match the researcher's understanding of events with participants' understanding of events, checking meanings with participants, and reviewing any data that seem atypical or discrepant.

Discussing the Results

Probably the most important aspect of research is the conclusions drawn from the study. This conclusion, is based on the data and information collected. The researcher can present his or her theories about the meaning of the study results.

Although discussions allow for some leeway, the researcher should not take giant leaps in an effort to present "the truth." For instance, in Table 8.1, one can easily see that a much larger number of individuals attended individual counseling compared with group, family, or couples counseling. However, any discussion about why this is the case should be worded carefully and tentatively because the researcher should not make major interpretive statements regarding the data.

Using Research in Human Service Work

Knowledge of basic research techniques is valuable for human service professionals. First, such knowledge enables human service professionals to understand professional journal articles and to make conclusions concerning what might be the most effective interventions for their clients. Second, research can validate what we are doing; at other times, it might suggest new ways of approaching client change (Lambert, Ogles, & Masters, 1992). Third, research might suggest new avenues to explore and is often the basis for future research. Finally, use of basic research techniques can be valuable for program evaluation.

PROGRAM EVALUATION

Although many research concepts are used in evaluation, the purpose of **program evaluation** tends to be different (Krathwohl, 1998). Whereas research tends to examine new paradigms to expand understanding and knowledge and to learn how such knowledge can be applied to practice, program evaluation has to do with whether or not a program has achieved its goals and objectives and has been shown to have worth and value (Halley, Kopp, & Austin, 1998; Leary, 2001; Sanders, 1994). Two types of evaluation are process evaluation and outcome evaluation.

Process Evaluation

When presenting a program, workshop, or conference, assessing effectiveness through an ongoing evaluation process is important. **Process evaluation,** sometimes called **formative evaluation,** involves the assessment of a program during its implementation to gain feedback about its effectiveness and to allow for change in the program as needed.

You can perform process evaluation in several ways. Probably the most basic way is to ask for verbal feedback from your audience. In this case, presenters need to be open to feedback, especially any negative criticism, and be willing to change their programs midway. A little less threatening, and sometimes more revealing, is to have participants write down reactions to the program while it is occurring. Doing this anonymously allows participants to express their feelings openly, without fear of repercussions. Along these same lines, participants can be asked to complete rating forms during the program so researchers can obtain ongoing feedback. The advantage of rating forms is that you can easily collate the data and get a sense of how the whole group feels about aspects of the program. The disadvantage is that rating forms do not allow for feedback outside the questions being asked. Of course, rating forms could be created that include room for written feedback.

Outcome Evaluation

Outcome evaluation, sometimes called **summative evaluation,** involves assessment of the total training program after it is finished. Like process evaluation, outcome evaluation may involve asking for verbal feedback, written feedback, and responses to rating scales (see Box 8.4). However, some programs also require a more systematic evaluation process that involves the use of research techniques. For instance, you might want to examine the effectiveness of two differing programs on attainment of effective parenting skills. You might randomly assign 20 parents to one group and 20 to a second group, run your training programs, and measure the effectiveness of the two programs. You can then contrast the effect of one program with the other, trying to determine if one type of training is more effective than another.

In some cases, you might expect training programs to have some far-reaching effects. For instance, I received a grant to train helpers in a local school system to identify, assess, and intervene with students at risk for drug and alcohol abuse. Some of the long-term outcome measures that we hoped to see from this training included the reduction in alcohol and drug use by students, a decrease in the dropout rate (chemical abuse has been shown to be related to dropout rate), and an increase in the age of first use of drugs or alcohol. To obtain information like this would be a major undertaking and would involve a large-scale assessment of students. Though not an easy project, these behaviors are measurable and could be an indication that our program was effective.

The Human Service Professional
and Program Evaluation

At some point in your career as a human service professional, you will be asked to run a program for your clients. It may be a self-esteem program, a job-awareness program, a parenting program, or simply a program that explains the services of your agency to your clients. Whatever program you run, you will want to receive feedback about its effectiveness. To improve the program while it is occurring or to improve it for the next time that it might be given, process and outcome evaluation measures should be undertaken: "Without ongoing evaluation, it is difficult to know whether you are helping. If change seems to be occurring, you may not know what actually is helping the consumer" (Halley et al., 1998, p. 373). Program evaluation also has an important place in examining the effectiveness of job-related behaviors at your agency. A responsible agency is willing to look at the effectiveness of its employees and its programs. Such evaluation can greatly assist in understanding what works and what needs to be changed.

In these times of fiscal conservatism, the issue of accountability of programs and agencies has become extremely important. No longer can programs and

---

BOX 8.4   Outcome Evaluation of a Drug and Alcohol Training Program

The following is an outcome evaluation measure that was used during a drug and alcohol awareness workshop (Project TRUST) for mental health professionals in a school system in Virginia. The numbers on the right under "Mean" represent the average score, on each item, for all participants. The presenters were generally rated very high, as was the workshop itself. Based on this information, in which areas would you want to see improvement in the future?

Workshop Evaluation (N = 52)
Describe your reaction to each of the following statements in terms of this scale.

1. Never	3. Sometimes	5. Always
2. Seldom	4. Usually	

Workshop presenters	*Mean*
1. Were well prepared.	4.7
2. Delivered material in a clear, organized manner.	4.7
3. Stimulated intellectual curiosity.	3.9
4. Showed respect for questions and opinions of participants.	4.6
5. Allowed for relevant discussion when appropriate.	4.7
6. Were concerned that participants understood them.	4.6
7. Were accessible for individual and group concerns.	4.6

Workshop TRUST	
8. Offered information applicable to one's field.	4.0
9. Was presented in a comfortable, conducive environment.	4.4
10. Provided a beneficial, educational experience.	4.1

---

agencies deliver services without some account that what they are doing is working. The use of evaluation techniques is an important step in the accountability process and assures the public and funding agencies that you are performing essential and effective services for your clients (Leary, 2001).

TESTING

As a human service professional, you will be involved with testing. You may be administering tests and will likely be called to interpret some tests. You may be a consultant about tests to clients, parents of clients, or other professionals. You may use tests in research and in evaluation, and you will read about tests in the professional literature. Tests have permeated many aspects of our society, and they are an intricate part of the work of the human service professional. Let's examine some of the different kinds of tests we may encounter.

Norm-Referenced Tests and Criterion-Referenced Tests

Generally, tests are either norm-referenced or criterion-referenced. **Norm-referenced tests** are those instruments in which the examinee can compare his or her score with a peer or norm group. This means that an individual's score can be compared with conglomerate group scores of his or her peers. Many tests that are sold by national publishing companies are norm-referenced.

Criterion-referenced tests are those tests in which the examinee has specific goals to meet based on his or her rate of learning. This allows the individual to move at his or her own pace in accomplishing those goals. Criterion-referenced testing is used with the learning disabled because they may need additional time to meet learning goals compared with other students in their grade levels.

Standardized Tests and Informal Tests

Standardized tests are assessment instruments that are given in a standard fashion; that is, each test administration, regardless of where and when it is given, is given by the examiner in the exact same fashion. **Informal tests** are assessment instruments that are not necessarily compared with a **norm group,** and the way they are administered may vary during each test-taking situation. Teacher-made tests and rating scales are two examples of informal types of tests. Teacher-made tests measure what students have learned in the classroom. Because they are based on the teacher's sense of what students have learned, they are somewhat subjective. Rating scales are often used for evaluation purposes or for a quick overview of an individual's personality style.

Tests can be standardized and norm-referenced, standardized and criterion-referenced, informal and norm-referenced, or informal and criterion-referenced. Sometimes, criterion-referenced tests may also be norm-referenced. Some examples follow:

1. A standardized, norm-referenced test might be an individual intelligence test in which the test is given the exact same way across the country, and the individual's score is then compared with national scores of his or her peer group.

2. A standardized, criterion-referenced test might be an individual achievement test given to a student who is learning disabled. The test is given the same way across the country, but the student will take only those parts of the test in which he or she has likely reached individualized learning goals.

3. An informal, norm-referenced test might be a rating scale devised by a researcher to measure the amount of cynicism among a national group of human service professionals and educators. The test could be sent to all members of the National Organization for Human Service Education (NOHSE), and a score received by one human service professional can then be compared with the larger population of human service professionals.

4. An informal, criterion-referenced test might be a teacher-made test that has targeted learning goals for students.

5. A criterion-referenced test that is also norm-referenced might be an individual diagnostic test that assesses for a possible learning disability in math. Being criterion-referenced, it has individualized learning goals. However, because it is also norm-referenced, it allows the examiner the opportunity to compare the individual with a norm group.

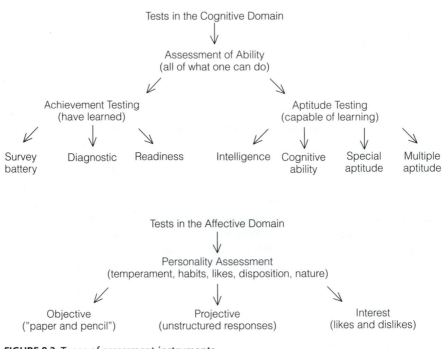

FIGURE 8.2 Types of assessment instruments

Types of Tests

Ability Testing (Tests in the Cognitive Domain) Tests in the cognitive domain are generally called **ability tests.** These tests measure an individual's cognitive capabilities (Anastasi & Urbina, 1997; Thorndike, Cunningham, Thorndike, & Hagen, 1997). Two major categories of ability tests include **achievement tests,** tests that measure what you have learned, usually in school; and **aptitude tests,** tests that measure what you are capable of learning (see Figure 8.2).

Achievement Tests Three major types of achievement tests include **survey battery tests**, **diagnostic tests**, and **readiness tests**. Survey battery tests measure general achievement and are usually given in large-group settings in schools. You are probably familiar with this type of test through your own education. The **Iowa Test of Basic Skills (ITBS)** and the **Stanford Achievement Test** are two examples of survey battery tests. The uses of survey battery tests are many and include the assessment of a student's ability level, the determination of teaching effectiveness, and the examination of the general level of ability throughout a school system.

Diagnostic tests delve more deeply into suspected problem areas and are often given one-on-one by an experienced examiner, usually a school psychologist or learning disabilities specialist. Following the results of a diagnostic test and in consultation with parents and teachers, it may be decided that a student has a learning disability; that is, in one or more specified areas, the student's ability is suspected to be much lower than his or her average ability in other areas (see Box 8.5).

Readiness tests assess an individual's ability to advance to the next educational level. One major use of readiness tests is to determine if a child is developmentally ready to enter first grade. Because children at kindergarten age develop at different rates, some children need additional time in kindergarten before they are ready to enter first grade. Readiness at this age does not imply innate ability but simply reflects differing stages of development at an early age in life. For instance, a very bright child may be developmentally too immature to enter first grade.

Aptitude Tests Four major kinds of aptitude tests include **individual intelligence tests, cognitive ability tests, special aptitude tests**, and **multiple aptitude tests** (see Figure 8.2). Individual intelligence tests, such as the **Stanford-Binet**, are individually given to measure general intellectual ability and are usually administered by highly trained examiners, most often psychologists. These tests have a broad range of use; they help identify individuals who have learning disabilities or developmental disabilities, or those who are gifted. Usually, when a comprehensive assessment of an individual is requested, an individual intelligence test is included.

Cognitive ability tests are paper-and-pencil tests used to measure general cognitive ability. These tests, which are often given in groups, assess an individual's ability to do well in school. Therefore, they are sometimes used for placement in school, as part of determining learning disabilities and giftedness and as predictors of ability for college (for example, the **Scholastic Aptitude Test, or SAT**), graduate school (for example, the **Graduate Record Exam, or GRE**), and so forth.

Special aptitude tests measure a specific, clearly defined segment of ability (for example, spatial ability, hand-eye coordination, mechanical ability). Special aptitude tests are sometimes used as part of the criteria for job placement and acceptance into specialty schools (for example, the use of a hand-eye coordination test to determine ability for operating complex machinery in a factory). Multiple aptitude tests measure a number of clearly defined segments of ability and often help an individual understand his or her broad range of abilities and how those abilities might be associated with occupational choice. The **Armed Services Vocational Aptitude Battery (ASVAB),** which is given by the military (often for free in the schools), and the **General Aptitude Test Battery (GATB),** which is given by an employment security office, are two examples of multiple aptitude tests.

Although both achievement tests and aptitude tests may be standardized, informal, norm-referenced, or criterion-referenced, most testing of this kind tends to be norm-referenced and standardized. A standardized test ensures that the comparisons with the norm group are of high quality and the use of norm groups allows for comparisons with large groups of examinees.

Personality Testing (Tests in the Affective Realm) The assessment of personality includes the examining of one's temperament, attitudes, values, likes and dislikes, emotions, motivation, interpersonal skills, and level of adjustment (Anastasi & Urbina, 1997; Drummond, 1996; Gibson & Mitchell, 1990). Three

---

BOX 8.5   Public Law 94-142 and the IDEA

In 1975, the **Education for All Handicapped Children Act (PL94-142)** was passed (Federal Register, 1977). This landmark legislation ensured the right to an education within the least restrictive environment for any individual between the ages of 3 and 21 who had a disability. The importance of this law for individuals with a disability, particularly a learning disability, was enormous. To implement this law, diagnostic testing has become one of the main ways of determining who might have a

disability. Subsequent laws have enhanced this landmark legislation (Gable & Hendrickson, 1990).

PL94-142 was recently updated with the passage of the **Individuals with Disabilities Education Act (IDEA).** The IDEA, along with section 504 of the **Rehabilitation Act** and parts of the **Americans with Disabilities Act (ADA),** are all important laws that help children with disabilities gain an education within the least restrictive environment.

---

types of personality assessment most frequently used today are **objective tests**, **projective tests**, and **interest inventories** (see Figure 8.2).

Objective Tests Objective tests are often multiple choice or true-false paper-and-pencil measures that allow us to compare the individual's personality with his or her norm group. Therefore, individuals can compare personality traits such as depression, anxiety, interests, and introversion with individuals who exhibit such behavior or with the "normal" population. Objective tests are given in groups or on an individual basis. Some of these tests, like the **Minnesota Multiphasic Personality Inventory-II (MMPI-II)**, can measure psychopathology, whereas others, like the **Myers–Briggs Type Indicator**, measure common personality characteristics. The use of objective tests are many and include helping make a clinical diagnosis, helping an individual understand his or her personality style, and determining emotional stability for certain types of jobs (for example, working in a nuclear missile silo).

Projective Tests Projective tests allow an individual to make an unstructured response to a stimulus with the purpose being to uncover hidden and unconscious aspects of the client. For instance, the **Rorschach**, a major projective test, consists of showing ten inkblots to an individual and asking the individual to state what he or she sees in the blots. (See Figure 8.3.) Other types of projective tests include **sentence completion**, where the end of a sentence is omitted and the client completes it with the first thought that comes to mind; drawings, where the client is asked to make a specific drawing (for example, a drawing of the client's family all doing something together); and tests in which the individual is asked to develop stories from pictures that are presented. In all of these, based on the client's responses, a highly trained clinician makes judgments about the client's personality style.

Interest Inventories Interest inventories measure an individual's likes and dislikes as well as his or her personality orientation toward the world of work. These paper-

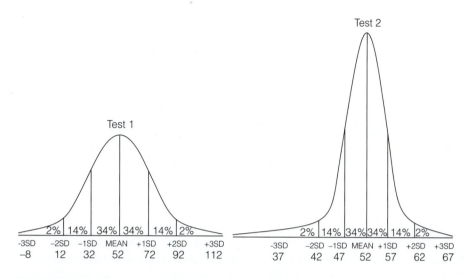

FIGURE 8.3 Comparison of the variability of two different normal curve distributions

and-pencil assessment instruments are most frequently used to help individuals discover those occupations and careers to which they would most likely have a good fit. The **Strong Vocational Interest Inventory** and the **Self-Directed Search (SDS)** are two of the more common interest inventories used today.

The Nature of Tests

Relativity of Scores John receives a score of 47 on a test. How did he do? Jill receives a 95 on a different test. How did she do? If John's test score was 47 out of 50, he probably did pretty well. But, if 1,000 people take the test and all but John receive a score of 50 out of 50, we might view his test score a little differently.

What about Jill's score? Is a score of 95 good? If the best possible score is 100, perhaps it is a good score. But what if the best possible score is 200, or 550, or 992? If 1,000 people take the test and Jill's score is the highest, we might say that she did well, at least compared with this group. But if her score is at the lower end of the group of scores, then comparatively she did not do well. To make things even more complicated, what if a high score represents more of an undesirable trait (for example, cynicism or depression)? Then clearly, the higher Jill scores compared with her peer or norm group, the worse she has done comparatively. What's important here is the concept that scores on tests—particularly norm-referenced, standardized testing scores—are relative, and an individual's raw score makes sense only in its relative position to his or her group.

Measures of Central Tendency and Measures of Variability When comparing an individual's test scores with his or her norm group, understanding measures of central tendency and measures of variability of the test become very important. **Measures of central tendency** include the **mean**, the average of all the scores; the **median**, the middle score representing the point where 50% of the examinees score above and 50% fall below; and the **mode**, the most frequent score. Two important **measures of variability** include the **range**, which represents the spread of scores from the highest to the lowest score, and the standard deviation, which represents how much, on average, scores vary from the mean. For instance, one test has a mean of 52 and a standard deviation of 20. This means that most scores (about 68%) on this test range between 32 and 72 ($\pm$ 1 standard deviation, or 52 plus 20 and 52 minus 20) (see Figure 8.3). Another group of scores also has a mean of 52, but this test has a standard deviation of 5. This means that most of the scores (about 68%) range between 47 and 57 ($\pm$ 1 standard deviation, or 52 plus 5 and 52 minus 5). Clearly, even though the two tests have the same mean, the range of scores around the mean varies considerably. An individual's score of 40 would be in the average range on the first test but well below average on the second test. If you know the central tendency and the measures of variability of the group of scores, you can compare your scores to these measures.

Qualities That Make a Good Test Four qualities that are particularly important in establishing the worthwhileness of a test are (1) **validity**, whether or not a test measures what it is supposed to measure; (2) **reliability,** the ability of a test to accurately measure a trait or ability; (3) **practicality**, the ease of administration and interpretation of the test; and (4) **cultural fairness**, whether or not the test measures what it is supposed to measure in a consistent manner for all subgroups for which the test is given. Let's take a closer look at these qualities.

Validity Test validity involves a systematic method of showing that a test measures what it purports to measure. A test's validity is a function of how it is created. To create a valid test, one should do a thorough analysis of the literature concerning the test content, consult with experts about the test content, and compare the test with other tests of a similar nature. Often, a statistical analysis is used to show test validity. Some of the more popular types of validity are content validity, concurrent validity, predictive validity, and construct validity. Regardless of the method used, it is important to remember that validity is attempting to show that the test is indeed measuring the quality it purports to measure. Validity is a statement about the test, not about the people taking the test.

Reliability The second quality that is examined in determining the adequacy of an assessment instrument is reliability. Whereas validity is used to show that a test is measuring what it's supposed to measure, reliability examines the accuracy of test scores. If a test were reliable, one could assume that an individual's score would remain about the same even if that individual were to take the test a number of times (assuming the person did not change, that is learn, between testings). As with validity, reliability is measuring the adequacy of the test and is not making a statement about the people taking the test. Some of the more common types of reliability are called internal consistency, split-half reliability, parallel forms reliability, and test-retest reliability.

Practicality Suppose I have a test that can accurately assess mental health diagnoses but each administration costs $1,000. This test may be good at what it does, but the cost may be prohibitive for most people. Or, suppose we have an instrument than can accurately measure learning disabilities but takes a school psychologist two days to administer. These are some of the questions that we must struggle with when deciding whether a test is practical.

Practicality examines whether or not the test is realistic to give. It includes issues related to the cost of testing, the ease of administration, the length of the test, and the ease of interpretation. A test can have good validity, good reliability, be cross-culturally fair, yet not be a practical test to give.

Cross-Cultural Fairness of Tests

> [T]ests must be used in ways that, as far as possible, take advantage of the tremendous utility of test and other assessment data, while also facilitating optimal understanding and nurturance of a wide range of individual and cultural differences. (Walsh & Betz, 1995, p. 423)

The last quality important in determining the worthwhileness of a test is whether it is cross-culturally fair. Although it is impossible to eliminate all bias from tests, one should expect that the bias is small enough to allow for justifiable interpretations of any individual's score. When examining cultural bias, test publishers should have exhaustively reviewed the extent to which the content of a test has cultural bias. For those instruments that are used to predict future behavior, the test should be shown to be predictive for minority groups. This does not mean that it will predict in the same manner for all groups, but that the predictive validity of each subgroup was examined and that the test was shown to predict accurately for each subgroup (Anastasi, 1992; Anastasi & Urbina, 1997). In fact, the U.S. Supreme Court case of **Griggs v. Duke Power Company** (1971) asserted that tests used for hiring and advancement at work must show that they can predict job performance for all groups.

Cross-cultural bias in testing is an important issue whenever assessment instruments are used with minorities. Examiners need to be aware of bias in testing, ethical issues related to assessment and multiculturalism, and state and national laws related to the use of tests with minorities (see Box 8.6). Some related issues will be discussed later in this chapter.

Who Can Administer Tests?

The American Psychological Association (APA) defines three levels of test complexity that are associated with who can administer tests:

- Level A tests are those that can be administered, scored, and interpreted by responsible nonpsychologists who have carefully read the test manual and are familiar with the overall purpose of testing. Educational achievement tests fall into this category.

**BOX 8.6   The Use of Intelligence Tests with Minorities:
Confusion and Bedlam**

The use of intelligence tests with minorities has always been an area of controversy. Some states have found intelligence tests biased and have banned their use in certain circumstances with some minority groups (Swenson, 1997). Other states have not found widespread evidence of bias. If intelligence tests are used with minority clients, the examiner needs to know the proper way to administer and score them.

The concern for bias in testing has gone so far in some circles that if the situation weren't so serious, it would almost be comical. Take the case in California of Mary Amaya, who was

concerned that one of her sons was being recommended for remedial courses he did not need. Amaya had an older son who was found not to need such assistance after he was tested. Amaya requested intelligence testing for her other son. However, since the incident with her first son, laws had been changed, and California decided that intelligence tests were culturally biased and thus banned their use for certain minority groups. Despite the fact that Amaya was requesting the use of an intelligence test, it was found that she had no legislative right to have it given to her son.

- Level B tests require technical knowledge of test construction and use and appropriate advanced coursework in psychology and related courses (e.g., statistics, individual differences, and counseling).

- Level C tests require an advanced degree in psychology or licensure as a psychologist and advanced training/supervised experience in the particular test. (APA, 1954, pp. 146, 148)

Generally, the associate's- or bachelor's-level human service professional who has some course work in tests and measurement can give a Level A and, under some circumstances, a Level B test. Level C tests require at least a master's degree along with advanced training in the test in question.

The Human Service Professional's Use of Tests

With literally thousands of tests in use today, the responsible use of assessment instruments can be a great adjunct to our work with clients: "Psychological tests and inventories, derived from and refined by scientific research, contribute to responsible practice by providing an empirical basis . . . for assessment and intervention" (Claiborn, 1991, p. 456).

Although the human service professional may not have the advanced training needed to administer many tests, it is not uncommon for a client to have taken some assessment instruments as a means of providing adequate goal setting. For example, tests are commonly used in many settings: the unemployment office where vocational assessments help clients find jobs, the community-based mental health center where assessment is useful for diagnosis and treatment, or schools where assessment helps identify children with special needs as well as measure students' progress. Tests have become an integral part of our lives.

Even though human service professionals will probably not be administering and interpreting most tests, consultation with examiners is a crucial step in working with our clients. Usually, examiners will provide a written test report that summarizes their results, and human service professionals should be able to use these results in working with their clients. Therefore, basic knowledge of how tests are used is essential to our work with clients.

ETHICAL AND PROFESSIONAL ISSUES

Informed Consent

Informed consent involves the client's right to know the purpose and nature of all aspects of client involvement with the helper. In reference to research and testing, clients have the right to know the general purposes of the research in which they are involved as well as how any tests they are taking are going to be used. Except in special cases (for example, court referrals for testing), clients also have the right to refuse to take part in any testing and research. Corey et al. (2003) note that when a client is not fully informed, the helper is open to liability concerns. Most ethical guidelines speak directly to the issue of informed consent. For instance, the *Ethical Standards of Human Service Professionals* states,

> Human service professionals negotiate with clients the purpose, goals, and nature of the helping relationship prior to its onset as well as inform clients of the limitations of the proposed relationship. (See Appendix B, Statement 1)

Today, an increasing number of authors are recommending that clients sign informed-consent forms indicating that they are fully aware of any therapeutic, testing, or research procedures in which they are participating (Cottone & Tarvydas, 1998; Thorndike et al., 1997). As testing and research become more prevalent, and within this increasingly liability-conscious society, the issue of informed consent has become paramount (Bennett, Bryant, VandenBos, & Greenwood, 1995).

Use of Human Subjects

Stanley Milgram's "shocking" research on obedience (1965, 1974) dramatically affected the way research has been conducted in the United States. Recruiting subjects through a local newspaper ad, he told them that they would be participating in research on the effects of punishment in learning. Assigning them to the role of teacher, he told the subjects that they would be administering an electrical shock to a learner every time the person did not complete a task properly. In actuality, the equipment was not hooked up, and the learner was an actor who would respond every time a "shock" was administered. As the experiment continued, the teacher was told to increase the voltage, and the learner, who initially was making mild grunting sounds following the shock, began to respond more strongly, eventually screaming. Despite the fact that many of the teachers protested what they were doing, with prodding by the experimenter, 65% of the subjects ended up administering 450 pseudo-volts to the learner, potentially enough to harm or kill a person had it been electricity. Although an interesting study, Milgram's research was much criticized for its potential psychological harm to the participants.

As a result of this study, as well as other research that had the potential to cause psychological or even physical harm to subjects, many restraints have been placed on the type of research in which people can participate. In fact, research like Milgram's could not legally be done today, and restraints on research that might cause physical or psychological harm are now guided by ethical standards and by legislation. For instance, most ethical guidelines now limit the amount of deception allowed in the use of research. In addition, federal legislation now requires that all organizations that conduct research supported by federal funds have a human subjects committee or institutional review board whose purpose is to ensure that there is little or no risk to research participants. Today, many institutions have adopted human subjects committees even if they do not receive federal funds.

Proper Interpretation and Use of Test Data

Human service professionals are not experts in test administration and test interpretation. Therefore, they must rely on those who are. However, effective human service professionals can use the results of test data in their work with clients. Therefore, they should carefully read the results of test reports and consult with experts in the field to understand how such data can best serve their clients. As noted earlier in this chapter, the proper use of test data involves sensitivity to clients, knowledge of informed consent, and awareness of the cultural biases that are inherent in some tests. Finally, human service professionals should understand that testing is one small aspect of a broader analysis of the individual that is called assessment. A test should never be used only to make predictions. If one test is helpful, two will be more helpful. And, if two tests are helpful, then two tests and a clinical interview will even be better! And, if two tests and a clinical interview are better, then what about interviewing others who know the individual being assessed? Whenever important decisions are being made, a careful assessment that is reliable, valid, and cross-culturally fair should be undertaken.

THE DEVELOPMENTALLY MATURE HUMAN SERVICE PROFESSIONAL

Understanding the Changing Face of Research, Program Evaluation, and Testing

The main purpose of research, program evaluation, and testing is to benefit our clients. Research helps us understand those interventions that are most effective with our clients, program evaluation helps us understand whether the programs we are offering benefit our clients, and help clients better understand themselves. Research, as Kuhn (1962) notes, is an ever-evolving process that continually adds new knowledge to the field. Tests are always improving, giving us better insights into the clients with whom we work. Because the evaluation process relies heavily on research and testing, it too is an evolving process. Developmentally mature human service professionals do not view research, evaluation, and testing as a stagnant process. Mature human service professionals understand that new ideas, new tests, and new programs will be devised, and they are flexible enough to adopt those concepts that will best benefit their clients.

SUMMARY

In this chapter, we examined the nature and purpose of research, program evaluation, and the use of tests in the work of the human service professional. We noted that research adds knowledge to our field and therefore helps us make wise decisions concerning treatment plans for our clients. Two broad categories of research we studied in this chapter included quantitative research and qualitative research. Quantitative research, we stated, relies on controlled research designs and can be applied in a laboratory setting or in the field. Quantitative research tests hypotheses or clarifies research questions. Qualitative research is generally field research that relies on the researcher to carefully observe and describe phenomena and to interpret the phenomena within a social context. This kind of research bases itself on the research question.

We briefly reviewed four kinds of quantitative research, specifically examining true experimental research, causal-comparative (ex post facto) research, correlational research, and survey research. We also explored two kinds of qualitative research called ethnographic research and historical research. We explained that in qualitative research, the researcher goes through a rigorous process of reviewing the data, synthesizing results, and drawing conclusions and generalizations. The researcher needs to be careful to not get caught up in his or her point of view and should be open to offering opinions that both support and contradict the ultimate findings. In contrast, the quantitative method attempts to carefully control the study and uses statistical analysis to come to conclusions. Regardless of the type of research you are doing, certain steps must be followed in implementing research, including reviewing the literature, developing a hypothesis or research question, designing the study, finding ways to analyze the data, and discussing the results.

The second major topic of this chapter was program evaluation. We discussed process (or formative) and outcome (or summative) evaluation. We noted process evaluation takes place during the activity being measured, whereas outcome evaluation takes place at the conclusion or after an activity has occurred. We noted that program evaluation ensures that the services we are offering our clients are of high quality. Basic research designs are sometimes helpful in evaluating our programs. Other times, we employ process or outcome evaluation techniques to examine the efficacy of our programs. In either case, evaluation ensures that we are ever vigilant in our efforts to improve services.

Testing was our third major topic in this chapter. We discussed the differences between norm-referenced and criterion-referenced tests, as well as standardized and informal assessments. In addition, we defined the varying types of ability tests, including achievement tests—such as survey battery, diagnostic, and readiness tests, and aptitude tests—such as cognitive ability, individual intelligence, special aptitude, and multiple aptitude tests. In the area of personality assessment, we briefly reviewed the differences among objective tests, projective tests, and interest inventories.

Relative to testing we next discussed the qualities of validity, reliability, practicality, and cross-cultural fairness, four attributes that should be examined in determining whether a test should be used. We also discussed the importance of understanding the concepts of measures of central tendency and measures of variability in the interpretation of tests. We noted that although human service professionals do not generally have enough training to give many of the more in-depth tests, they will be constantly exposed to test reports and test data. Therefore, it is important to be in close consultation with supervisors and experts in test administration.

Whether doing research or testing, the importance of fully informing our clients of the purpose and nature of their involvement is crucial. Clients have a right to informed consent concerning all aspects of their treatment. Finally, whether human service professionals are involved in research, the evaluation process, or testing, it is important that these processes are seen as evolving; that is, as more knowledge is gained through research and evaluation and as tests are improved, developmentally mature human service professionals must be willing to examine and adapt these new concepts and materials in ways that will benefit their clients.

EXPERIENTIAL EXERCISES

1. Critiquing a Journal Article

Obtain a research article from a human service journal and, using the following criteria, critique the article.

1. Have the authors used quantitative or qualitative research methods?
2. What kind of quantitative (e.g., true experimental, causal-comparative, correlational, survey) or qualitative (e.g., historical, ethnographic) methods have been used?
3. Was the hypothesis or research question based on an adequate literature review?
4. What results were found?
5. What are the implications of the results for the human service professional?
6. What future research might arise out of this research?
7. Generally, what did you think of the article?

2. Designing a Research Study

Have the instructor divide the class into groups of four or five students. Each group is to design a research study concerning the effectiveness of human service professionals with their clients. Each group is to design one of the following types of studies: a true experimental study, a causal-comparative, a correlational study, a survey study, a historical research study, or an ethnographic study. In designing your study, make sure you address the following issues:

1. Literature review
2. Hypothesis or research question
3. Research design
4. Results
5. Discussion

3. Developing Evaluation Instruments

In small groups or as a class, develop a process and an outcome evaluation instrument for your class.

4. Evaluating an Evaluation Form—Part 1

Most colleges and universities have some form of course evaluation that is completed at the end of the semester. Obtain a copy of the evaluation form that is used at your college and discuss any positive and negative aspects of that form.

5. Evaluating an Evaluation Form—Part 2

Visit a local social service agency and see whether the agency has any evaluation forms that are used to assess client satisfaction, the effectiveness of programs, or the overall effectiveness of the agency. Share these instruments in class.

6. Sharing Experiences with Testing

In class, discuss any positive or negative experiences you have had relative to taking a test.

7. Advantages and Disadvantages of Testing

In small groups, discuss the following issues, pick a spokesperson, and report back to the class. Have the instructor write on the board the advantages and disadvantages that are noted by the groups.

1. The advantages and disadvantages of the SATs
2. The advantages and disadvantages of individual intelligence testing
3. The advantages and disadvantages of personality assessment

8. Using Tests with Clients

Refer to the differing types of tests listed in the chapter and discuss the possible use of educational and psychological assessment for each of the following scenarios:

1. Johnny is a 12-year-old child in seventh grade. His grades have always been average, but recently his math scores have dropped considerably. In addition, he tells you that he found out not long ago that his parents are getting divorced.

2. William is 35 years old and recently separated. A few months following the separation, his wife accused him of molesting their 4-year-old child. He vehemently denies this accusation and states that she is "just saying those things in order to gain custody."

3. Judy is applying for a high-security job with the CIA. Following a background check, as a matter of course, they give her a number of assessment instruments.

4. Juanita is in lower management at a major computer firm. Her supervisor is thinking of recommending her for a promotion. Her new job would involve making quick decisions, and it requires a stable personality.

5. Jason is considering changing careers. He is not sure what career options are open for him and is unclear about what he likes to do. He is also unclear about what he is good at.

9. Evaluating the Passion Test

Using the following "Passion Test," discuss the following.

1. How might you show that this test is or is not valid?

2. How might you show that the test is or is not reliable?

3. Are any of the test questions cross-culturally biased? Explain.

4. What assumptions does this test make about men, women, and sexual orientation?

Passion Test

1. I like to have romantic dinners:
   a. very much
   b. somewhat
   c. a little bit
   d. not at all

2. I think Halle Berry (or Brad Pitt) is very hot:
   a. very much
   b. somewhat
   c. a little bit
   d. not at all

3. I like to have flowers sent to me:
   a. very much
   b. somewhat
   c. a little bit
   d. not at all

4. I prefer spicy food to bland food:
   a. very much
   b. somewhat
   c. a little bit
   d. not at all

5. I would like to spend a week on the Riviera:
   a. very much
   b. somewhat
   c. a little bit
   d. not at all

6. To me, romance is all in the head:
   a. very much
   b. somewhat
   c. a little bit
   d. not at all

7. I make love at least once a day:
   a. very much
   b. somewhat
   c. a little bit
   d. not at all

8. I would rather have a steamy conversation than have sex:
   a. very much
   b. somewhat
   c. a little bit
   d. not at all

9. I believe that passion is related to how much a person cares about you:
   a. very much
   b. somewhat
   c. a little bit
   d. not at all

10. I exercise at least three times a week
    a. very much
    b. somewhat
    c. a little bit
    d. not at all

10. Ethical and Professional Vignettes

Discuss the ethics of the following scenarios:

1. Recently, there has been some research on the effectiveness of various drugs to combat HIV. To test if there is any effect, a drug company obtains permission to randomly assign individuals who have tested HIV-positive to two groups. One group will get a new drug, and the second group will get a placebo (a sugar pill). Individuals do not know to which group they belong. Is this ethical? Professional? Legal?

2. Based on the available research, a human service professional, who works at a 30-day rehabilitation center for chemically dependent individuals, develops a program on confrontation and humiliation. Although individuals can theoretically leave at any time, in this program, those who do not admit to their addictions and who do not begin to make major changes in their lives are heavily confronted by the whole group, are forced to shave their heads, and during "social time" are made to sit in their rooms and think about their lives. Is this ethical? Professional? Legal?

3. To become more familiar with a local community religious group, a human service professional decides to become a participant observer and spends a week with the community at their retreat center. Part of their ritual is to smoke marijuana during their meditation times. Following the week at the center, he reports them to the local law enforcement agency for the illegal use of drugs. Is this ethical? Professional? Legal?

4. After receiving negative feedback concerning a workshop on communicating with teenagers, a human service professional decides, "They really didn't want to learn how to communicate with their kids. I simply won't do workshops on this topic for 'those people' any more." Is this reasonable? Ethical? Professional?

5. During the taking of some routine tests for promotion, it is discovered that, based on the results of the tests, there is a high probability that one of the

employees is abusing drugs and is a pathological liar. The firm decides not to promote him and instead fires him. Is this ethical? Professional? Legal?

6. An African–American mother is concerned that her child may have an attention problem. She goes to the teacher who supports her concerns and they go to the assistant principal requesting testing for a possible learning problem. The mother asks if the child could be given an individual intelligence test that can screen for such problems and the assistant principal states, "Those tests have been banned for minority students because of concerns about cross-cultural bias." The mother states that she will give her permission for such testing, but the assistant principal says, "I'm sorry, we'll have to make do with some other tests and observation." Is this ethical? Professional? Legal?

7. A test that has not been researched to show that it is, or is not, predictive for minority graduate students in social work is used as part of the program's admission process. When challenged on this, the head of the program states that the test has not been proven to be biased and that the program does have other criteria that it uses for admission. Is this ethical? Professional? Legal?

8. A social worker with no training in career development is giving interest inventories as she counsels individuals for career issues. Can she do this? Is this ethical? Professional? Legal? If this social worker were a colleague of yours, what, if anything, would you do?

9

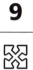

The Human
Service Professional
and the World of Work

When I was a young child, my father, a building contractor, took me around to various construction sites, and I would watch buildings slowly get built. As a teenager, during the summers, I would help a carpenter or general laborer at the sites. I remember getting picked up at five o'clock in the morning, being crammed half-asleep into the cab of a well-seasoned truck, to be taken on a bumpy ride to work. I would think to myself, "Is this what I want to do for the rest of my life?" Luckily, because I did well in school, I knew I'd be going on to college, but to do what?

Majoring in biology and thinking I was not bright enough to get into medical school, I chose dentistry as my eventual career path. My mind was made up, but something did not feel right. Although a part of me said, "Go to professional school in a medical-related field," another distant voice said, "This is not for you; you have other things to do in your life, other things that involve helping people." These divergent feelings and thoughts were certainly an outgrowth of many things, including my family values, my placement in my family, my interests, my own emerging values, and my abilities. Although it was a tough decision, I eventually chose to listen to my distant voice, and I switched majors to psychology. Eventually, mostly through selected trial and occasional error, I ended up in the field of counseling and human services. No doubt my life would have been made much easier if someone with training had assessed my likes and dislikes, my values, and my abilities; had helped me understand my personality style as it relates to the world of work; and helped me match these qualities with possible careers.

As I proceeded on my career journey through life, I continue to be faced with a number of choices. Should I go on to graduate school? Should I go toward clinical work or toward academia? Should I switch occupations totally? Again, my choices often seemed to be a product of trial and error. I would try something out to see if I liked it, if I was good at it, and would then make a decision about my future career direction. After working in a number of social service agencies, and after teaching for a number of years, I slowly settled into academia as a profession.

Despite the fact that I have been pretty satisfied at my work, there were times when my life did not feel complete. Therefore, other activities began to fill in some of the spaces. In my mid-twenties, I began to jog. As the years continued, running and aerobics became a focal point in my life. They offered an outlet for my stress, a place to meet other people, and an activity that took me away from my work. When I entered my early forties, I married and soon had two children. My life became filled with new joys and more responsibilities. With these changing life roles, I had to adapt to new ways of living in the world.

Now, as I enter my fifties, I think differently about my future. I now rarely think about changing jobs; instead, I think about how I can maximize my current job situation. And, where I thought I would never slow down or retire, I now look forward to a slower pace. Things have definitely changed in my career path.

I have found that my story, with its twists and turns, is common. And all of these —including my jogging, being a counselor, teaching, marrying, and having children—are part of my career development because they all define my life roles.

This chapter will attempt to explain how we define ourselves through our career roles. We will do this by defining important terms, reviewing prevalent models of career development, and exploring career resources. Perhaps most important, in this chapter we will learn the importance of making purposeful choices in our lives—choices that are made from understanding our personalities, abilities, and interests. We will learn that choosing our life roles is possible and better than letting fate make choices for us.

SOME DEFINITIONS

Perhaps more than any other subject in the helping professions, the career development process is the most misunderstood. Therefore, it is particularly important to start out with some basic definitions. The following are definitions of terms related to the career development process (Gysbers, Heppner, & Johnson, 2003; Herr & Cramer, 1996; Niles & Harris-Bowlsbey, 2002; Sears, 1982; Super, 1976; Wise, Charner & Randour, 1978). Keep in mind that some of these definitions may not be the same as our common, lay definitions.

Avocation—A chosen activity, not necessarily pursued for money, that gives the individual satisfaction and fulfills an important aspect of the person's life.

Career—The totality of work and life roles that a person takes on in life through which the individual expresses himself or herself. A career not only represents one's efforts at occupations but how all life roles are expressions of self.

Career Awareness—One's consciousness about career-related decisions, which can be facilitated through a self-examination of one's values, abilities, preferences, knowledge of occupations and life roles, and interests.

Career Counseling—Individual or group counseling with a focus to increase career awareness and to foster decision making relative to career goals.

Career Development—All the psychological, sociological, educational, physical, economic, and other factors that are at play in shaping one's career over the life span.

Career Guidance—A program, designed by helping professionals, that offers information concerning career development and facilitates career awareness for individuals.

Career Path—The sequence of positions or jobs, that typically signifies potential advancement, available to persons within an organization or business.

Jobs—Positions within a work environment (e.g., school, agency, business) that are similar in nature.

Leisure—Time taken from required effort (for example, job or occupation) to pursue self-chosen activities that express one's abilities and interests.

Occupation—Jobs of a similar nature that can be found within several work environments and connote the kinds of work a person is pursuing.

Occupations are definable outside of the person; careers are defined by the person's total work and life roles.

Work—Effort expended in pursuit of a job, occupation, or avocation to produce or accomplish something.

THE IMPORTANCE OF CAREER DEVELOPMENT

Many authors have highlighted the importance of career education and career counseling in facilitating one's career development. Work, a potentially important aspect of one's career development, serves a number of economic, social, and psychological needs for the individual (Herr & Cramer, 1996) (see Table 9.1).

Lack of adequate career planning has been associated in numerous studies with job dissatisfaction, whereas a good match between one's personality and chosen occupation has been shown to lead to job satisfaction (Assouline & Meir, 1987; Jagger, Neukrug & McAuliffe, 1992; Spokane, 1985). In a similar vein, Niles and Harris-Bowlsbey (2002) note that career uncertainty and occupational dissatisfaction have been shown to be related to psychological and physical stress. These factors highlight the importance of adequate career counseling for the clients of the human service professional.

Despite the importance of work and other career-related activities in our lives, our career development happens all too often by trial and error or hit or miss. Therefore, after reviewing some history of the career development process, we will examine some of the more prevalent theories that help us understand the career development process. In addition, we will explore sources of information that help us make informed choices. You will have the opportunity to examine the kinds of choices you have made in your life path and learn how you can apply some of these concepts to your clients. Finally, we will examine how human service professionals can optimize career choices for their clients and how developmentally mature human service professionals view the career development process from a life-span perspective.

A LITTLE BIT OF HISTORY

The Industrial Revolution of the late 1800s brought about many demographic changes throughout the United States. Almost overnight, thousands of people moved from rural areas to the cities, numerous immigrants settled mostly in urban areas, and, with this, a great number of children enrolled in city schools. Shifts in the types of available jobs were also evident, as was the need to assist these new city dwellers and students in their vocational development. In addition, social reform, as evidenced by the settlement houses and charity organization societies, reflected the new focus on helping individuals determine their futures. All these

Table 9.1 Different Purposes Work Can Serve

Economic	Social	Psychological
Gratification of wants or needs	A place to meet people	Self-esteem
Acquisition of physical assets	Potential friendships	Identity
Security against future contingencies	Human relationships	A sense of order
Liquid assets to be used for investment or deferred gratifications	Social status for the worker and his/her family	Dependability, reliability
Purchase of goods and services	A feeling of being valued by others for what one can produce	A feeling of mastery or competence
Evidence of success	A sense of being needed by others to get the job done or to achieve mutual goals	Self-efficacy
Assets to purchase leisure or free time	Responsibility	Commitment, personal evaluation

SOURCE: From *Career Guidance and Counseling through the Lifespan*, Fifth Edition, p. 70, by E. Herr and S. H. Cramer. 1996 by Pearson Education. Reprinted by permission of Addison Wesley Educational Publishers, Inc.

changes led to the beginnings of the vocational guidance movement, which represented one of the first attempts to help individuals make vocational decisions.

One of the first persons credited with a systematic approach to vocational guidance was Frank Parsons (McDaniels & Watts, 1994). Parsons suggested that vocational guidance involves a three-step process: knowing oneself, knowing job characteristics, and making a match between the two through "true reasoning" (Parsons, 1909, 1989). Although undergoing some changes over the years, this **trait-and-factor approach** to vocational guidance has continued to be prominent in assisting individuals in the career counseling process. Today, the trait-and-factor approach states (Savickas & Walsh, 1996; Zunker, 2002),

1. Individuals have unique traits that can be measured, and they seek out environments for those traits.

2. Occupations require workers with certain traits.

3. The better the fit between the person and the occupation is, the better the outcome (e.g., job satisfaction, productivity, etc.) will be.

4. As assessment procedures of the individual and the environment improve, the helper will be more effective at helping clients make choices that will ultimately lead to job satisfaction.

In 1913, the increased emphasis on vocational guidance led to the founding of the National Vocational Guidance Association (NVGA). This association was a forerunner to the American Counseling Association (ACA). In the 1920s and 1930s, vocational guidance was offered mainly in the schools and by the U.S. Department of Labor, and the testing movement began. The merging of vocational guidance with testing was a natural consequence because assessment offered a relatively quick and reliable means of determining individual traits. At about the same time, the U.S. Department of Labor published the **Dictionary of Occupational Titles (DOT),** which represented one of the first attempts at organizing career information. Now individuals could assess their traits and match these traits to existing jobs.

In the 1950s, a shift from vocational guidance to career development began (Niles & Harris-Bowlsbey, 2002). No longer was there an emphasis simply on making a job choice; instead, emphasis was placed on one's lifelong career patterns. In addition, with this new definition, postvocational patterns related to retiring were now included in the definition of career guidance. Donald Super, with his developmental approach to career guidance, was one of the leaders in changing the focus from vocational guidance to developmental career counseling.

With the emergence of the humanistic approach to the helping relationship and government initiatives such as the National Defense Education Act (NDEA) of 1958, which stressed career guidance in the schools, new comprehensive models of career guidance were developed in the 1960s and 1970s. These models viewed career guidance in the broadest sense and included focusing on lifelong patterns of career development, helping individuals make choices that reflected their self-concepts, defining career guidance as not only occupational choices but also as leisure and avocational options, and allowing for flexibility and change in one's lifelong career process (Herr & Cramer, 1996). In addition, these models emphasized the individual, not the helper, as the career decision maker.

During the 1980s, 1990s, and into the 21st century, viewing career development as a life-span process has been increasingly emphasized. Within this framework, career development models have been expanded to assist individuals in their lifelong pursuits. In addition, the computer age has brought about a wealth of accessible information that allows for quick exploration of the world of work. The evolution of career development models in conjunction with this new technology makes career exploration an exciting and in-depth process.

MODELS OF CAREER DEVELOPMENT

When I ask students how they chose their college major, I often get a response such as, "Well, it was something I thought I'd like to do." Similarly, when I ask an individual how he or she ended up in a job, I find responses such as, "The job was available" or "I always wanted to be a . . ." Also, it is not unusual for a returning student to say to me, "I always knew I was in the wrong field; I don't know why I did that for so many years." These responses show me how little reflection and self-assessment have taken place when many people make one of the most significant decisions in their lives. If individuals had a broader understanding of their likes and dislikes, abilities, and personality characteristics, the reasons why they make these important choices would be clearer. Greater awareness of individual traits, along with an understanding of the career development process, would probably lead many individuals in different directions from those in which they settled—directions that would yield greater career and life satisfaction.

Since the beginning of the vocational guidance movement, and particularly during the past 25 years, a number of career development models have been devised that have a common focus of helping individuals understand their career choices. However, despite this common theme, there are some major differences among the models. For instance, **self-efficacy theory** states that career choices are based on our *beliefs* about our ability in specific areas, even if there is evidence to the contrary (a successful student who believes she cannot go onto graduate school because of fears she will not be able to do well in a research course) (Albert & Luzzo, 1999; Bandura, 1997; McAuliffe, 1992). **Decision-making theory,** on the other hand, views the individual's decision-making process as crucial in successfully making career choices (Tiedeman & Miller-Tiedeman, 1984; Tiedeman & O'Hara, 1963), and **constructivist theory** suggests that how we make sense of and derive meaning from the world is basic to the kinds of career decisions we make (McAuliffe, 1993, 1999; Peavy, 1994). Finally, **situational theory** states that career choices are sometimes out of our control (for example, unavailability of jobs because of a recession) (Warnath, 1975). However, probably the two models that have been most prevalent in the field are the **developmental** and **personality approaches to career development.**

The Developmental Perspective

Like the developmental perspectives studied in Chapter 5, career development, from a life-span viewpoint, involves a series of stages through which individuals pass. Two of the major developmental theories are those of **Eli Ginzberg** (1972) and **Donald Super** (Super, Savickas, & Super, 1996). Super, in particular, has extensively researched his career development theory, and this will be presented in brief form.

Super's Developmental Self-Concept Theory Super views career development as a lifelong process in which we attempt to make choices based on our view of self. He stated that individuals differ in their abilities, interests, and personalities and that, despite these differences, each person can fit into a number of occupations. He further noted that as we pass through the life stages, our perceptions of self may change and we may therefore shift our orientation toward the world of work.

Super's developmental self-concept theory describes career development as a five-stage process. The **growth stage** (from birth to 14 years of age) involves the development of career self-concept through identification with others and beginning awareness of interests and abilities related to the world of work. Included in this stage is the very young child's beginning awareness of the world of work and the middle school youth who compares his or her abilities and interests with those of his peers. In the **exploration stage** (ages 14–24 years), we begin to test out our occupational fantasies tentatively through work, school, and leisure activities. At the later part of this stage, the individual begins to crystallize his or her vocational preferences by choosing an occupation or further professional training. The **establishment stage** (ages 24–44 years) involves stabilizing our career choices and

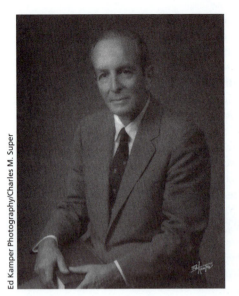

Ed Kamper Photography/Charles M. Super

Donald Super, with his developmental approach to career guidance, was one of the leaders in changing the focus from vocational guidance to developmental career counseling.

advancing in our chosen fields, and the **maintenance stage** (ages 44–64 years) encompasses the preservation of our current status in the choices we have made and avoidance of stagnation. In the **deceleration stage** (ages 64 to death), we begin to disengage from our chosen fields and focus more on retirement and leisure and avocational activities. Later in his life, Super added a minicycle in which he suggests that we can cycle through the five stages at any point in our careers.

Personality-Based Theories of Career Development

Roe's Psychodynamic Approach In 1956, Ann Roe developed a rather elaborate psychodynamic theory that based career choice partially on the kinds of early parenting received (Roe, 1956). **Roe's psychodynamic approach** suggests that parents can be classified as either warm or cold and that these two styles result in one of three types of emotional climates: emotional concentration on the child, acceptance of the child, or avoidance of the child. The type of emotional climate in the home, said Roe, will result in one of six types of parent–child relationships, which influences the kinds of occupational choices the child will eventually make (Roe & Siegelman, 1964). Parenting style, said Roe, ultimately results in the individual having one of the following eight orientations toward the world of work: service, business, organization, technology, outdoor, science, general culture, and arts and entertainment. Despite the fact that her theory has not been supported by research, it was one of the first attempts to link early history with eventual career choices.

Holland's Personality Type and Occupational Code Approach Although John Holland did not directly address how our personalities were formed, his vocational choice theory states that people express their personalities through the types of career choices that they make. Holland proposes that there are six personality types, which he calls **realistic, investigative, artistic, social, enterprising**, and **conventional**. By taking an assessment instrument such as the Strong Vocational Interest Inventory (Consulting Psychologists Press, 1994) or the Self-Directed Search (SDS) (Holland, 1994), an individual can determine which type of work best fits his or her personality orientation. This is done by rank ordering the top three personality codes and then matching one's personality orientation (code) to the jobs that best express those personality traits. Then an individual can generate a list of jobs to which he or she might be best suited.

Holland stated that, regardless of ability, we can fit into a number of work environments based on our personality. For example, although I may not have the ability to be a physician, I still might enjoy working in the medical field. Much research has found that the better the fit between an individual's personality type and his or her chosen field, the more likely that person would be satisfied in his or her career (Assouline & Meir, 1987; Jagger, Neukrug, & McAuliffe, 1992). Although it is not as valid as taking one of the instruments just described, Activity 9.1 will give you a sense of your personality code.

Now that you have examined your personality type, let's look at some of the work environments that fit various personality types. For example, some work environments for the various personality types include the following: (1) realistic type: a filling station, a machine shop, a farm, a construction site, and a barber shop; (2) investigative type: a research laboratory, a diagnostic case conference, a library, and work groups of scientists, mathematicians, or research engineers; (3) artistic type: a play rehearsal, a concert hall, a dance studio, a study, a library, and an art or music studio; (4) social type: a school classroom, counseling offices, mental hospitals, religious settings, educational offices, and recreational centers; (5) enterprising type: a car lot, a real estate office, a political rally, and an advertising agency; (6) conventional type: a bank, an accounting firm, a post office, a file room, and a business office (Brown, 2003). Appendix F contains a more detailed description of the codes and some occupations that match them.

To obtain a more comprehensive examination of the work environments, Holland and his colleagues have written a book called the **Dictionary of Holland Occupational Codes** (Gottfredson, Holland, & Ogawa, 1996). This book lists, by **Holland code,** thousands of jobs. After an individual discovers his or her top three codes by going through the book, he or she can make a list of possible jobs that are of interest. This is where the work begins. After making a list of potential jobs, the person needs to obtain information about them, which can be accomplished in a number of ways. First, the individual can use many sources to obtain information about specific jobs (see the section entitled "The Use of Informational Systems in Career Development"). Second, once the list has been narrowed, the person can go on informational interviews to hear firsthand about those jobs.

Integrating Models of Career Development

When working with clients, most career development experts use an integrative approach to career counseling. Let's use, as an example, a 17-year-old who is in the exploration stage of her career. You decide that it would be appropriate to give

ACTIVITY 9.1   What Planet Do You Come From?

Imagine that you are on a space ship traveling to another solar system. When you get to this solar system, you see six planets, each of which is occupied by people who share similar qualities. Which planet would you land on first? Then if you left that planet, which would you go to next, and so forth.

Assessment: Take the letter that corresponds to the groups that you picked and place them, one after another, in the order that you picked them. For instance, I picked the Social group first, the Artistic group second, and the Enterprising group third. Therefore, placing them in order we find "SAE." This is my code. After you have determined your code, read the Appendix F, *Understanding Your Holland Code*.

Planets

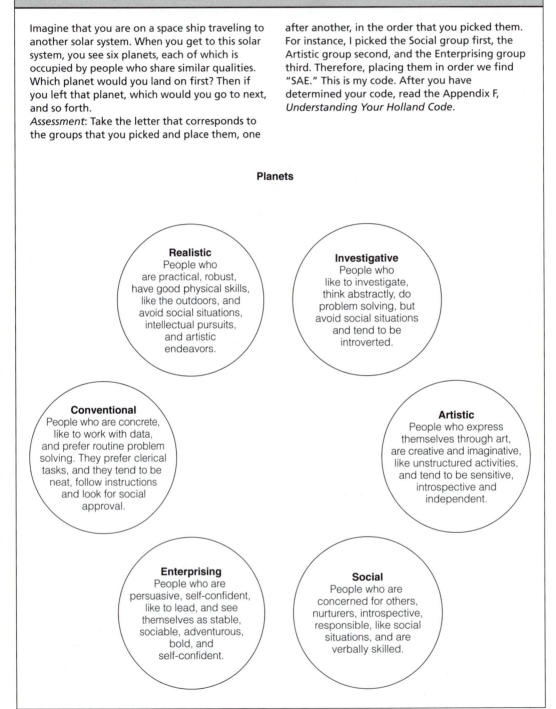

Realistic
People who are practical, robust, have good physical skills, like the outdoors, and avoid social situations, intellectual pursuits, and artistic endeavors.

Investigative
People who like to investigate, think abstractly, do problem solving, but avoid social situations and tend to be introverted.

Conventional
People who are concrete, like to work with data, and prefer routine problem solving. They prefer clerical tasks, and they tend to be neat, follow instructions and look for social approval.

Artistic
People who express themselves through art, are creative and imaginative, like unstructured activities, and tend to be sensitive, introspective and independent.

Enterprising
People who are persuasive, self-confident, like to lead, and see themselves as stable, sociable, adventurous, bold, and self-confident.

Social
People who are concerned for others, nurturers, introspective, responsible, like social situations, and are verbally skilled.

career interest inventories and aptitude tests to understand the occupations in which her personality might best fit. Upon giving the Self-Directed Search and the Strong Vocational Interest Inventory, you discover that your client has high realistic, investigative, and enterprising codes. One possible occupation would be engineering. You offer varying choices to the student, including engineering, at which point she says, "Oh, I always thought about doing that, but I know I couldn't make the grades in college." Because this student has done well in high school and scored high on her aptitude test in the areas associated with engineering, there seems to be no objective evidence that this is true. Instead, it appears that this student's beliefs about herself are deterring her from at least one possible career. Therefore, working on examining and possibly changing her beliefs (self-efficacy theory) could help her find a satisfactory career, possibly in engineering.

After an involved career assessment, our client decides to enter college and major in engineering. However, just before our client graduates from high school, her mother suddenly becomes chronically ill (situational factor), funds for college become depleted, and this young woman has to decide between going to college and taking out massive loans or delaying college and helping care for her ailing mother. At this point, the helper, having a good decision-making model, can assist this young woman in this very difficult decision. It is important that the helper understand the world of the client, for how the client makes meaning of her current predicament is crucial for the kinds of decisions she eventually makes (constructivist theory).

This example shows the importance of knowing a client's strengths and interests, understanding and being able to implement developmental and personality theories, being able to apply self-efficacy theory, recognizing the importance of situational factors, helping the client understand how he or she makes meaning of the world, and how decision-making theory is important when struggling with major choices in life.

To understand further how knowledge of the various theories can help us work with clients, read the excerpt in Box 9.1. Consider Roger's passage through Super's exploration, establishment, maintenance, and deceleration stages, how personality theory (for example, Holland and Roe) would explain the choices he made, how situational factors affected his career decisions, and how the way he made sense of the world led him to his various occupations.

THE USE OF INFORMATIONAL SYSTEMS
IN CAREER DEVELOPMENT

An extensive amount of information on all aspects of occupational information is available in the field of career development. In the career counseling process, using some of these resources as a method of understanding the nature of different jobs, as well as examining long-range job forecasts, is usually important. In this section, we will examine some of the more prevalent informational resources available to helpers and their clients.

BOX 9.1   Roger: An Integrative Understanding of Career Development

Sixty-one-year-old Roger is about to retire as coordinator of field-placement and certification services at a College of Education and Human Services. Roger places teacher education students, human services students, and school counseling students into the local public schools and assists with getting students credentialed in their respective fields. However, his route to this occupation was by no means direct.

When Roger first started college, he had an interest in becoming a minister; however, because he was totally turned off by religious courses, he gave up that idea. Although he considered veterinary medicine, he decided not to pursue this interest because he would have to transfer schools; he instead majored in math education and joined ROTC for the financial aid afforded by the GI Bill. Although Roger wanted to enter pilot training, he was told that he would have to commit to the air force for five years, a commitment he did not wish to make. Therefore, he took a job in meteorology, which required only a three-year commitment. Roger so enjoyed meteorology that he began to think that a career in the air force, being a meteorologist, might not be so bad. He became enthused about the field, received his master's degree, and traveled the world. Continually promoted, Roger practiced meteorology in the air force for 18 years. Wanting a change, Roger then took a job as head of ROTC at a large midwestern university and later worked at officer assignment in personnel.

Then after 24 years in the air force, promotion to colonel, and having seen some friends become bitter and others start drinking too much, Roger began to feel that the air force was not fun any more. So, he changed occupations in midstream.

In his mid-40s, Roger retired from the air force but not from work. He pursued a master's degree in business administration (M.B.A.) and subsequently took a position at the financial aid office at the university where he now works. However, feeling a lack of fit, he stopped pursuing his M.B.A. and eventually took a position in freshman advising. Finding he really enjoyed academic advising and wanting skills to match what he was doing, he started his master's degree in counseling. Although Roger considered pursuing a career as a school counselor, he decided to stay in academic advising and eventually took on his current position as coordinator of field-placement and certification services. Then, after 10 years in this job, Roger decided to retire and move on to other interests and activities.

Roger has had a full life. He has fallen into some jobs, chosen others, gotten tired of some, fully immersed himself in others, and is now ready to retire. Is this the end of his career? Well, hardly. He may be ending this job, and perhaps he will not take on a new one. But until he dies, he will continue to work and will pursue leisure activities and avocations.

Dictionary of Occupational Titles

The Dictionary of Occupational Titles (DOT), which is published by the U.S. Department of Labor (1999), is a comprehensive classification system for occupations. The DOT provides a short description for each of approximately 30,000 occupations and offers a nine-code classification system for each job. The first three numbers of the classification system describe jobs in general occupational groups, and the second series of three numbers presents the complexity of worker traits related to the use of data on the job, the type of interactions with people at work, and the use of different types of things on the job (for example, equipment, food). Each of the second series of numbers ranges from 0 to 9, with the level of complexity decreasing as you approach 9. The last three digits distinguish jobs that have the same first six digits. For instance, psychiatric social worker and school social worker have the same first six digits but are distinguished by the last three digits (see Box 9.2).

> **BOX 9.2   An Example from the DOT: Social-Services Aide (DOT Number 195.367.034)**
>
> Assists professional staff of public social service agency, performing any combination of following tasks: interviews individuals and family members to compile information on social, educational, criminal, institutional, or drug history. Visits individuals in homes or attends group meetings to provide information on agency services, requirements, and procedures. Provides rudimentary counseling to agency clients.
>
> Oversees day-to-day group activities of residents in institution. Meets with youth groups to acquaint them with consequences of delinquent acts. Refers individuals to various public or private agencies for assistance. May care for children in client's home during client's appointments. May accompany handicapped individuals to appointments. (U.S. Department of Labor, 1999, p. 163)

The Enhanced Guide for Occupational Exploration

The **Enhanced Guide for Occupational Exploration (GOE)** (Maze & Mayall, 1995) was originally published in 1979 as a companion volume to the DOT. The GOE offers job descriptions based on skills, abilities, physical requirements, environment, salary, and job outlook. Although the Guide only focuses on 2800 jobs, these jobs represent 95 percent of the workforce. The GOE can still be used with the DOT and is a quicker and easier way to examine job possibilities.

Occupational Outlook Handbook

The **Occupational Outlook Handbook** (OOH) (2002–2003a) includes information on the outlook for selected occupations, the nature of the work of those occupations, the type of training that is needed for the job, and wage and employment conditions. Although the handbook examines only approximately 250 jobs, and is not always perfect in its predictions, it is a good source of information concerning general categories of work.

Interest and Aptitude Testing in Career Counseling

Over the years, a number of assessment instruments have been developed to assist in the career exploration process of individuals. Probably the most important of these have been the interest inventories. Inventories like the **Strong Vocational Interest Inventory** (Consulting Psychologists Press, 1994), the **Career Decision–Making System (CDM)** (Harrington & O'Shea, 2000), and the **Career Assessment Inventory (CAI)** (Johansson, 1996) generally compare an individual's interests in areas such as school subjects, types of people, types of occupations, amusements, and personal characteristics with those of people in varying occupations. Therefore, one can obtain a sense of whether a client might share similar interests with people in those occupations. Other interest inventories like the **Self-Directed Search (SDS)** (Holland, 1994) and the Strong Vocational Interest Inventory (again) examine an individual's personality orientation toward the world of work and usually provide occupations in which the client might find a good fit.

Aptitude testing has also been a valuable aid in the career assessment process. These tests allow an individual to examine whether occupational preferences match the individual's ability. For instance, an individual who has interest in becoming a researcher but has little math ability may have a difficult time achieving his or her occupational goals. Some of the aptitude tests that include this type of career assessment program include the **Differential Aptitude Test (DAT)** and the **General Aptitude Test Battery (GATB),** which is published by the U.S. Department of Labor, Employment and Training Administration.

Computer-Assisted Career Guidance

The expansion in the use of personal computers has made career information systems available to a vast array of individuals. Computers offer an easy and quick method of accessing large amounts of career information. Today, numerous computer programs allow us to assess abilities, interests, values, and skills and let us obtain all kinds of occupational information. Following are some of the ways that the computer is used today in career guidance.

Comprehensive Computer-Based Programs Increasingly, computer-based programs are being developed that allow the individual to examine his or her values, interests, and skills and contain information on such things as occupations, college and trade schools, college majors, job availability, and financial aid. Many of these computer programs can be found in schools, colleges, business and industry, public employment and labor-related agencies, and private career counseling agencies. Some of the more popular programs include the **Guidance Information System (GIS)** (Riverside Publishing Company, 1997), Discover (ACT Discover Center, 1998), and the System of Interactive Guidance and Information-Plus (SIGI-Plus) (Educational Testing Services, 1998–1999).

Computerized Testing It is now possible to offer many interest and ability tests on computer and, increasingly, helpers will no longer have to send tests out to be scored or spend a lengthy amount of time hand scoring an instrument. Many of the traditional assessment instruments are rapidly being developed for computer usage.

The Internet Occupational information is increasingly being found on the Internet. Today, the DOT and the OOH can be downloaded, for a price, from the Internet. More recently, **O★NET**, developed by the U. S. Department of Labor (2002), has come on line. This resource is intended to eventually replace the DOT, and it offers comprehensive information on job skills and job requirements. Also, most publishing companies have now begun to sell software on the Internet, and in some cases, you can download the software directly from the Internet—for a price, of course. As the Internet is increasingly used, we will see an explosion of career information that can be found on it.

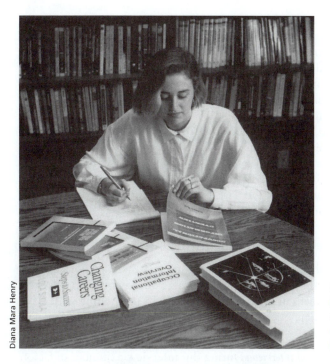

Diana Mara Henry

Sources of occupational information can greatly aid an individual's understanding of his or her career choices.

Other Sources of Occupational Information

The amount of occupational information that is available is enormous, and much of it is free. For instance, materials can be obtained from a number of government agencies, commercial publishers, professional associations, educational institutions, and periodicals. In addition, many colleges and trade schools have career centers available for student use and sometimes for the general public. Finally, even your local bookstore is often filled with career counseling information. One excellent paperback that can assist you or a client in the career exploration process and that gives a rather comprehensive list of available career resources is *What Color Is Your Parachute?* (Bolles, 2002).

CHOOSING A CAREER
IN THE HUMAN SERVICE PROFESSION

Am I in the Right Field?

How do you know if the human service field is a good choice for you? After reading this text, you should have a sense if you are the type of person who has or wishes to strive for the personality characteristics considered important in human service work (for example, empathy, caring, being nondogmatic, relationship builder, competent, etc.). However, you may still be wondering, "Is this something I really want to do?" The job characteristics of the human service professional (discussed in the next section) might help you decide if you want to enter the field; however, you might also want to examine your abilities and interests to see if there is a fit between your personality type and the work environment of the human service field. You did this to a small degree in Activity 9.1. However, if you want a more comprehensive understanding of your personality style, see if the career services center at your college or university can help you understand your career aspirations. Roger, in our example earlier, did not have the opportunity to have a comprehensive career assessment for himself. Perhaps such an assessment might have assisted him in his career search through life. In addition to self-knowledge, such assessments can be a valuable exercise in helping you understand how to work with clients who are wondering about their career direction. Finally, as you read the next section, consider applying the strategies to your own career development.

Helping Clients Choose a Career

Between the numerous theories of career counseling and the enormous amount of occupational information available to professionals, you may be asking, "Where do I start when doing career counseling with clients?" To make some sense of all that we have discussed, let me offer some strategies when doing career counseling with adults.

1. *Conduct a thorough clinical interview:* During this interview a number of factors can be assessed that are crucial to the client's career development process, including the following:
    a. *Early childhood:* Assess how early childhood issues have affected the client's propensity toward certain careers
    b. *Socioeconomic status:* Assess how socioeconomic status of one's family of origin has affected the client's aspirations
    c. *Parent's career development:* Assess how the career development of parents has affected the client's aspirations
    d. *Emotional problems:* Assess how emotional problems could interfere with career decision making
    e. *Situational issues:* Assess situational issues that could interfere with career decision making
    f. *Developmental level:* Assess the developmental level (for example, Super) of the client
    g. *Worldview:* Assess how the individual understands his or her world, and how does the client's construction of reality affect the choices he or she makes
2. *Conduct testing:* Measure clients' abilities, interests, and personality characteristics (for example, review of school records, aptitude testing, Holland Code, the CAI, the Strong).
3. *Develop treatment strategies:* Based on your clinical interview, the developmental stage of the client (for example, Super), and your assessment

of your client thus far, in collaboration with your client, devise treatment strategies that are congruent with client developmental readiness.

4. *Offer resources:* Make available appropriate informational resources that can be used in conjunction with your treatment plan.

5. *Raise awareness:* Assist the client in understanding the world of work and factors that could potentially affect career choice (economic conditions, market saturation, etc.).

6. *Facilitate decision making:* Have the client make tentative career decisions.

7. *Examine choices:* Explore the practicality of the career decisions chosen and begin to crystallize a choice.

8. *Facilitate choice making:* Have the client take preliminary steps toward choosing a career path by doing such things as informational interviews with individuals who have taken a similar path, shadowing people at a job, and reading literature about the client's potential career path.

9. *Follow-up:* Follow-up with client to ensure satisfaction and closure of the career development process.

10. *Recycle:* If the client is unsatisfied with his or her progress, start the process over and reexamine issues.

As you can imagine from this list, a thorough career assessment can be a rather lengthy process. However, using such a process creates career choice rather than career happenstance.

ETHICAL AND PROFESSIONAL ISSUES

Optimizing Career Options—Being All That You Can Be

Over the years, I have heard many discouraging stories related to the career development process. For instance, a successful college student told me that her high school counselor said she would never succeed in college and that she should find a job in a technical occupation. A 55-year-old man told me, upon losing his management job, that he was convinced he did not have the skills to make a career shift. A number of female students in the helping professions have not pursued graduate school, particularly doctoral programs, because of fears of math. What do these scenarios have in common? They all speak to the limited focus that many of us have about our abilities or the abilities of others.

One should never tell another that he or she cannot succeed in a field. Although it is reasonable to tell a client specific qualifications for a field and to explore whether the client currently has those qualifications, it is condescending to assume that another person cannot succeed in a certain occupation. As mental health professionals, we should try to optimize the choices that individuals have. Although a person may not currently have the ability, if he or she is motivated, we need to encourage the client to reach for his or her potential. As good helpers, the best we can do is to point out an individual's strengths and weaknesses, listen carefully, and help the client decide what options seem best.

We do a service for clients when we facilitate their career exploration by expanding the choices they have for their career development. After expanding options, clients can make better-informed choices about the direction they want to take in their lives. We would be violating our ethical guideline related to "competence" if our biases and actions limited our clients' choices.

THE DEVELOPMENTALLY MATURE HUMAN SERVICE PROFESSIONAL

Viewing Career Choice as a Life-Span Process

Developmentally mature human service professionals see the career development process from a life-span perspective. They view this process as a flowing river that twists and turns, with parts that seem shallow, dangerous, and scary and parts that are deep, still, and stable. Developmentally mature human service professionals see this river as starting to flow in young childhood when youngsters wonder about the world of work; picking up speed in adolescence when teenagers begin to explore their interests, values, and abilities; moving more rapidly and dangerously in young adulthood when individuals tentatively choose careers; becoming deep but sometimes twisting and turning in mid-adulthood when middle-aged workers feel established in their careers or individuals decide to take a fresh look at career choices; and finally slowing down in later life when individuals move out of work and into leisure activities or shift the type or amount of work they are doing. Developmentally mature human service professionals are willing to flow, for a short while, along this river with their clients; perhaps, if helpers are good navigators, they can help guide the client down the river along the most direct and stable route.

SUMMARY

In this chapter, we examined the career development process and looked at the important position that career plays in our lives. We started by offering some basic definitions of avocation, career, career awareness, career counseling, career development, career guidance, career path, jobs, leisure, occupation, and work. After defining some basic terms, we talked about the importance of work in our lives. In particular, we noted how work fills economic, social, and psychological needs.

In the next section of this chapter, we explored the beginnings of the career counseling and career education movements. We discussed the role that the Industrial Revolution played in bringing on the vocational guidance movement and highlighted the important role Parsons played. We described Parsons' trait-and-factor theory and noted how educators first used it. We discussed the beginning of the NVGA as well as some of the early occupational information systems that were developed. Next, we showed the historical importance of the developmental models of Super and others in helping us understand career development, as well as the beginnings of the personality theories of Roe and Holland.

As we continued in this chapter, we discussed how the career development process today tends to be viewed from a developmental perspective. We also highlighted the importance of understanding one's abilities, values, and interests when making decisions relating to occupational choice. We examined the career development theories of Super, Roe, and Holland. More specifically, we discussed the developmental stages of Super, including the growth, exploration, establishment, maintenance, and deceleration stages. And, we examined the Holland codes: realistic, investigative, artistic, social, enterprising, and conventional. We also discussed the importance of Roe's psychodynamic perspective in understanding the person. In addition, we mentioned some other approaches to understanding the career development process including decision-making theory, self-efficacy theory, constructivist theory, and situational factors.

In this chapter, we also noted that there is a vast amount of informational material in the area of career development. We highlighted the *DOT,* the *OOH,* the Enhanced *GOE, O*NET,* the use of interest and aptitude testing, and the use of computer-assisted career guidance such as comprehensive computer-based programs, testing, and the Internet. Finally, we described specific steps you might take when doing career counseling.

Near the end of this chapter, we noted that professionally astute human service professionals optimize and expand job options for their clients. These human service professionals do not assume clients cannot be successful in certain fields. Instead, effective human service workers point out the qualifications required for various occupations; note the skills, values, and interests of the client; and help clients make wise choices for their future. Along these lines, we stated that developmentally mature human service professionals can optimize client choices throughout the life span, whether it be helping the 5-year-old in his first awareness of the world of work or in assisting the 85-year-old in deciding what activities would give her the most pleasure in this part of her life.

EXPERIENTIAL EXERCISES

1. Work, Avocations, Leisure Activities: What Are They?

Define the words *work, avocations,* and *leisure activities.* How are they the same? How are they different?

2. Satisfaction of Needs

Using the following chart, give examples of how work, avocations, and leisure activities may satisfy some of the needs listed:

	Work	Avocations	Leisure Activities
Income			
Ego/Pride			
Self-Esteem			
Meaning in Life			
Social Interaction			
Sense of Identity			

3. Personality Development and Career Choices

Describe how each of the following has influenced your career choices:

1. Early child-rearing practices by your parents or guardians
2. Modeling by parents or guardians
3. Position in your family
4. Personality factors of siblings
5. Other early influences that may have affected your personality formation

4. Situational Factors and Career Choices

Describe how the following situational factors may have influenced your career choices:

1. Economic factors
2. Geographical factors
3. Health factors
4. Social factors
5. Other factors

5. Self-Efficacy, Decision Making, and Constructivist Factors in Career Decision Making

Discuss how each of the following factors might have affected your career decision-making process. Note that the theory that underlies the factor is in parentheses.

1. Your self-evaluation of your abilities (self-efficacy theory).
2. Your ability at making important decisions in life (decision-making theory).
3. How you understand and make sense out of the world of work (constructivist theory).

6. Developmental Career Strategies

Divide the class into small groups, assigning each group to one of Super's five developmental stages. Each group should develop ways to assist individuals in their career development on the basis of developmental stages.

7. Finding Out About an Occupation

Interview an individual in an occupation about which you would like more information. Ask the following questions as well as any others you might find interesting:

1. Do you view your current job as part of your career or as a transitory job?
2. How long have you held this job?
3. If you view this job as part of your career, when did you first start to think about doing what you are doing?
4. What early family factors affected your eventual career choices?
5. What situational factors affected your career choice?
6. What interests, abilities, and values do you hold that seem to fit with your career choice?

8. Exploring the DOT and OOH

Gather the following information and discuss the varying information you received in small groups in your class.

1. From the DOT, choose one occupation to examine. Copy the general description of the job, along with information about the level of skills needed for people, data, and things (the middle three digits of the nine-digit code).
2. From the OOH, choose one occupation to examine. Copy the job's DOT nine-digit code, information about job characteristics, job forecast, and earning power. Then examine the job characteristics in the DOT.

9. Assessing Your Developmental Stage

1. Box 9.3 is a checklist of the Exploration Stage of Super's developmental theory and was developed by Harris-Bowlsbey, Spivack, and Lisansky (1991, p. 175). In this checklist, Super's exploration stage is broken down into crystallization, specification, and implementation tasks. Go through the checklist and identify those areas in which you have not completed a task leading to eventual career choice. Or, if you believe you have successfully passed through the exploration stage, give this checklist to a client or friend to complete.

2. Greenhaus (1987) has taken Super's Establishment Stage and broken it down into what he calls Early Establishment, and Achievement or Late

BOX 9.3 Exploration Stage Checklist

	Not Yet Completed	Already Completed
Crystallization Tasks		
Realizing that I need to crystallize my alternatives.	☐	☐
Knowing how to organize occupations and programs of study in a meaningful way.	☐	☐
Knowing what interests me.	☐	☐
Knowing what my abilities/skills are.	☐	☐
Knowing what my values are.	☐	☐
Knowing how to use information about myself to focus my exploration of occupations and educational programs.	☐	☐

	Not Yet Completed	Already Completed
Applying the steps of a planful decision-making process to my vocational and educational choices.	☐	☐
Knowing which life roles I want to play.	☐	☐
Identifying several occupations for detailed exploration.	☐	☐
Identifying several educational programs for detailed exploration.	☐	☐
Specification Tasks		
Selecting criteria that will assist in narrowing my occupational alternatives.	☐	☐
Gathering detailed information about high-priority occupations and educational programs.	☐	☐
Using information and criteria to make a tentative selection of occupational and educational programs.	☐	☐
Declaring a major or choosing a program of study.	☐	☐
Drafting plans to "reality test" three or more occupations.	☐	☐
Implementation Tasks		
Drafting a plan for the implementation of possible educational or occupational choices.	☐	☐
Learning and using job interviewing skills.	☐	☐
Learning and using networking skills (to identify available jobs).	☐	☐
Finding a full-time job in the chosen occupation.	☐	☐

Establishment. Box 9.4 is a checklist I created based on these substages. Go through the checklist, and identify those areas in which you have not completed a task leading to eventual career choice. Of, if you believe you have successfully passed through the establishment stage, give this checklist to a client or friend to complete.

BOX 9.4 Establishment Stage Checklist

	Not Yet Completed	Already Completed
Early Establishment Tasks		
I have settled in fairly well to my career.	☐	☐
I fit in at my work setting pretty well.	☐	☐
I feel a sense of belonging to my organization.	☐	☐
I would rarely "rock the boat" at my work setting.	☐	☐
At my work setting, I am learning what I am good at.	☐	☐
I often reflect on how well I perform at work.	☐	☐
To some degree, my sense of self depends on how I achieve at work.	☐	☐
I often look to others for approval about how well I am doing work.	☐	☐
Achievement Tasks (Late Establishment Tasks)		
I am definitely "moving up" in my work setting.	☐	☐
I am a creative and independent thinker at work.	☐	☐
I add more than my share to the work environment.	☐	☐
I feel good about who I am in my work setting.	☐	☐
I am self-confident about my ability at work.	☐	☐
I consciously attempt to take on positions of authority at work.	☐	☐
I seek to satisfy myself, not others at work.	☐	☐

---

10. The Internet

Using a search engine, enter words such as *career, interest inventories, aptitude tests,* and whatever else you like. Share some of your results with others in class. You should find some rather interesting career-related sites.

11. Ethical and Professional Vignettes

Review the following vignettes and share your thoughts about them in class. Refer to the Ethical Standards of Human Services Professionals in Appendix B when necessary.

1. It is not unusual for individuals who have little or no training in career development to be offering workshops on career issues, testing for career decision making, and even conducting career counseling. What do you think of this practice? Is it ethical? Professional? Legal?

2. A social worker you know tells you that he is doing career counseling with some of his clients. You know that social workers rarely, if ever, get specific training in career counseling. What should you do? Is this ethical? Professional? Legal?

3. A human service professional tries to strong-arm her clients into taking jobs in which they are not interested. You can often hear her saying things like, "Don't you want to work?" "Are you lazy?" "At least you'll be doing something." What do you think of this practice? Is it ethical? Professional? What, if anything, should you do?

4. A human service professional working with a minority client on career development issues tells you that she thinks the client is making excuses for not finding a job. The client, she says, insists that there is little upward mobility for a "lower-class, undereducated, black client." Would you say anything to this helper? Is she acting ethically? Professionally?

5. An elementary school counselor you know continues to use gender-specific language when referring to certain occupations (for example, "fireman" rather than "firefighter"). In addition, he tends to push girls toward traditionally female occupations and boys toward traditionally male occupations. You mention that you think he might want to change his language and ways of acting with the students, and he says, "This is how the world is. Why should I give them a false image?" What should you do? Is he acting ethically? Professionally?

6. A student assistance worker insists on having students make career decisions despite the fact that developmentally they should be exploring their strengths and weaknesses and examining the different kinds of occupations in the world of work. How should you approach this situation? Is the helper acting ethically? Professionally?

7. A high school counselor you know spends considerable time assisting the high achieving students with college-bound issues. He spends little time working on career and vocational counseling for other students. What should you do? Is this ethical? Professional?

8. Your supervisor at the "Career Management Center" where you work has insisted that no helpers should be spending more than two, one-half-hour sessions with clients. She says that all the information for finding jobs these days is on computers, and helpers should simply help students learn how to use the computer. You believe that career counseling is an intensive career development process that needs to be facilitated in a face-to-face helping relationship. What should you do?

9. You work at a day treatment center at a mental health clinic. Your supervisor insists that all issues with your clients have deep-seated roots. Thus, he does not want you to advocate for getting work for your clients. He says that these clients are too damaged to find and be successful at work. Does the supervisor have a point? Has the supervisor acted ethically? Professionally? Legally? What should you do?

10

✛

A Look to the Future

Trends in the Function and Roles of the Human Service Professional

A student asked a question in class that I thought I had answered a number of times. She asked it on a day that I had a cold and was not feeling well. I remember responding somewhat belligerently, saying something like "I've answered this question four times before!" After class, I saw that she looked angry so I asked her what was going on. She stated, "I thought you were condescending toward me, and it makes me feel like not asking any more questions." I realized she was right, and I also knew that sometimes I get like that. I try my best to be accepting of students, but I know that sometimes I just "lose it." This has been a constant struggle for me to try to hear each question and comment for what it is and not to lose my patience. This student reminded me again that I still have issues to work on. Change for me is not easy, and when I think of my clients attempting to make change and having difficulty, I try to remember that in certain areas of my life I, too, have difficulty.

I sometimes joke with my colleagues about the trends in the titles of conferences that have been held within recent years. Every conference seems to have a theme like "Human Services in the 21st Century and Beyond," "Transformation of the Counseling Profession," "The New Millennium and Beyond: Change in Human Services" and "Change, Metamorphosis, and Trends for the Future." No question, change is on people's minds. Some workshops at these conferences are exciting because they present new, cutting-edge information about innovative ways to work with clients and systems. However, I find that more often than not, the changes aren't implemented or, at the very least, are implemented very slowly. This is because the tendency to maintain the status quo is great, whether it be within ourselves, in our family, in social systems, or in organizations.

Despite the tendency to keep things the way they are, there is some inner sense in all of us that change keeps us alive. In this chapter, we will examine what changes and adaptations seem imminent in the future of the human service profession. Some of these changes will assuredly take place, and others may fall by the wayside. Thus, in this chapter we will examine some of the likely changes in the human services profession in the 21st century. First, we will explore current trends in working with some special populations including the incarcerated, their families, and the victims of crime; those who are HIV-positive; the homeless and the poor; older people; individuals who are chronically mentally ill; people with disabilities; and individuals at risk for chemical dependence. Next, we will note how technology, especially the use of the computer, is changing the way that the human service professional will be doing business. We will also focus on how a greater emphasis on standards in the profession, in the areas of program accreditation, ethical codes, skills standards, and credentialing, will affect our work in the future. This will be followed by an examination of the recent developmental focus in human services and how such a focus encourages a greater emphasis on providing primary prevention. A discussion about how changes in managed health care will affect the kinds of jobs available for the human service professional will be discussed next, and this will be followed by an examination of how medical breakthroughs are likely to affect the work of the human service professional.

Although stressed throughout the text, we will again note the continued importance multicultural issues will play in the upcoming years. How stress, cynicism,
and burnout affect the work of the human services professional and what we can
do about it will be discussed next. The chapter will then shift to looking at your
future in the human services as we examine trends in the job market and issues
related to going to graduate school. Finally, the chapter concludes with a discussion of the importance of continuing education in one's future as a human service
professional and how the effective human service professional is willing to deal
with the changes that come.

TRENDS IN CLIENT POPULATIONS

Discussed in relationship to counseling skills in Chapter 7, the human service professional will increasingly find himself or herself working with a number of
unique groups of individuals. These include those who are incarcerated, their families, and the victims of crime; those who are HIV-positive; the homeless and the
poor; older people; individuals who are chronically mentally ill; people with disabilities; and individuals at risk for chemical dependence. Let's take a brief look at
why these groups will be so important in the 21st century.

The Incarcerated, Their Families,
and the Victims of Crime

In 1999, 6.3 million people were in jail, on probation, or on parole—more than
3% of all U.S. adults (U.S. Department of Justice, 2001). With most prisoners being
undereducated, abused as children, abusing drugs and alcohol, and coming from
dysfunctional families, the need for social services is paramount. As a result,
human service professionals will find themselves providing a wide range of social
services for those who are incarcerated, their families, and the victims of crime
(Hagen, 2001; Hicks-Coolick & Millsap, 2001; King, 2001; Miller, 2001). With the
many needs of these clients, a multisystem approach that addresses this broad range
of services will need to be implemented (Hicks-Coolick & Millsap, 2001). Unless
there is a drastic reduction in crime in the United States, many human service
professionals will find themselves working within the criminal justice system well
into the 21st century.

Individuals Who Are HIV-Positive

Between 800,000 and 900,000 Americans are HIV-positive, and almost one-half
million have died of the disease (Centers for Disease Control, 2002). Worldwide,
approximately 42 million children and adults are HIV-positive or have AIDS
(UNAIDS, 2002). With some U.S. insurance companies dropping individuals who
become chronically ill, and with drug companies fighting to ban easy access to
AIDS drugs in third world countries, it is clear that this epidemic has had a personal and economic cost to people throughout the world (see Box 10.1).

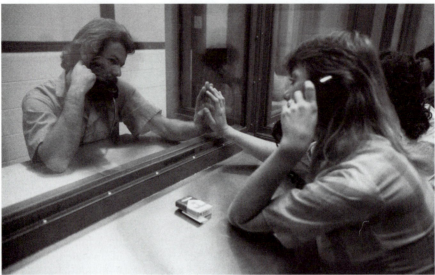

Ed Kashi/CORBIS

Families and friends of the incarcerated, victims of crime, and our communities are all affected by crime and its aftermath.

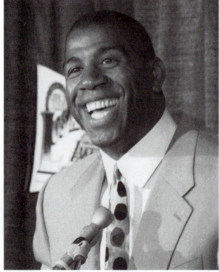

AP/Wide World Photos

Magic Johnson has an upbeat attitude and finds ways of helping the underpriviliged despite his HIV-positive status.

Mental health professionals have responded to the disease by providing individual and group counseling, support groups for HIV-positive individuals and their families, needle exchange programs, programs for children who have AIDS, prevention and education programs, condom distribution programs, and hotlines to respond to questions about AIDS (Britton, 2000; Britton, Rak, Cimini, &

BOX 10.1   Legal Problems to Health Care Access

Thirty-nine of the world's major pharmaceutical companies sued South Africa, which was attempting to have other drug companies manufacture expensive AIDS drugs at a much reduced cost. Because the drug companies received so much negative press about their lawsuit, the lawsuit was dropped. However, the ability to manufacture the drugs is still in doubt because of legal issues and economic problems in South Africa (Jetter, 2001).

Meanwhile, the Supreme Court denied an appeal that would have prevented insurance companies from dropping health insurance coverage for individuals who had AIDS or other catastrophic illnesses. The obvious result of this decision is that many individuals who have serious illnesses may find themselves without medical coverage (Savage, 1992).

Shepherd, 1999; Kain, 1989). In addition, workshops and articles about the AIDS virus are now commonplace at conferences and in professional journals. Until a cure to this disease is found, AIDS will continue to be a major focus for many mental health professionals. Finally, as sexual activity with an HIV-positive individual is potentially life threatening, professionals who are in a helping relationship with HIV-positive clients may face a new challenge: the ethical dilemma concerning confidentiality with their clients versus the duty to warn those who could be unknowingly exposed to the virus (Cohen, 1990).

> A counselor who receives information confirming that a client has a disease commonly known to be both communicable and fatal is justified in disclosing information to an identifiable third party, who by his or her relationship with the client is at a high risk of contracting the disease . . . (ACA Ethical Standards, B.1.d, ACA, 1995)

The Homeless and the Poor

> Now we can walk on the moon and thousands of dying people cannot walk to a cup of food or clean drinking water. (Dykeman, 1997)

Today, more than 32 million Americans (11.8%) are poor (U.S. Census Bureau, 2000d). As a function of race, we see that minorities are disproportionately represented (see Figure 10.1) (U. S. Census Bureau, 2000e). The homeless today include children who have run away from home, intact families, single-parent families, poor single men and women, those who have minimum paying jobs but cannot afford shelter, and the deinstitutionalized mentally ill.

Despite legislation like the **McKinney Act** of 1987 that provides a wide range of services for the poor, the negative results of homelessness and poverty are great and include being at greater risk of being abused, developing AIDS, tuberculosis, and other diseases; being more likely to have retarded language and social skills, and have delayed motor development; and having higher rates of depression, hopelessness, and mental illness (Blasi, 1990; Dykeman, 1997; Nooe, 2001). The human service professional of the 21st century will undoubtedly be faced with

286

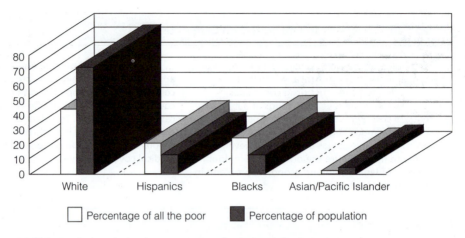

Percentage of all the poor   Percentage of population

FIGURE 10.1 Comparison of poverty rates of select racial/ethnic groups

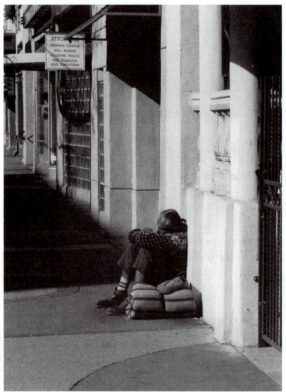

© Michael Siluk

Many of the homeless in America have little hope for the future.

BOX 10.2   An Interview with Al

Al is a 41-year-old homeless man in Norfolk, Virginia. Although raised in New York City, he and his family of origin now live in Norfolk. Having some college credits and growing up with modest means, he notes, "My dad grew up in the Depression. I never thought that I would be in this situation." He goes on to state that being homeless can suddenly happen to anybody. Until recently, Al was staying with his parents, adopted sister, and her three children. However, after his father had a mild stroke, he felt that he was a burden on his family, so he took to the streets. He states that he believes things have become much worse during the past 10 years and notes that he made more money as a teenager than he does now.

Although Al is homeless, he usually has a roof over his head at night. Generally, he stays at one of the local church shelters or at the Union Mission. Every morning Al goes to a temporary job-placement service with the hope of finding work. Al states that obtaining food is usually not a problem because local religious groups and shelters provide some food daily. Al has a 23-year-old daughter and 4-year-old twin boys. He says, "It hurts that I don't have a job—hurts that I can't support them."

Al's sense of the homeless is that about one-third would work if employment was available, that some of the homeless are those who have been institutionalized for mental illness and are probably incapable of working, and that some of the homeless have developed attitudes from years of hopelessness. He says the street term for such people is "ate up." Being on the streets, according to Al, has a domino effect. A homeless person has few resources, no nice clothes, no place to keep personal things and records, and little hope. The result: Pulling oneself out of the situation is difficult. Al, however, seems to keep a positive attitude and states, "Sometimes I slip into a blue funk, but I don't lose hope." He says that keeping a positive attitude is like a mental volley.

---

individuals who are poor, homeless, and destitute and must have the knowledge and skills to work with this population in the 21st century.

Older People

In 1900, 4.1% of the United States was over 65, by 1996, the percentage had grown to 12.8%, and it is estimated that by 2030, 20% will be over 65 (Special Committee on Aging, U.S. Senate, 1997; U.S. Administration on Aging, 1999). The median income of older persons in 1995 was only $16,684 for males and $9,626 for females.

As the population of individuals over 65 years old continues to rise, so does their need for increased social services in such areas as income assistance, health care, housing, employment, leisure activities, and environmental assistance (e.g., large print books) (Clubok, 2001; Russell-Miller, 2001). (See Box 10.3.) It is therefore not surprising that across the country we have seen an increase in day-treatment programs for the elderly at community mental health centers, long-term care facilities such as nursing homes, housing settings that are specifically geared toward older persons, foster care settings for the elderly, senior centers, and programs for the elderly offered through religious organizations and social services agencies (Clubok, 2001; Myers & Schwiebert, 1996). With the growing number of elderly people in the United States, along with more programs to service

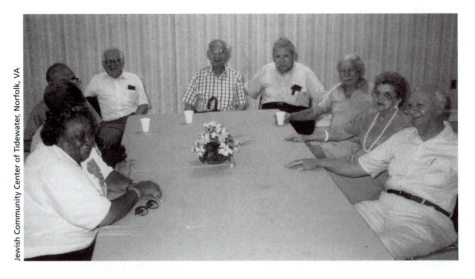

Jewish Community Center of Tidewater, Norfolk, VA

Seniors at a community center discuss some of the problems they face in older age.

this population, more human service professionals will undoubtedly be needed to work with the elderly in the 21st century.

Individuals Who Are Chronically Mentally Ill

It is now estimated that 22% of the adult population is affected by a mental disorder every year, and almost 3% of adults have a chronic mental disorder (NIMH, 1998). Also, estimates are that almost 11% of the population seeks mental health treatment each year.

Since the 1950s, a number of dramatic events have greatly reduced the number of individuals needing psychiatric inpatient care while sharply increasing the number of individuals needing ongoing outpatient support. First, the development of new psychotropic medications has made the management of severe emotional conditions possible outside the inpatient setting. Second, the Community Mental Health Centers Act of 1963 funded hundreds of mental health centers that provide free or low-cost short-term inpatient care, outpatient care, partial hospitalization, emergency services, and consultation and education services (Burger & Youkeles, 2000, 1997). Third, the proliferation of social service programs, introduced through the Great Society Initiatives of the Johnson presidency, created a myriad of other types of social service agencies. Finally, in 1975, the U.S. Supreme Court decision *Donaldson v. O'Connor* stated that a person who is not dangerous to self or others could not be confined in a psychiatric hospital against his or her will (Box 10.4). This case and others were instrumental in the eventual **deinstitutionalization** of mental hospitals (Swenson, 1997).

One result of these events is the proliferation of services for the mentally disabled—services often staffed by human service professionals. Undoubtedly, the

---

BOX 10.3   Needs of Older Americans

In an effort to understand some of the needs of older Americans, I visited a local community center that had organized senior services. These included meals at reduced prices, educational activities such as guest speakers on a variety of topics, and social activities such as movies and trips to local theater productions. At the center, I had lunch with Irving, Lasard, Izzi, Jeanette, Max, Joe, and some other senior citizens; their average age was about 80 years old. We had an informal discussion about a number of issues facing older Americans. Although there was some debate concerning the amount of federal subsidies that should be given to seniors, some of their major issues seemed clear. For instance, all felt that seniors are entitled to safe and secure housing, good medical care, transportation, healthy meals, and federal assistance in the delivery and implementation of these programs. Most of the group felt that they had spent a lifetime at hard work and now deserved something in return. Finally, it was clear that many of these seniors were dealing with losses of spouses, friends, and relatives in their lives. This psychological component was clearly not being attended to by any of the existing available services.

---

human service professional of the 21st century will be intimately involved in the future of social services for individuals who are chronically mentally ill.

People with Disabilities

Today, nearly 1 in 8 individuals identifies himself or herself as having a disability and 1 in 5 as having a severe disability. Of the 53 million Americans with disabilities, 5 million are under 15 years old, and only 1 in 6 of these individuals is born with their disability (U.S. Census Bureau, 2001e). Some of the most common disabilities include mental retardation, learning disabilities, emotional problems, and speech impairments, whereas some other disabling conditions include hearing impairment, visual impairment, orthopedic impairment, multiple disabilities, and other health impairments.

A number of federal laws have affected the ability of individuals with disabilities to receive services. The Education for All Handicapped Children Act of 1975 (PL94-142) and the subsequent Individuals with Disabilities Education Act (IDEA) ensure the right to an education within the least restrictive environment for all children who are identified as having a disability that interferes with learning. The Rehabilitation Act of 1973 ensures vocational rehabilitation services for adults with disabilities who are in need of employment. The Americans with Disabilities Act of 1992 updated these laws and ensures that qualified individuals with disabilities cannot be discriminated against in job applications procedures, hiring, firing, advancement, compensation, fringe benefits, job training, and other terms, conditions, and privileges (U.S. Department of Labor, 1992).

As new medical procedures make it possible for individuals to live with disabling and chronic health conditions, we may see an increase in the number of individuals with disabilities. This will result in additional needed services for these individuals, services in which we may find the human service professional taking an increasingly active role. Finally, let us remember that we are all only temporarily able-bodied.

BOX 10.4 **Donaldson v. O'Connor: The Deinstitutionalization of Mental Hospitals**

In 1975, the U.S. Supreme Court decided a case that dramatically affected the status of mental hospitals in the United States. Kenneth Donaldson, who had been committed to a state mental hospital in Florida and confined against his will for 15 years, sued the hospital superintendent, Dr. J. B. O'Connor, and his staff for intentionally and maliciously depriving him of his constitutional right to liberty. Donaldson, who had been hospitalized against his will for paranoid schizophrenia, said that he was not mentally ill, and that even if he was, the hospital had not provided him adequate treatment.

Over the 15 years of confinement, Donaldson, who was not in danger of harming himself or others, had frequently asked for his release; relatives had stated they would attend to him if he were released. Despite this, the hospital refused to release Donaldson, stating that he was still mentally ill. The U.S. Supreme Court unanimously upheld lower court decisions stating that the hospital could not hold him against his will if he was not in danger of harming himself or others. This decision led to the large-scale release of hundreds of thousands of individuals across the country who had been confined in mental hospitals against their wills and who were not a danger to self or others.

Individuals at Risk for Chemical Dependence

With nearly 15 million Americans using illicit drugs, 45 million people being binge drinkers, and 12 million being heavy drinkers, substance abuse services are necessary (U.S. Department of Health and Human Services, 2000). Drug and alcohol abuse today can be found in the inner cities and in middle-class America, affecting not only the users but also family members and society. Estimates suggest that as many as 1 out of 7 Americans are **children of alcoholics** (COAs) (Black, 1979; Woititz, 1983), and substance abuse is related to many of the problems facing our nation, including violent crime, problems on the job, and changing morals. Thus, the widespread abuse of substances, unfortunately, provides an array of places for counselors to work, including hospital detoxification (detox) units, halfway houses, and drug and alcohol treatment centers (Field, 2000). Unfortunately, the 21st century will likely bring an increased need for human service professionals to be working with those who abuse drugs and alcohol.

TECHNOLOGY IN HUMAN SERVICE WORK

In the United States today, more than 61% of homes have a computer and more than 42% have Internet access (Department of Commerce, 2000). And in business, this figure is considerably higher. These are truly amazing statistics, especially given that only 20% of households had a computer in 1992, only 20% had Internet access in 1998, and the first PCs were sold about 22 years ago.

Mental health professions have quickly adapted to the use of computers and to other new technologies (Dipietro & Nelson, 2001; Guterman & Kirk, 1999;

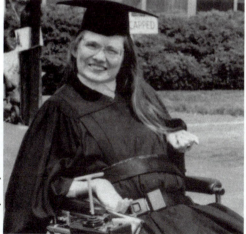

Courtesy Lisa Lyons

Despite being born with cerebral palsy and later having an accident that resulted in quadriplegia, Lisa Lyons obtained her master's degree in counseling.

Wilson, 1995). For instance, mental health professionals now use computers and other technologies such as interactive videos and CD-ROMs in case management, record keeping, clinical assessment and diagnosis, personality assessment of clients, comprehensive career counseling, documentation of client records, billing, marketing, and assisting clients in learning new skills (e.g., parenting skills, assertiveness training, and vocational skills for specific jobs).

Computers have also been shown to be successful in training helping professionals (Casey, 1999; Haney & Leibsohn, 1999; Hohenshil, 2000; Neukrug, 1991). But perhaps the greatest change in the use of technology has been the Internet. The Internet has brought us home pages of our professional associations (e.g., see www.NOHSE.org), emails to colleagues, distribution lists and Listservs of professionals who have common interests, video streaming for professional conferencing, Web-based courses, search engines for research, downloadable files on just about any counseling-related subject you might think of, and the controversial topic of counseling online. In fact, *Ethical Guidelines for Internet On-Line Counseling* have even been developed (see ACA, 1999). The Internet holds much potential, and mental health professions have not lagged behind in getting online (Granello, 2000; Sampson, Kolodinsky, & Greeno, 1997; Wilson, 1995).

STANDARDS IN THE PROFESSION

Professionalism, however, is an attitude that motivates individuals to be attentive to the image and ideals of their particular profession. (VanZandt, 1990, p. 243)

Standards raise a profession to its highest level. Four standards that have taken prominence in the human services field recently, and will likely be crucial in the

21st century, are program accreditation, credentialing, ethical codes, and skills standards. Although these standards were discussed in detail in Chapters 1 and 2, I will briefly highlight their importance for the future.

Program Accreditation

A major thrust of the Council for Standards in Human Service Education (CSHSE) is to provide an accreditation process for human service programs. Although a limited number of programs have so far acquired accreditation, such accreditation will likely become increasingly important, if not essential, for human service programs of the future. The two main goals of accreditation are to provide a curriculum that prepares generic human service professionals and to provide for the personal development of the student in areas related to human service work, "including personal values, motivation, orientation towards human services work, interpersonal relationships, and communication skills." (CSHSEa, 2002, Goal Two Section, ¶1, see www.cshse.org to obtain a copy of the accreditation standards). Thus, accreditation helps ensure that a program is educationally sound and focused on improving personality skills needed to be an effective human service professional.

Ethical Guidelines

> The development of the Ethical Standards was a necessary step in the growth of the profession. (*Ethical Standards of Human Service Professionals*, 1996, p. 12)

The *Ethical Standards of Human Service Professionals* were approved in 1995 (see Appendix B). Ethical standards are an important mark of a profession and indicate that there is a unique body of knowledge to which standards can be applied (see Chapter 2). In the future, we will increasingly see these standards used by human service professionals, and as we continue to develop and change, we will see these standards revised.

Skills Standards

During the 1990s, competencies for human service professionals and the skills needed to implement them were established through a national effort that included feedback from educators and practitioners (Taylor, Bradley, & Warren, 1996). These standards "define the competencies used by direct service workers in a wide variety of service contexts in community settings across the nation [see Chapter 1]. Designed to be relevant to diverse direct service roles (residential, vocational, therapeutic, etc.), the standards are based upon a nationally validated job analysis involving a wide variety of human service workers, consumers, providers and educators." (Community Support Skills Standards, 2002, ¶1). The new millennium will undoubtedly see a more highly qualified human service professional as a result of these standards.

Credentialing

Although a certification process for human services professionals does not now exist, there are discussions about such a possibility occurring (Diambra, 2000). Certification ensures that individuals with such a credential are minimally qualified (see Chapter 2). It is likely that certification for human service professionals will become a reality in the near future.

A DEVELOPMENTAL AND PRIMARY PREVENTION EMPHASIS

The mental health professions have increasingly highlighted the importance of understanding the developmental level of the client, and this is likely to continue in the upcoming years. The focus on developmental issues has been evidenced in many ways, including the adoption of a developmental approach to counseling in the schools (Hughey, 2001), the increased focus on wellness throughout the life span (Gladding, 2000), and the recent proliferation of developmental models of counseling (Ivey, 1993; McAuliffe & Eriksen, 2000). This developmental emphasis tends to have a wellness focus and views client growth or stagnation in terms of uncompleted developmental stages. In addition, it helps us determine a client's **developmental readiness** to move on to higher stages.

There is a natural marriage between knowledge of development and **primary prevention** activities because if we are knowledgeable about what is likely to occur developmentally, we can prepare activities and workshops to help ease individuals through stages in their lives (Baker & Shaw, 1987). This contrasts with **secondary prevention,** which focuses on the control of nonsevere mental health problems, and **tertiary prevention,** which concentrates on the control of serious mental health problems (Burger & Youkeles, 2000). Examine the continuum of Figure 10.2 and compare it with the focus of the human service professional as delineated in Table 1.1 (see p. 5). Clearly, primary prevention fits in naturally with the existing focus and training of the human service professional.

During this century, human service professionals will increasingly be asked to do something that comes naturally to them—primary prevention. No doubt, the human service professional will be seen as an expert in wellness and prevention programs.

MANAGED HEALTH CARE

Within the past 20 years, the cost of mental health services has skyrocketed, and **managed health care** has become one method of controlling it (Carroll, 1996; Wylie, 1995). In the past, when individuals sought mental health services, they

Primary → **Secondary** → **Tertiary**

Short term	→	→	→	Long term
Modifying behavior	→	→	→	Personality reconstruction
Wellness focus	→	→	→	Focus on pathology
Before problem occurs	→	→	→	After problem occurs
Preventive	→	→	→	Restorative

FIGURE 10.2 Comparison of the focus of professionals who provide primary, secondary, or tertiary prevention.

almost always sought private counseling from private practice practitioners or from mental health agencies, and, usually, an employee health care package would include a certain amount of coverage toward individual, group, or family counseling. However, in an effort to contain the cost of mental health services, many employers now provide medical coverage through **Health Maintenance Organizations (HMOs)** (Medical Economics Staff, 2001). In addition, **Employee Assistance Programs (EAPs)** are now offered as an additional cost-reduction effort. HMOs are managed health care systems that limit accessibility to providers while strictly overseeing diagnosis and treatment. EAPs are programs run by business and industry to provide primary prevention and early referral for treatment.

To keep costs down, managed mental health care programs will likely have an increased emphasis on primary prevention and early detection of problems. In the past, private practice practitioners were the primary deliverers of services (Wylie, 1995); with this change in focus, however, less highly trained professionals, who will be paid at lower salaries, will likely be employed to offer some of the primary prevention services. Bachelor's- and even associate's-level human service professionals will also likely be hired to do some of this work (Carroll, 1996).

MEDICAL BREAKTHROUGHS
AND MENTAL HEALTH

Organ transplantation is no longer considered experimental. By the middle of the 21st century, it is likely that most people will meet someone who is waiting on a transplant; someone who has received a transplant; or someone who, themselves, may need a transplant. (Eidson-Claxton & Bridges, 2001)

This quote speaks to the tremendous advances we have had in keeping people alive. However, it also raises a number of other issues that will directly affect the work of the human service professional. As individuals are increasingly faced with complex decisions about their health, a number of mental health issues will arise. Some of these include making medical decisions that might prolong life but deleteriously affect one's quality of life, the affects of medical procedures on families, decisions about whether one wants to know if he or she is likely to acquire a disease (e.g., genetic testing), decisions about whether to become pregnant with children who are likely to acquire a disease, and how the use of medication might affect one's way of interacting in the world (Mulkey, 2001; Neukrug, 2001). These medical breakthroughs will lead to difficult and complex decisions by the consumer. If the human service professional is to adequately assist individuals with these tough decisions, he or she will need to be versed on the medical aspects of diseases and disabilities and the ethical concerns related to them (Eidson-Claxton & Bridges, 2001; Mulkey, 2001). Clearly, the 21st century will bring some new challenges to the human service professional in the realm of medical breakthroughs.

INCREASED FOCUS
ON MULTICULTURAL ISSUES

Multicultural counseling is a hot topic, and it seems evident that we will, and must, see (1) increased training in multicultural counseling, (2) new theories and models of multicultural counseling, and (3) increased research on the efficacy of varying counseling approaches with diverse clients (Conwill, 2001; Hanna, Bemak, & Chung, 1999; Holcomb-McCoy & Myers, 1999; Lucas, 2001).

Chapter 7 introduced us to multicultural counseling, and we noted the importance of having (1) knowledge about other cultures, (2) the skills necessary in working with diverse populations, and (3) the proper attitudes when working with individuals of varying cultural backgrounds. As we move into the 21st century, the human service professional will continually be challenged to meet the needs of an increasingly diverse client population. In fact, some authors think that the increasing diversity in the United States and its impact on the mental health professions might represent a new forefront in the helping professions (Essandoh, 1996).

Finally, in the 21st century, we will likely see agencies that increasingly focus on providing a multicultural environment in their attitude, in whom they employ, and in the types of clients they attract. This new focus will greatly change the way we understand our own backgrounds as well as the cultures of others and positively affect our ability to work with clients of diverse backgrounds.

STRESS, CYNICISM, AND BURNOUT:
UNDERSTANDING AND COMBATING IT

Human service professionals often witness the saddest side of humanity, such as when they work with clients who are homeless, hungry, or dealing with a recent loss. As a result of this difficult work, some human service professionals develop what has recently been called **compassion fatigue/vicarious traumatization syndrome** (Slater & Spetalnick, 2001). In addition to working with difficult clients, the intense overseeing of many human service professionals by funding sources and the subsequent perceived loss of autonomy yields stress levels that are probably higher than in other professions (Arches, 1997). No wonder many human service professionals who are payed poorly, deal with high-stress situations, and receive minimal reinforcement for their work eventually choose to change careers.

Unfortunately, stress, cynicism, and burnout are likely to continue to be major concerns of human service professionals in the 21st century. **Hans Selye** (1956, 1974), one of the leading researchers on stress, stated that stress is an adaptive response to a changing situation. **Stress** therefore can be seen as a healthy response that enables a person to handle new or highly charged situations (Pritts et al., 2000). However, too much stress has been associated with a myriad of psychological states as well as a wide range of illnesses (Fava & Sonino, 2000).

With the human service profession being such a high stress field, it is important to find ways of ameliorating such stress. Evidence now suggests that meditation and other mind-altering experiences can reduce levels of stress, be helpful in recovery from alcoholism and other addictions, reduce or alleviate physical symptoms that are associated with stress-related illnesses, and even have a positive effect on the immune system, thus potentially being an adjunct therapy for such diseases as cancer and AIDS (Benson & Klipper, 2000; Neukrug, 2001; Pollak, Levy, & Breitholtz, 1999).

Some authors have suggested that human service professionals must be ever-vigilant in attending to their physical, emotional, behavioral, interpersonal, and attitudinal domains (Kahill, 1988a, b). Attending to each of these can help the mental health professional remain emotionally and physically healthy. For instance, healthy professionals are aware of their physical well-being and attend to it by eating well and taking care of their bodies through exercise, meditation, or other related activities. Such professionals also care about their emotional health by seeking out, when necessary, counseling for themselves and by having supportive relationships. In addition, the activities in which healthy mental health professionals involve themselves are indicative of a positive lifestyle, one in which they take responsibility for their actions and attend to the important relationships in their lives.

One method of assessing your level of health is through what Myers, Sweeney, and Witmer (2000) describe as the **Wheel of Wellness.** This model, intended for client use, is easily applied to mental health professionals and asks individuals to assess their level of health in the areas of spirituality, work and leisure, friendship, love, and self-direction, which is further divided into twelve subtasks (see Figure 10.3). You may want to complete an informal assessment on each of the tasks and subtasks to determine what areas you might decide to work on. For instance, give yourself a ranking from 1 to 5 on each of the tasks and subtasks. The closer your ranking is to "5," the more you need to focus on that area. Then, write down ways you can better yourself in those areas where you gave yourself a score of 3, 4, or 5. (For a more involved analysis, see Myers, Sweeney, & Witmer, 2000.)

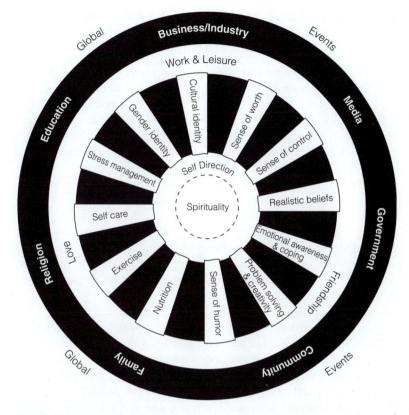

FIGURE 10.3 Wheel of Wellness

Finally, Carl Whitaker (1976) suggests a number of ways of keeping oneself healthy. Noting his points and adding a few thoughts of my own, one can

1. Place yourself as a priority

2. Learn how to love

3. Listen to your impulses

4. Listen to your inner voice, listen to others

5. Enjoy your significant other more than anyone else

6. Fracture role structures and challenge authority

7. Challenge yourself—you're not always right

8. Build long-term relationships so you feel safe and grounded enough to express your feelings

9. Act "crazy" and whimsical

10. Face the fact that you must grow until you die

YOUR FUTURE IN HUMAN SERVICES

Trends in Jobs and Earnings

In 2000, there were 271,000 jobs in the human services professions (OOH, 2002–2003b). This figure is about 100,000 more than only four years earlier in 1996 (U.S. Department of Labor, 1998–99). The Occupational Outlook Handbook (OOH) has some optimistic job forecasts for the future. In fact, between 2000 and 2010 the number of social and human service assistants is projected to grow much faster than the average for all occupations ranking it among the most rapidly growing occupations.

Approximately 50% of human service professionals work for private agencies, providing such services as counseling, job training, adult day care, crisis intervention, counseling, and job training. Another 25% work in local and state governments, usually in public welfare agencies or with the mentally and developmentally challenged. In addition, many work in mental health clinics, detox centers, psychiatric hospitals, sheltered workshops, and day-treatment programs. Finally, many human service professionals can be found supervising individuals in group homes and halfway houses (OOH, 2002–2003b, see "Employment," ¶1).

Some of the best opportunities in the field will be in the areas of "job-training programs, residential care facilities, and private social service agencies, which include such services as adult day care and meal delivery programs. . . . In addition, social and human service assistants will continue to be needed to provide services to pregnant teenagers, the homeless, the mentally disabled and developmentally challenged, and those with substance-abuse problems." (OOH, 2002–2003b, see "Job Outlook" section, ¶1). Four books that list dozens of additional jobs and other information about the human service field include Burger and Youkeles' (2000) *The Helping Professions: A Careers Sourcebook;* Collison and Garfield's (1996) *Careers in Counseling and Human Development;* Baxter, Toch, and Perry's (1997) *Opportunities in Counseling and Development, Careers;* and Garner's (2001) *Careers in Social and Rehabilitation Services.*

In the 21st century, human service professionals will have to have at least an associate's degree, with many employers requiring a bachelor's degree or even a master's degree, especially if one wants to advance in the field. Increasingly, some kind of on-the-job experience or internship will be required for employment. Although salaries in the human services tend to be on the low end compared with other professions, they have gone up considerably. In 2000, the median salary was $22,330, and the middle 50% of professionals earned between $17,820 and $27,930 (OOH, 2002–2003b), with government jobs usually offering the highest salaries. Today, those who obtain a master's degree and an administrative position can earn well above $40,000.

Finding a Job/Applying to Graduate School

If you intend to have a career in human services, in a short amount of time you will either be looking for a job or applying to graduate school. Perhaps both. Regardless of which you are doing, you should consider the following to make the process a little easier.

Networking Whether you are looking for a job or going on to graduate school, networking will help you in that process. Networking puts you in the "loop" to meet the right people and helps you hear about potential jobs and opportunities for graduate school. However, networking is not something you do just to get a job or to get into graduate school. Networking means that you are involved, interested, and active in your field. It means you are committed to your field. (See Box 10.5).

Some ways to network include joining and getting involved in your local, state, and national professional associations; assisting faculty in their research; doing volunteer work at an agency; and getting involved in a human service student association. Whatever method you use, networking is a good way to build your résumé and increases your chances of being accepted into the graduate school of your choice or obtaining your dream job.

Developing a Résumé A good résumé is essential for finding a job, and it can assist in getting you into graduate school. Whether it be for a job or for acceptance into graduate school, résumés should be readable, attractive, and to the point. Although some advocate a one-page résumé, my philosophy is to not worry about how long it is. It should be as long as is necessary to show your important qualifications, *without causing the reader confusion*. Do not put anything on the résumé that might prevent you from getting an interview (for example, marital status or a goal statement that is too focused), and make sure it is grammatically correct and neat.

Don't underestimate what you have done. For example, so often a person's skills from one job or activity are transferable to another job or activity. A person who was secretary for a college human service organization may very well have writing skills, planning skills, and organizational ability. These **transferable skills** are important to mention on a résumé, particularly if your work experience is limited. And don't forget to add your networking experiences, such as membership in professional associations. Employers and graduate schools love to see that you have been involved. Relative to graduate school, strongly consider sending a résumé even if a graduate program hasn't asked for one. Résumés help admission committees know your strengths. For a more detailed look at résumés, get a good book on résumé writing (for example, see Biegeleisen, 1991; Donaho & Meyer, 1990).

Developing a Portfolio Besides a good résumé, other materials may strengthen your chances of being admitted to graduate school or obtaining a wanted job. For instance, a paper or Web-based portfolio can furnish the prospective employer or graduate program with a broad survey of your knowledge and skills (Cobia, Carney, & Shannon, 2000; French, 1993). Portfolios may include such things as transcripts, papers you have written, your counseling philosophy, and outlines of workshops you might have presented (Baltimore, Hickson, George, & Crutchfield, 1996).

Looking Good and the Interview When interviewing for a job or for graduate school, make sure that you look good and present yourself well. I have often seen potentially good employees or graduate students who are applying for a position present themselves poorly. I am not necessarily talking about getting dressed

---

**BOX 10.5   Randy: Getting Networked, Getting Involved,
and Getting a Job**

Randy is a former student of mine who was enthusiastic about the human service field. He joined the professional associations, worked on research with me, and participated in professional activities whenever possible. Because Randy was so involved, he had the opportunity to present a workshop at a state professional association conference. His enthusiasm showed during the workshop. At the end of the workshop, one woman who attended the presentation was so impressed with him that she offered him a job right there. Thus, we see the importance of getting involved and being enthused.

---

in a business suit. I mean dressing appropriately so that you will impress, rather than offend, your potential employer or graduate school. It is generally better to be overdressed than underdressed.

In addition to looking good, have a strong sense of what you are going to say in an interview. Of course, you cannot predict all the questions that may be asked of you, but you probably can have a pretty good sense. How do you get a sense of what will be asked? Well, first find out about the agency or graduate school. Talk to people who are employed there or students who have been admitted. Next, have friends and colleagues help you practice with a mock interview. Doing this will help you feel much more confident about the kinds of questions that may be asked and how you might respond. Some of the more common questions that are asked follow:

1. Why are you interested in this position or graduate school?
2. How did you hear about this position or graduate school?
3. What are your strengths and weaknesses?
4. How do you see yourself working with clients?
5. What is your theoretical orientation to working with clients?
6. What can you bring to this agency (or graduate school) that no one else can bring?
7. Why should I hire you (or admit you)? Why shouldn't I hire you (or admit you)?
8. Have you any work experience? What have you done, and how will it help you at this job (or in this graduate school)?
9. Let me give you a situation and tell me how you would respond.
10. Do you have anything else you would like to add?

These are just a sample of potential questions. Also, note that it is generally illegal to ask questions of a personal nature. Usually, an employer or graduate school cannot ask about a potential employee's cultural or ethnic background, if the employee is single or married, has a family, or other such questions. If they do, you can politely refuse to answer the question. And, if you think they blatantly asked an inappropriate question, you can contact the Equal Opportunity Office or a supervisor of the interviewer.

Going on Informational Interviews Whether you are looking for a job or applying to graduate school, gathering information about a potential place of employment or school can help you in this process. Chances are you have identified a few different types of jobs in the human service field or have chosen potential graduate schools to which you want to apply. Find some people who have these jobs or who work at these schools and go on some informational interviews. These interviews will allow you to get a closer look at exactly what people do in these jobs or give you the "inside scoop" on potential graduate schools. This will help you make a decision regarding whether you would really want to pursue a particular position or apply to a particular school. Although you should not expect this, sometimes through informational interviews you can learn of specific job openings or get some information on ways that you might be able to increase your chances of getting into a specific graduate school.

Other Methods of Finding a Job If you have tried these techniques and are still looking, you can use a number of other methods to obtain a job. For instance, apply directly to an employer. If a phone call and résumé get to the right person at the right time, you may be hired. Some other methods include responding to or placing an ad in a newspaper or professional journal, going to a private or state employment agency, and using your college or university placement office.

Points to Consider When Applying to Graduate School Don't go blindly into a graduate program. Although there is much in common from one counseling program to another, there are differences. If you are considering applying to a program, Baxter et al. (1997) suggest that you should consider the following points in making your decision:

- Program accreditation (e.g., CACREP, APA, NASW)
- Client emphasis
- Philosophical orientation
- Counseling specialties offered
- Degree requirements
- Correlation of degree requirements with certification requirements
- Degree granted
- Entry requirements
- Location
- Size
- Faculty-student ratio
- Location of field experience

- Placement of recent graduates
- Cost
- Availability of scholarships and loans (pp. 87–88)

Locating a Graduate Program A number of resources are available to assist the potential graduate student in locating a graduate school (see Baxter et al., 1997; Burger & Youkeles, 2000; Collison & Garfield, 1996; Garner, 2001). If you have freedom of movement and can travel, there are numerous options open to you. Even if you cannot travel, often there are two, three, four, or more programs in your vicinity. Check them out! Following is a list of where you can find graduate programs in a number of mental health areas.

- For lists of master's and doctoral programs in counseling:
  Council for Accreditation of Counseling and Related Educational Programs (CACREP)
  5999 Stevenson Avenue
  Alexandria, VA 22304
  (703) 823-9800
  Web site: www.counseling.org/cacrep

- For detailed information on master's- and doctoral-level graduate programs in counseling:
  Hollis, J. W., & Dodson, T. A. (2000). *Counselor preparation 1999–2001: Programs, faculty, trends* (10th ed.). Philadelphia: Taylor & Francis.
  1-800-222-1166
  Web site: www.taylorandfrancis.com/

- For a list of doctoral programs in counseling psychology:
  American Psychological Association (APA)
  750 First Street, NE
  Washington, DC 20002
  (202) 336-5500
  Web site: www.apa.org/ed/doctoral.html

- For information on accredited rehabilitation counseling programs:
  National Council on Rehabilitation Education
  Rehabilitation Counseling Program, California
  State University–Fresno, 5005 North Maple Avenue, M.S. 3
  Fresno, CA 93740-8025.
  (559) 278-0325
  Web site: www.rehabeducators.org

- For information on accredited marriage and family therapy programs:
  Commission on Accreditation of Marriage and Family Therapy Education
  American Association for Marriage and Family Therapy
  1133 15th Street, N. W., Suite 300
  Washington, DC 20005-2710
  (202) 452-0109
  Web site: www.aamft.org/about/coamfte/aboutcoamfte.htm

- For accredited clinical pastoral programs:
  Association for Clinical Pastoral Education, Inc.
  1549 Clairmont Road, Suite 103
  Decatur, GA 30033
  (404) 320-1472
  Web site: www.acpe.edu

- For accredited graduate programs in social work:
  Council on Social Work Education
  1725 Duke St., Suite 500
  Alexandria, VA 22314
  (703) 683-8080
  Web site: www.cswe.org/

- For accredited art therapy programs:
  American Art Therapy Association
  1202 Allanson Road
  Mundelein, IL 60060
  (847) 949-6064 or (888) 290-0878
  Web site: www.arttherapy.org

Some Specifics for Applying to Graduate School There are usually a number of items to consider when applying to graduate schools. Following is a listing of some of the more important concerns. Read them carefully before applying.

1. *Meeting deadlines:* Meet your application deadlines! Become aware of the deadlines and make sure you follow them. If you do not, the program has a right and is likely to not review your application.

2. *Completing forms:* Make sure that you have completed all the necessary forms for graduate school. Type them! Make sure they look neat. When your application is reviewed, the presentation of it may be taken into account.

3. *Taking a cognitive ability test (for example, Graduate Record Exam [GRE], Miller Analogy Test [MAT]):* You will likely be asked to take some type of cognitive ability test when applying to graduate school. Your scores will probably be weighed fairly heavily in the application process, so prepare yourself for the test. At the very least, obtain a test review book. Also, consider taking a review course. People who make decisions regarding graduate school want to see the best score you can obtain, not your worst!

4. *Writing an essay:* As unbelievable as it might sound, I have received essays that were handwritten and replete with spelling and grammatical mistakes. If you are asked to write an essay, speak to the question asked, check your grammar and spelling, and have someone review it.

5. *Interviewing:* See pages 299–301

6. *Submitting a résumé:* See page 299

7. *Submitting a portfolio:* See page 299

8. *Being admitted, being denied:* Programs vary dramatically in their admission rates. Should you be denied admission, ask for feedback about your

application. Although it is sometimes hard to not take a denial personally, remember that this is your opportunity to discover what you can do to improve your application. Once you know what was amiss, you can either reapply to the same school or look for a different school to which to apply.

ETHICAL AND PROFESSIONAL ISSUES

Continuing Education

Education never ends. Although you obtain a degree and work hard for it, to be effective throughout your career as a human service professional, you must continue your learning. Once you are in the field, you will find that there are gaps in your education—things that were not stressed that seem essential for you to know at work. Therefore, continuing education beyond your degree is crucial. You can accomplish this through a variety of means. By joining the appropriate professional associations, you can participate in workshops that keep you current regarding the most recent advances in the field. You can take additional course work, perhaps to earn an advanced degree. Sometimes agencies will have staff development workshops aimed at increasing skills in areas deemed important. Increasingly, boards of registration, certification, and licensing are requiring continuing education to maintain professional credentials. This ensures that the professional is continuing to learn and that he or she can offer the best services possible to his or her clients.

THE DEVELOPMENTALLY MATURE
HUMAN SERVICE PROFESSIONAL

Anxious about Change, Desirous
of Change, Hopeful about the Future

As noted in earlier chapters, change is often not an easy process. It usually requires giving up an old system and accommodating to a new way of viewing the world. However, effective human service professionals, even though they may be anxious about the future, are willing and want to take on new challenges; they look at change as crucial to their own process of living and crucial to the evolution of the profession. Human service professionals who are stressed, burned out, cynical, and stagnant do little for themselves, probably provide poor services to their clients, and generally are not involved in positive ways with professional associations. On the other hand, human service professionals who are positive, forward looking, and desirous of change are probably the people who work best with their clients and offer the most to the future of the field.

Who is the effective human service professional? It's my friend Bob, who is attending workshops, has a positive attitude toward the future, takes care of himself by going to aerobics and meditating, and always has a positive attitude toward his clients. It's Rivers, who is encouraging of all people he meets, is a person you always want to hug, is warm, is caring, and is a great listener. It's Maggie, who is always willing to take a stand, a people's advocate, and a person who is able to love. And, it's Steve, who is a leader of others, is willing to confront his colleagues, even those to whom he is close, is constantly working on self-growth, and is always thinking about what he can do differently in the future. And it's you. Each of you has it within yourself to be caring, loving, reflective, energized, an advocate, a risk taker, a leader, and a doer!

SUMMARY

This chapter focused on the future. In it, we examined some possible changes in the roles of the human service professional and discussed, in particular, some of the client populations with whom the human service professional will most likely work in the upcoming years. These included the incarcerated, their families, and the victims of crime; those who are HIV-positive; the homeless and the poor; older people; individuals who are chronically mentally ill; people with disabilities; and individuals at risk for chemical dependence.

In addition to focusing on special populations, we also highlighted some important issues facing the human service professional during the 21st century. For instance, we noted how changes in technology have already affected and will continue to affect the human service professional as computers and other technologies such as interactive videos take on a more prominent role in human service work. We went on to discuss how the 21st century will bring a greater focus on a number of standards in the profession, including program accreditation, ethical guidelines, skills standards, and credentialing.

The chapter went on to highlight how the recent developmental emphasis in the human service profession has changed the manner in which many mental health professionals work, especially in reference to the importance of offering a primary prevention focus. We next examined how managed health care has greatly affected the social service field and the likelihood that human service professionals may be increasingly employed by HMOs. This was followed by a discussion about medical breakthroughs and the impact they will have on individuals. We noted that the human service professional must be well-versed in medical aspects of diseases and disabilities if he or she is to meet the new challenges that medical breakthroughs will bring. Although discussed in many parts of the text, we next highlighted how multicultural issues will continue to be particularly important in the 21st century.

The fact that the human service profession is a particularly high stress occupation was next discussed, and we noted some ways that human service professionals could live healthier lives. As the chapter continued, we discussed your future in the human services. We noted that the job outlook in the human services seems particularly good. We showed how there is much in common to applying for a job or applying to graduate schools, such as the importance of networking, knowing how to write a résumé, developing a portfolio, presenting yourself well, looking good when interviewing, and going on informational interviews. We then highlighted some specific suggestions for finding a job and listed a number of addresses where you can find information on graduate degrees in the social services. We suggested a number of points to consider when you apply to graduate schools.

As we neared the end of the chapter, we highlighted how the developmentally mature human service professional looks toward the future and is willing and eager to continue learning by joining professional associations, taking courses, and attending workshops.

EXPERIENTIAL EXERCISES

1. Interview a Person from a Special Population

Interview an individual in one or more of the following special populations, and ask the accompanying questions (and any other questions you think would be appropriate).

A Person Who Is Incarcerated:

1. Why were you incarcerated?
2. What's it like for you to be in jail (or prison)?
3. Do you believe you had a fair trial?
4. What prejudices have you experienced?
5. What social services have you used?
6. What social services would you like to have available?
7. Is there anything you would like to have changed about your life related to your current status?

A Person Who Has Been Victimized by Crime:

1. What is the nature of your victimization? (What happened to you?)
2. What's it like being a victim of crime?
3. Have you experienced any unusual reactions or prejudices from people as a result of your victimization?
4. What social services have you used?
5. What social services would you like to have available?
6. What changes in society, including the social service system, would you like to see related to those who are victims of crime?

An Individual Who Is HIV-Positive:

1. How did you become HIV-positive?

2. What unique experiences have you had related to being HIV-positive?

3. What prejudices have you experienced?

4. What social services have you used?

5. What social services would you like to have available?

6. What changes would you like to see take place in society related to your HIV-positive status?

A Poor Person or Homeless Person:

1. How did you become homeless or poor?

2. What unique experiences have you had related to your current life situation?

3. What prejudices have you experienced?

4. What social services have you used?

5. What social services would you like to have available?

6. How do you make it financially day-to-day?

7. What financial resources are available to you?

An Older Person:

1. How do you feel about being an older person?

2. What unique experiences have you had related to your age?

3. What prejudices have you experienced?

4. What social services have you used?

5. What social services would you like to have available?

6. What attitudes related to aging would you like to see changed in society?

An Individual Who Struggles with Mental Illness:

1. When do you first remember having to deal with your mental health problems?

2. What unique experiences have you had related to your mental illness?

3. What prejudices have you experienced?

4. What social services have you used?

5. What social services would you like to have available?

6. Has medication assisted you with your mental health problems?

7. What changes in the mental health care delivery system would you like to see?

An Individual Who Has a Disability:

1. How did you become disabled?

2. What unique experiences have you had related to your disability?

3. What prejudices have you experienced?

4. What social services have you used?

5. What social services would you like to have available?

6. Is there anything you would like to have changed about your life related to your current status?

An Individual Who Is (or Was) Chemically Dependent:

1. What led you to become chemically dependent?

2. What drugs or alcohol do (have) you use(d)?

3. What unique experiences have you had related to your substance abuse?

4. What prejudices have you experienced?

5. What social services have you used?

6. What social services would you like to have available?

7. How do you currently expect to handle your addiction to drugs or alcohol?

2. The Use of Computers

E-mail

1. In small groups, discuss how email has changed the way the helping professions offer services.

2. Talk to faculty and fellow students, and contact professional associations and find any newsgroups that exist for helping professionals.

The Use of PCs with Clients and in Research

Your instructor will distribute publisher catalogues and ask you to discuss, in small groups, the trend toward using computers for tests, programs to assist in diagnosis, billing programs, programs to assist in case report writing, and other software programs that are used on the PC. Discuss, in small groups, the use of these kinds of programs on the PC.

Counseling Online

Already, some professionals are offering free, or for a fee, counseling services online. Your instructor can make available the *Ethical Standards for Internet On-line Counseling* (ACA, 1999). Review these guidelines and in small groups discuss the ethical, professional, and legal implications of this new trend.

Web Pages

1. Professional organizations, faculty, and any individuals who are online can now create their own home pages. Discuss the implications of this for the helping profession.

2. Your instructor will divide the class into groups of seven students. He or she will then ask each group to take one or more of the following professional

organizations and examine its Web page. After you have reviewed it, report what you found to the class.

AAMFT: www.aamft.org (American Association of Marriage & Family Therapy)

ACA: www.counseling.org (American Counseling Association)

APA: www.psych.org (American Psychological Association)

APA: www.apa.org (American Psychiatric Association)

APNA: www.apna.org (American Psychiatric Nurses Association)
NASW: www.nasw.org (National Association of Social Workers)

NOHSE: www.nohse.com (National Organization for Human Service Education)

3. Standards of Practice

Discuss, in small groups, how you think the following standards could become more important.

1. Program approval
2. The use of ethical standards
3. Competency and skills standards
4. Credentialing

4. Health Maintenance Organizations (HMOs), Preferred Provider Organizations (PPOs), and Employee Assistance Programs (EAPs)

In small groups, research an HMO, PPO, EAP, or traditional health insurance plan. Compare and contrast these mental health delivery systems in the following ways:

1. What services are offered by each?
2. Does an individual need to go through a primary care physician to receive services?
3. Is preventive care covered?
4. How is specialty care dealt with?
5. Are mental health services covered?
6. What are the limitations of mental health services?
7. What is the payment for services, if any?
8. What are the job opportunities for an individual who has a degree in human services?

5. Medical Breakthroughs

1. In small groups, discuss the mental health implications for an individual who is faced with the following medical problems:

a. An individual who is waiting for an organ transplant and will die if it is not received.

b. An individual who might have the gene for a debilitating disease and has the opportunity, through genetic testing, to discover if he or she has the disease.

c. An individual who carries a gene for a debilitating disease and is considering having a child.

d. An individual who refuses medical treatment for himself or herself because of religious beliefs.

e. An individual who refuses medical treatment for his or her child because of religious beliefs.

2. What are the implications for the families of the individuals noted in number 1?

3. What are the ethical, legal, and professional implications of working with the individuals noted in number 1?

6. Developmental Emphasis and Primary Prevention Emphasis

For each of the following theories, develop a primary prevention activity that could assist an individual through any stage of the theory (you may want to refer back to Chapter 5 for assistance).

1. Piaget's Theory of Cognitive Development
2. Kohlberg's and/or Gilligan's Theory of Moral Development
3. Erikson's Theory of Psychosocial Development
4. Kegan's Constructive Development Model

7. Trends in Multiculturalism

Answer the following questions concerning muticulturalism:

1. What changes do you foresee in the future of the human service profession if, as predicted, multicultural issues continue to be stressed?

2. What are some positive and negative aspects to having same-culture helpers work with same-culture clients?

3. How do you think you will be personally affected by a more diverse group of human service professionals?

8. Dealing with Stress and Burnout

Discuss the various ways that you deal with stress and burnout.

1. Are the ways that you deal with stress working for you?

2. Are there other ways that you might find to deal effectively with your stress?

3. What would you do if you noticed a colleague of yours was burned out and was working poorly with clients?

4. What would you do if you were burned out and were working poorly with clients?

5. Have your instructor distribute the Wheel of Wellness article (Myers, Sweeney, & Witmer, 2000) and examine what areas in your life you might work on. Share in small groups.

9. Finding Potential Jobs

Do one or more of the following activities and make a list of all of the potential occupations that you might like:

1. Take an interest inventory and have it interpreted.

2. Look through the newspaper want ads and write down all jobs that seem interesting to you.

3. Do Activity 9.1 and make a list of all jobs that seem interesting to you. If you can obtain a copy of the *Dictionary of Holland Occupational Codes* (check your library or career services office), expand your list of potential jobs by looking up your three-letter code in the book.

4. Spend some time looking through the *Dictionary of Occupational Titles* (DOT) to identify possible jobs you might like.

5. Include in your list any jobs about which you have fantasized, regardless of whether you think you could do that job.

6. Go on an informational interview and obtain information about a job.

10. Narrowing Your List of Potential Occupations

Take the top 10 or 20 jobs you listed in Exercise 9 and rank-order your list; that is, make a list, starting with the job you like best and ending with the job you like least.

11. Identifying Skills Needed for Your List of Occupations

From the list in Exercise 10, starting with your top-ranked occupation, write down the jobs on the left side of the page and then, to the right of the job, identify the skills needed for those jobs (use the DOT or OOH if needed). Then ask yourself if you currently have the skills needed for the job and if not, what you can do to obtain the skills. See the example that follows:

Job	Skills Needed	Do I Have the Skills	How Can I Obtain the Skills?
Social services professional	Interviewing	Yes	
	Empathy	Partly	Practice sessions, role-play
	Record Keeping	No	Take course, obtain information from agency
	Supervising Clients	No	Internship
	Counseling	Partly	Role-play with feedback from others, internship
	Consulting	No	Course, internship, speak with consultants about what they do, reading materials

12. Developing a Résumé

Based on the points in this chapter, and any others noted in class, develop a résumé. Bring it to class and share it with other students. Give feedback to one another concerning the strengths and weaknesses of each other's résumés.

13. Focus on Continuing Education

List some continuing education activities in which you would like to get involved when you are working in the human service field and answer the following questions:

1. Do you think continuing education should be mandatory for human services professionals? Why or why not?

2. If you think continuing education should be mandatory, discuss the number of hours per year you think should be required for each human service professional to undertake?

14. Ethical and Professional Vignettes

Review the following vignettes and discuss in class. When appropriate, refer to the ethical standards in Appendix B.

1. A colleague of yours tells you that he is working with an individual who just discovered that she carries the gene for a fatal disease. Although she will not get the disease, any child of hers has a 50% chance of developing the disease. She has told you that she has decided to "have my tubes tied and not tell my husband." What ethical, professional, or legal obligation, if any, do you have?

2. A classmate tells you that she sells flower extracts to clients to help them heal. She states this is the "wave of the future." Is this ethical? Professional? Legal? Is this reasonable? What, if anything, should you do?

3. A colleague of yours, who has a bachelor's degree in human services, decides to set up her own Web page where individuals can ask personal questions to which she will reply by email. Is this ethical? Professional? Legal?

4. You are aware that a colleague of yours is no longer effective with his clients because he is burned out. He does not realize this. What is your responsibility to the colleague? To his clients?

5. A colleague of yours refuses to become involved in any professional associations, read any journals, or keep up with any advances in the field. She states, "I do what has been shown to be tried and true." Does she have a point? Is what she's doing ethical? Professional? What is your responsibility in this situation?

6. One of your faculty never acknowledges differences in clients as a function of cultural background. When a student notes this in class, her only response is, "Every helping relationship is a cross-cultural one, so why should I discuss any one culture in particular?" Does she have a point? Do you have any responsibility in this situation?

7. Your human services program is not approved by CSHSE. Do you have a responsibility to advocate for approval? Why or why not?

8. A colleague of yours often uses ethical guidelines from a related social service profession when the *Ethical Standards of Human Service Professionals* does not offer guidance in the direction he anticipates. Is this ethical? Professional?

9. A colleague of yours offers a primary prevention workshop on avoiding the use of drugs and alcohol. Your colleague used to take drugs and drink heavily but has not taken any coursework or workshops, or read the literature on substance abuse. She notes, "I have my own experience, that's why I can do this workshop." Is this ethical, legal, professional?

10. You have decided to take a job with an HMO despite hating the way the company does business. However, they are offering you a good salary and you will be able to run psychoeducational workshops for adolescents and adults. Is it a good idea that you take the job? Why, or why not?

Appendix A

✦

Select Web Sites of Organizations

AAMFT (American Association of Marriage and Family Therapy): www.aamft.org

AAPC (American Association of Pastoral Counselors): www.aapc.org

AATA (American Art Therapy Association): www.arttherapy.org

ACA (American Counseling Association): www.counseling.org

ACPA (American College Personnel Association): www.acpa.nche.edu

ACPE (Association for Clinical Pastoral Education): www.acpe.edu

ACSW (Academy of Certified Social Workers): www.naswdc.org /credentials/acsw.asp

AMCD (Association for Multicultural Counseling and Development): www.amcd–aca.org

AMHCA (American Mental Health Counselors Association): www .amhca.org

APA (American Psychiatric Association): www.psych.org

APA (American Psychological Association): www.apa.org

APNA (American Psychiatric Nurses Association): www.apna.org

APsaA (American Psychoanalytical Association): www.apsa.org

ARCA (American Rehabilitation Counselor Association): www.nchrtm.okstate.edu/ARCA/index .html

ASCA (American School Counselor Association): www.schoolcounselor.org

ASWB (Association of Social Work Boards): www.aswb.org

CACREP (Council on Accreditation of Counseling and Related Educational Programs): www.counseling.org/cacrep

COAMFTE (Commission on Accreditation for Marital and Family Therapy Education): www.aamft.org/about /COAMFTE/AboutCOAMFTE.htm

CORE (Council on Rehabilitation Education): www.rehab.org

CRCC (Commission for Rehabilitation Counselor Certification): www. crccertification.com

CSHSE (Council on Standards in Human Service Education): www.cshse.org

CSWE (Council on Social Work Education): www.cswe.org

IAMFC (International Association of Marriage and Family Counselors): www.iamfc.org

NACFT (National Academy of Certified Family Therapists): www.iamfc.org /nacft.htm

NASP (National Association of School Psychologists): www.nasponline.org

NASW (National Association of Social Workers): www.naswdc.org

NBCC (National Board for Certified Counselors): www.nbcc.org

NCRE (National Council on Rehabilitation Education): www. nchrtm.okstate.edu/ncre

NOHSE (National Organization of Human Service Education): www.nohse.com

NRA (National Rehabilitation Association): www.nationalrehab.org

NRCA (National Rehabilitation Counseling Association): www.nationalrehab .org/website/divs/nrca.html

Appendix B

⌘

Ethical Standards of Human Service Professionals

PREAMBLE

Human services is a profession developing in response to and in anticipation of the direction of human needs and human problems in the late twentieth century. Characterized particularly by an appreciation of human beings in all of their diversity, human services offers assistance to its clients within the context of their community and environment. Human service professionals and those who educate them, regardless of whether they are students, faculty or practitioners, promote and encourage the unique values and characteristics of human services. In so doing human service professionals and educators uphold the integrity and ethics of the profession, partake in constructive criticism of the profession, promote client and community well-being, and enhance their own professional growth.

The ethical guidelines presented are a set of standards of conduct which the human service professionals and educators consider in ethical and professional decision making. It is hoped that these guidelines will be of assistance when human service professionals and educators are challenged by difficult ethical dilemmas. Although ethical codes are not legal documents, they may be used to assist in the adjudication of issues related to ethical human service behavior.

Used by permission of the National Organization for Human Service.

SECTION I—STANDARDS
FOR HUMAN SERVICE PROFESSIONALS

Human service professionals function in many ways and carry out many roles. They enter into professional-client relationships with individuals, families, groups and communities who are all referred to as "clients" in these standards. Among their roles are caregiver, case manager, broker, teacher/educator, behavior changer, consultant, outreach professional, mobilizer, advocate, community planner, community change organizer, evaluator and administrator (SREB, 1967). The following standards are written with these multifaceted roles in mind.

The Human Service Professional's
Responsibility to Clients

Statement 1
Human service professionals negotiate with clients the purpose, goals, and nature of the helping relationship prior to its onset as well as inform clients of the limitations of the proposed relationship.

Statement 2
Human service professionals respect the integrity and welfare of the client at all times. Each client is treated with respect, acceptance and dignity.

Statement 3
Human service professionals protect the client's right to privacy and confidentiality except when such confidentiality would cause harm to the client or others, when agency guidelines state otherwise, or under other stated conditions (e.g., local, state, or federal laws). Professionals inform clients of the limits of confidentiality prior to the onset of the helping relationship.

Statement 4
If it is suspected that danger or harm may occur to the client or to others as a result of a client's behavior, the human service professional acts in an appropriate and professional manner to protect the safety of those individuals. This may involve seeking consultation, supervision, and/or breaking the confidentiality of the relationship.

Statement 5
Human service professionals protect the integrity, safety, and security of client records. All written client information that is shared with other professionals, except in the course of professional supervision, must have the client's prior written consent.

Statement 6
Human service professionals are aware that in their relationships with clients power and status are unequal. Therefore they recognize that dual or multiple rela-

tionships may increase the risk of harm to, or exploitation of, clients, and may impair their professional judgment. However, in some communities and situations it may not be feasible to avoid social or other nonprofessional contact with clients. Human service professionals support the trust implicit in the helping relationship by avoiding dual relationships that may impair professional judgment, increase the risk of harm to clients or lead to exploitation.

Statement 7

Sexual relationships with current clients are not considered to be in the best interest of the client and are prohibited. Sexual relationships with previous clients are considered dual relationships and are addressed in Statement 6 (above).

Statement 8

The client's right to self-determination is protected by human service professionals. They recognize the client's right to receive or refuse services.

Statement 9

Human service professionals recognize and build on client strengths.

The Human Service Professional's
Responsibility to the Community and Society

Statement 10

Human service professionals are aware of local, state, and federal laws. They advocate for change in regulations and statutes when such legislation conflicts with ethical guidelines and/or client rights. Where laws are harmful to individuals, groups or communities, human service professionals consider the conflict between the values of obeying the law and the values of serving people and may decide to initiate social action.

Statement 11

Human service professionals keep informed about current social issues as they affect the client and the community. They share that information with clients, groups and community as part of their work.

Statement 12

Human service professionals understand the complex interaction between individuals, their families, the communities in which they live, and society.

Statement 13

Human service professionals act as advocates in addressing unmet client and community needs. Human service professionals provide a mechanism for identifying unmet client needs, calling attention to these needs, and assisting in planning and mobilizing to advocate for those needs at the local community level.

Statement 14

Human service professionals represent their qualifications to the public accurately.

Statement 15

Human service professionals describe the effectiveness of programs, treatments, and/or techniques accurately.

Statement 16

Human service professionals advocate for the rights of all members of society, particularly those who are members of minorities and groups at which discriminatory practices have historically been directed.

Statement 17

Human service professionals provide services without discrimination or preference based on age, ethnicity, culture, race, disability, gender, religion, sexual orientation or socioeconomic status.

Statement 18

Human service professionals are knowledgeable about the cultures and communities within which they practice. They are aware of multiculturalism in society and its impact on the community as well as individuals within the community. They respect individuals and groups, their cultures and beliefs.

Statement 19

Human service professionals are aware of their own cultural backgrounds, beliefs, and values, recognizing the potential for impact on their relationships with others.

Statement 20

Human service professionals are aware of sociopolitical issues that differentially affect clients from diverse backgrounds.

Statement 21

Human service professionals seek the training, experience, education and supervision necessary to ensure their effectiveness in working with culturally diverse client populations.

The Human Service Professional's
Responsibility to Colleagues

Statement 22

Human service professionals avoid duplicating another professional's helping relationship with a client. They consult with other professionals who are assisting the client in a different type of relationship when it is in the best interest of the client to do so.

Statement 23

When a human service professional has a conflict with a colleague, he or she first seeks out the colleague in an attempt to manage the problem. If necessary, the professional then seeks the assistance of supervisors, consultants or other professionals in efforts to manage the problem.

Statement 24

Human service professionals respond appropriately to unethical behavior of colleagues. Usually this means initially talking directly with the colleague and, if no resolution is forthcoming, reporting the colleague's behavior to supervisory or administrative staff and/or to the professional organization(s) to which the colleague belongs.

Statement 25

All consultations between human service professionals are kept confidential unless to do so would result in harm to clients or communities.

The Human Service Professional's
Responsibility to the Profession

Statement 26

Human service professionals know the limit and scope of their professional knowledge and offer services only within their knowledge and skill base.

Statement 27

Human service professionals seek appropriate consultation and supervision to assist in decision-making when there are legal, ethical or other dilemmas.

Statement 28

Human service professionals act with integrity, honesty, genuineness, and objectivity.

Statement 29

Human service professionals promote cooperation among related disciplines (e.g., psychology, counseling, social work, nursing, family and consumer sciences, medicine, education) to foster professional growth and interests within the various fields.

Statement 30

Human service professionals promote the continuing development of their profession. They encourage membership in professional associations, support research endeavors, foster educational advancement, advocate for appropriate legislative actions, and participate in other related professional activities.

Statement 31

Human service professionals continually seek out new and effective approaches to enhance their professional abilities.

The Human Service Professional's
Responsibility to Employers

Statement 32

Human service professionals adhere to commitments made to their employers.

Statement 33

Human service professionals participate in efforts to establish and maintain employment conditions which are conducive to high quality client services. They assist in evaluating the effectiveness of the agency through reliable and valid assessment measures.

Statement 34

When a conflict arises between fulfilling the responsibility to the employer and the responsibility to the client, human service professionals advise both of the conflict and work conjointly with all involved to manage the conflict.

The Human Service Professional's Responsibility to Self

Statement 35

Human service professionals strive to personify those characteristics typically associated with the profession (e.g., accountability, respect for others, genuineness, empathy, pragmatism).

Statement 36

Human service professionals foster self-awareness and personal growth in themselves. They recognize that when professionals are aware of their own values, attitudes, cultural background, and personal needs, the process of helping others is less likely to be negatively impacted by those factors.

Statement 37

Human service professionals recognize a commitment to lifelong learning and continually upgrade knowledge and skills to serve the populations better.

SECTION II—STANDARDS FOR HUMAN SERVICE EDUCATORS

Human Service educators are familiar with, informed by and accountable to the standards of professional conduct put forth by their institutions of higher learning; their professional disciplines, for example, American Association of University Professors (AAUP), American Counseling Association (ACA), Academy of Criminal Justice (ACJS), American Psychological Association (APA), American Sociological Association (ASA), National Association of Social Workers (NASW), National Board of Certified Counselors (NBCC), National Education Association (NEA), and the National Organization for Human Service Education (NOHSE).

Statement 38

Human service educators uphold the principle of liberal education and embrace the essence of academic freedom, abstaining from inflicting their own personal views/morals on students, and allowing students the freedom to express their views without penalty, censure or ridicule, and to engage in critical thinking.

Statement 39

Human service educators provide students with readily available and explicit program policies and criteria regarding program goals and objectives, recruitment, admission, course requirements, evaluations, retention and dismissal in accordance with due process procedures.

Statement 40

Human service educators demonstrate high standards of scholarship in content areas and of pedagogy by staying current with developments in the field of Human Services and in teaching effectiveness, for example learning styles and teaching styles.

Statement 41

Human service educators monitor students' field experiences to ensure the quality of the placement site, supervisory experience, and learning experience towards the goals of professional identity and skill development.

Statement 42

Human service educators participate actively in the selection of required readings and use them with care, based strictly on the merits of the material's content, and present relevant information accurately, objectively and fully.

Statement 43

Human service educators, at the onset of courses: inform students if sensitive/controversial issues or experiential/affective content or process are part of the course design; ensure that students are offered opportunities to discuss in structured ways their reactions to sensitive or controversial class content; ensure that the presentation of such material is justified on pedagogical grounds directly related to the course; and, differentiate between information based on scientific data, anecdotal data, and personal opinion.

Statement 44

Human service educators develop and demonstrate culturally sensitive knowledge, awareness, and teaching methodology.

Statement 45

Human service educators demonstrate full commitment to their appointed responsibilities, and are enthusiastic about and encouraging of students' learning.

Statement 46

Human service educators model the personal attributes, values and skills of the human service professional, including but not limited to, the willingness to seek and respond to feedback from students.

Statement 47
Human service educators establish and uphold appropriate guidelines concerning self-disclosure or student-disclosure of sensitive/personal information.

Statement 48
Human service educators establish an appropriate and timely process for providing clear and objective feedback to students about their performance on relevant and established course/program academic and personal competence requirements and their suitability for the field.

Statement 49
Human service educators are aware that in their relationships with students, power and status are unequal; therefore, human service educators are responsible to clearly define and maintain ethical and professional relationships with students, and avoid conduct that is demeaning, embarrassing or exploitative of students, and to treat students fairly, equally and without discrimination.

Statement 50
Human service educators recognize and acknowledge the contributions of students to their work, for example in case material, workshops, research, publications.

Statement 51
Human service educators demonstrate professional standards of conduct in managing personal or professional differences with colleagues, for example, not disclosing such differences and/or affirming a student's negative opinion of a faculty/program.

Statement 52
Human service educators ensure that students are familiar with, informed by, and accountable to the ethical standards and policies put forth by their program/department, the course syllabus/instructor, their advisor(s), and the Ethical Standards of Human Service Professionals.

Statement 53
Human service educators are aware of all relevant curriculum standards, including those of the Council for Standards in Human Services Education (CSHSE); the Community Support Skills Standards; and state/local standards, and take them into consideration in designing the curriculum.

Statement 54
Human service educators create a learning context in which students can achieve the knowledge, skills, values and attitudes of the academic program.

Appendix C

⌘

Overview of the Council for Standards in Human Service Education (CSHSE)

The Council for Standards in Human Service Education (CSHSE) is the only national level organization accrediting Human Service (HS) educational programs in the United States. Founded in 1979, over 60 colleges across the country have been CSHSE members at one time or another. However, in recent years there has been a decline in membership.

College administrators and HS faculty have questioned a need for joining CSHSE. Many ask, "Since accreditation is not mandated, why get it?" Many see the CSHSE self-study process as a cumbersome and burdening activity added on top of an already demanding workload with understaffed programs. Given all of these disadvantages for seeking CSHSE program accreditation, are there any advantages?

HS College programs that join CSHSE accrue, at least, six benefits:

1. **Accreditation:** Although program accreditation is voluntary, that is, there are no organizational bodies requiring this accreditation (like in nursing), a program can take pride in knowing it has met national norms for human service education. Their program courses do not only reflect the good thinking of local HS faculty but also, with CSHSE accreditation, a program demonstrates it is as good as the best programs in America. A program can document its quality by showing it meets national norms. Also, students in an accredited program can be confident of the quality of their program.

2. **Marketing:** Having obtained accreditation from CSHSE, an HS program can put the CSHSE logo on all of its publications. With this logo, HS programs can market their programs with confidence.

3. **Publications:** CSHSE provides its members with the Bulletin three times per year. The Bulletin cites educational innovations in HS education from across America, discusses current HS issues, profiles nationally known HS educators, and possesses a variety of other lively articles about HS education. Also, the Council distributes monographs to its membership. Past monographs have covered topics like fieldwork placements, the history of HS education, and diversity in human services. CSHSE has recently published its first textbook, *Human Service Challenges in the 21st Century,* eds. Tricia McClam and Marianne Woodside. Faculty members have adopted monographs and the "21st Century" book in their classes as required reading for their students. Finally, the HS Directory, which lists over 400 human service programs in the United States, is available to CSHSE members. Those doing research in the human services have used this invaluable resource.

4. **CSHSE Web site:** CSHSE members can access such information as Council standards, CSHSE Board members and regional directors, and links to other HS sites (soon to be added). Also, each member college will be listed on the site so anyone on the Internet can access their school's HS program, thus rendering national recognition to the HS program and its college at no cost to either of them.

5. **Technical Assistance:** CSHSE Board members have a wealth of HS information about HS education and practice on national, regional, and local levels. Any CSHSE member college has access to the competence on the CSHSE Board with their wealth of HS information that can be incorporated into research projects or included in HS program planning. For instance, they can give information about fieldwork placements, admit /retain/dismiss procedures and policies, and general curriculum development gleaned from self-study reports and site visits from all over the country.

6. **Professional Networking:** As a CSHSE member, HS educators have access to a variety of HS professionals across the nation. This access can provide contact for those developing their curriculum, doing research and sharing "war stories." Rather than feeling alienated in an "unloved profession" CSHSE members can be involved in a network of active and engaging HS educational professionals all over the country. Heapes, J. (2001). *CSHSE Bulletin,* 20. (See also: www.cshse.org/index.html)

Appendix D

Overview and Summary of Accreditation Standards

Overview of Standards (CSHSE, 2002b)

The Standards are organized in two sections: General Program Characteristics and Curriculum. Each standard, printed in italics, contains a principle. These standards apply to all three levels of human services training programs unless specifically noted otherwise.

The three levels of training programs are: the Technical Level (nondegree granting), the *Associate Degree Level,* and the *Advanced Degree Level.*

The statements preceding each italicized standard provide an instruction explaining the rationale for the standard. The statements following each standard are the specifications for that standard. These specifications are the criteria that are used for evaluating program compliance to the standards. They reflect the minimum acceptable level of compliance.

In the Curriculum section, differential specifications for each of the training levels are given following each standard. Each higher level specification presumes the inclusion of the knowledge, skills, or attitude content specified for the preceding level(s), i.e., all associate degree level specifications are in addition to those given for the technical level and all advanced level specifications are in addition to the specifications of both the technical and associate degree levels. It is the responsibility of each program to demonstrate that its curriculum meets the knowledge, skill and attitude specifications described for the lower level(s) in addition to the specifications of the training level for which program accreditation is sought.

Many programs will exceed the minimum specifications for certain of these curricular standards, depending upon their particular program emphasis. The purpose of the curricular specifications is to delineate the minimal level of compliance at each training level for each standard.

Curriculum content standards may be met in either traditional academic settings (class, lab, fieldtrips, etc.) or in field experience settings. It is the responsibility of each program to demonstrate where in their program each of the curricular standards is met.

Summary of Standards (CSHSE, 2002c)

Standard Number 1
The primary program objective shall be to prepare human service practitioners to serve clients or carry out other supportive human service agency functions. Human service competencies shall be the basis for the design of program goals, curriculum, and methodology.

Standard Number 2
The program description shall state explicitly the philosophical and knowledge base of the program.

Standard Number 3
The program shall conduct periodic assessments of community needs for kinds and numbers of human service workers.

Standard Number 4
The program shall use the community needs assessment, graduate follow-up studies, and evaluation of faculty and courses to determine how well the program is meeting community and student needs and to modify the program as necessary.

Standard Number 5
The program shall have written standards and procedures for admitting, retaining, and dismissing students.

Standard Number 6
The collective competencies of the core faculty staff for each program shall include both a strong knowledge base and practical experience in delivery of human services to clients.

Standard Number 7
The program shall adequately manage the essential training program roles and provide opportunities for faculty to learn the essential staff role and skills required for service training programs.

Standard Number 8
Faculty evaluations shall reflect the total role responsibilities as defined in the position description of that faculty member and shall be conducted at least every two years.

Standard Number 9
The program shall have adequate staff support and program resources to provide a complete training program.

Standard Number 10
Each program shall make efforts to increase the transferability of credits to other academic program and have a written policy on how student's credits and previous learning achievements will be evaluated and accepted for admission and transfer.

Standard Number 11
The curriculum shall provide knowledge of the historical development of human services.

Standard Number 12
The curriculum shall provide knowledge of human systems individual, group, family, organization, community, society and their interaction.

Standard Number 13
The curriculum shall address the conditions which promote or limit optimal human functioning and identify classes of deviation from desired functioning in the major human system.

Standard Number 14
The curriculum shall provide skill training in systematic analysis of a service problem situation; in selection of appropriate strategies, services, or interventions; and in evaluation of outcomes.

Standard Number 15
The curriculum shall provide skill training in information management.

Standard Number 16
The curriculum shall provide training in human service intervention skills that are appropriate to the level of training.

Standard Number 17
Learning experiences shall be provided for the student to develop his/her interpersonal skills with clients, co-workers and supervisors.

Standard Number 18

The curriculum shall provide skill training in the administrative aspects of the service delivery system.

Standard Number 19

The training program shall transmit the major human service values and attitudes to students in order to promote understanding of human service ethics and their application in practice.

Standard Number 20

The training program shall provide experiences and support to enable students to develop awareness of their own values, personalities, reaction patterns, interpersonal styles, and limitations.

Standard Number 21

The program shall provide each student field experience that is integrated with the rest of the training and education.

Standard Number 22

The program shall award academic credit for the field experience.

Standard Number 23

It is the responsibility of the college to ensure that field placement sites provide quality training experiences and supervision.

Appendix E

✠

Global Assessment of Functioning Scale

Global Assessment of Functioning Scale (GAF)

Code*	(Note: Use intermediate codes when appropriate, e.g., 45, 68, 72)
100	**Superior functioning in a wide range of activities, life's problems never seem to get out of hand, is sought out by others because of his or her many positive qualities.**
91	**No symptoms.**
90	**Absent or minimal symptoms** (e.g., mild anxiety before an exam), **good functioning in all areas, interested and involved in a wide range of activities, socially effective, generally satisfied with life, no more than everyday problems**
81	**or concerns** (e.g., an occasional argument with family members).
80	**If symptoms are present, they are transient and expectable reactions to psychosocial stressors** (e.g., difficulty concentrating after family argument); **no more than slight impairment in social, occupational, or school functioning**
71	(e.g., temporarily falling behind in schoolwork).
70	**Some mild symptoms** (e.g., depressed mood and mild insomnia) **OR some difficulty in social, occupational or school functioning** (e.g., occasional truancy, or theft within the household), **but generally functioning pretty well, has some**
61	**meaningful interpersonal relationships.**
60	**Moderate symptoms** (e.g., flat affect and circumstantial speech, occasional panic attacks) **OR some difficulty in social, occupational, or school functioning**
51	(e.g., few friends, conflicts with peers or co-workers).
50	**Serious symptoms** (e.g., suicidal ideation, severe obsessional rituals, frequent shoplifting) **OR any serious impairment in social occupational, or school**
41	**functioning** (e.g., no friends, unable to keep a job).

Global Assessment of Functioning Scale (GAF)

Code*	(Note: Use intermediate codes when appropriate, e.g., 45, 68, 72)
40 ⋮ 31	**Some impairment in reality testing or communication** (e.g., speech is at times illogical, obscure, or irrelevant) **OR major impairment in several areas, such as work or school family relations, judgment, thinking, or mood** (e.g., depressed man avoids friends, neglects family, and is unable to work; child frequently beats up younger children, is defiant at home, and is failing at school).
30 ⋮ 21	**Behavior is considerably influenced by delusions or hallucinations OR serious impairment in communication or judgment** (e.g., sometimes incoherent, acts grossly inappropriately, suicidal preoccupation) **OR inability to function in almost all areas** (e.g., stays in bed all day; no job, home, or friends).
20 ⋮ 11	**Some danger of hurting self or others** (e.g., suicide attempts without clear expectation of death: frequently violent; manic excitement) **OR occasionally fails to maintain minimal personal hygiene** (e.g., smears feces) **OR gross impairment in communication** (e.g., largely incoherent or mute).
10 ⋮ 1	**Persistent danger of severely hurting self or others** (e.g., recurrent violence) **OR persistent inability to maintain minimal personal hygiene OR serious suicidal act with clear expectation of death.**
0	**Inadequate information**

Appendix F

Understanding Your Holland Code

When an individual discovers which of the Holland code types most represents his or her personality, then the corresponding job environments that fit his or her personality type could easily be found. For instance, a person with an investigative personality would want to find investigative jobs (for example, scientist, mathematician).

A brief description of each of the personality types and some jobs that fit that type follow. Examine the description and the sample jobs to see if they seem to fit how you see yourself. Keep in mind that no description will perfectly fit any person. In reviewing each description, most likely it would benefit you to try to find a job that fits both your personality type and its corresponding work environment.

Realistic

Realistic persons like to work with equipment, machines, or tools, often prefer to work outdoors, and are good with manipulating concrete physical objects. These individuals prefer to avoid social situations, artistic endeavors, or intellectual tasks. They are often practical, robust, and have good physical skills. Realistic people tend to do well in work environments that promote the use of large motor skills, athletic and/or technical skills, and places where they do not have to take on leadership roles. Some settings in which you might find realistic individuals include filling stations, farms, machine shops, construction sites, and power plants. Some typical jobs include forester, locksmith, animal trainer, farmer, machinist, geologist, mechanical engineer, cook, bricklayer, electrician, plumber, automobile or airplane mechanic, photographer, draftsperson, machine operator, and/or surveyor.

Investigative

Investigative persons like to think abstractly, problem solve, and investigate. These individuals feel comfortable with the pursuit of knowledge and with dealing with the manipulation of ideas and symbols. They prefer scientific methodology and feel comfortable with foreign languages, reading, arithmetic, and the arts. Investigative individuals prefer to avoid social situations and see themselves as introverted. They tend to do well in work environments that promote independence, originality, and scholarly pursuits. Some settings in which you might find investigative individuals include research laboratories, hospitals, universities, and government-sponsored research agencies. Some typical jobs include microbiologist, biologist, dentist, physician, chemist, scientist, physicist, research psychologist, geneticist, biochemist, civil engineer, assistant to scientist, dietitian, veterinarian, nurse practitioner, geologist, researcher, mathematician, computer programmer, and/or laboratory technician.

Artistic

Artistic individuals like to express themselves creatively, usually through artistic forms such as drama, art, music, and writing. They prefer unstructured activities in which they can use their imagination and creative side. They tend to prefer work environments that allow them to express their independence, sensitivity, and emotional side. They crave originality and flexibility at the workplace. Some settings in which you might find artistic individuals include the theater, concert halls, libraries, art or music studios, dance studios, orchestras, photography studios, newspapers, and restaurants. Some typical jobs include comedian, actor, dancer, musician, conductor, designer, artist, writer, photographer, drama and art teacher, pastry chef, editor, sculptor, and/or music teacher.

Social

Social people are nurturers, helpers, caregivers, and have high concern for others. They are introspective and insightful and prefer work environments in which they can use their intuitive and caregiving skills. They tend to be responsible citizens and usually have good communication skills. They prefer work settings where there is much social interaction and where they can use their social and helping skills. Some settings in which you might find social people are government social service agencies, counseling offices, churches, schools, mental hospitals, reaction centers, personnel offices, and hospitals. Some typical jobs include counselor, psychologist, minister, speech therapist, social worker, psychiatric aid, social science teacher, chiropractor, nurse supervisor, human service worker, political scientist, nurse, sociologist, teacher, college professor, and/or educational administrator.

Enterprising

Enterprising individuals are self-confident, adventurous, bold, and sociable. They have good persuasive skills and prefer positions of leadership. They tend to dominate conversations and enjoy work environments in which they can satisfy their need for recognition, power, and expression. They tend to be good public speakers and appear emotionally stable. Some settings in which you might find enterprising individuals include life insurance agencies, advertising agencies, political offices, real estate offices, new and used car lots, sales offices, and in management settings. Some typical jobs include life insurance agent, realtor, politician, broker, hotel clerk, sales, politician, manager, business executive, sales manager, manager of personnel, car salesperson, and/or many jobs in which there is a need for management, supervision, or administration of programs.

Conventional

Individuals of the conventional orientation are stable, controlled, conservative, and sociable. They prefer working on concrete tasks and like to follow instructions. They like routine problem-solving and working with data. They would prefer a work environment that is orderly, neat, and in which their tasks are clear and spelled out. They value the business world, clerical tasks, and tend to be good at computational skills. Some settings in which you might find conventional people include banks, business offices, accounting firms, and medical records. Some typical jobs include keypunch operator, bookkeeper, accountant, stenographer, machine duplicator, receptionist, secretary, teller, banker, tax expert, credit manager, payroll clerk, file clerk, and/or a variety of other clerk positions. Often it is important to find a job that not only matches your highest personality type but has qualities of your second and third orientation also. For instance, an individual who has a fairly high social and artistic orientation might be interested in jobs like counselor, teacher, physical therapist, minister, and so on, for all of these jobs have both a social and artistic component to them.

Holland did research that supported the notion that the six personality types could be viewed on a hexagon, with those that are next to one another being similar and those on opposite sides being different from one another (see Figure F.1). If you would like to compare your code to thousands of jobs listed in the *Dictionary of Occupational Titles* (DOT) (U.S. Department of Labor, 1999), you can obtain a copy of the *Dictionary of Holland Occupational Codes* (Gottfredson, Holland, & Ogawa, 1996).

Probably in discovering your highest personality types you have found that they are adjacent on the hexagon. This would make sense because the orientations adjacent to one another share more in common with each other compared with the types that are opposite. Similarly, most jobs do not exclusively follow one personality type but also offer some of the qualities of the orientation closest on the hexagon. If, however, you found that your highest personality types are not adjacent to one another, it is likely that you will have fewer job settings from which to choose. In some cases, this will make your job search more difficult.

Keep in mind that there are approximately 30,000 jobs in this country, many of which might fit your personality type. If you would like to examine different jobs after taking the inventory, there are a number of things you can do. First, you can go to a career counselor who, using a number of sophisticated instruments, can further the identification of your Holland personality type. Secondly, you can

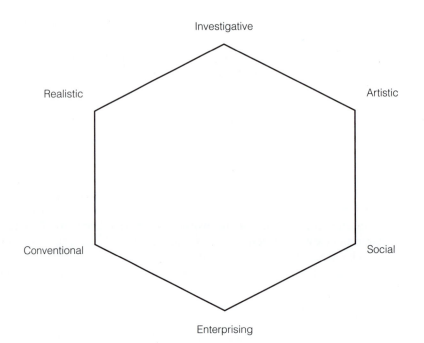

FIGURE F.1 The six Holland types can be viewed as a hexagon. Those closest to each other are more similar than those on opposite sides from one another.

go to the reference section of your local library and examine a book called the *Dictionary of Occupational Titles* (DOT) (U.S. Department of Labor, 1999). This important reference book, published by the U.S. Employment Service, offers a listing of all jobs in the United States, and you can cross-reference the list of jobs you found associated with your personality type with related jobs found in the DOT.

Glossary

AACD *See* American Association for Counseling and Development.

AAMFT American Association for Marriage and Family Therapy.

Ability test A test to measure an individual's cognitive capabilities. *See* Achievement test, Aptitude test.

ACA *See* American Counseling Association.

Academy of Certified Social Workers (ACSW) Established in 1960 by the National Association of Social Workers, this association sets standards of practice in the field for master's-level social workers.

Accommodate *See* Accommodation.

Accommodation The process of adapting new knowledge and experiences in a manner so that one's understanding of the world is altered.

Acceptance Respecting people's ideals, thoughts, and emotions. One of the eight characteristics identified as being related to counselor effectiveness.

ACES *See* Association for Counselor Education and Supervision.

Achievement test A type of an ability test that measures what has been learned. *See* Diagnostic test, Readiness test, Survey battery test.

ACSW *See* Academy of Certified Social Workers.

Actualizing tendency The inborn, positive inner qualities and inherent traits that arise in a person when placed in a nurturing and facilitative environment. *See also* Humanistic counseling and education.

Acute psychotic episode Short-term loss of reality.

ADA *See* Americans with Disabilities Act.

Addams, Jane A social activist who established Hull House in Chicago in 1899.

Adler, Alfred A student of Freud's who developed a humanistically oriented analytical theory known as Adlerian therapy.

Administrator A human service worker who supervises community service programs.

Advice giving   The offering of recommendations or suggestions pertaining to a decision for a given situation.

Advocate   A human service worker who champions and defends clients' causes and rights.

Affirmation   One method of helping to raise a client's self-esteem by reinforcing a client's existing way of being.

Al Hajj Malik al-Shabaz   The name adopted by Malcolm X following a pilgrimage to Mecca.

Almshouses   Established by the Poor Laws of 1601, these were shelters for individuals who could not care for themselves.

AMCD   *See* Association for Multicultural Counseling and Development.

American Association for Counseling and Development (AACD)   Formerly APGA, and currently ACA.

American Counseling Association (ACA)   The professional association for counselors.

American Personnel and Guidance Association (APGA)   A professional association for counselors formed out of the NVGA and other associations and established in the 1950s. A forerunner of the ACA.

American Psychiatric Association (APA)   The professional association for psychiatrists.

American Psychiatric Nurses Association (APNA)   The professional association for psychiatric nurses.

American Psychological Association (APA)   The professional association for psychologists.

Americans with Disabilities Act (ADA)   Enacted in 1992, ensures that qualified individuals with disabilities cannot be discriminated against in job application procedures, hiring, firing, advancement, compensation, fringe benefits, job training, and other terms, conditions, and privileges.

Anal stage   Sigmund Freud's second stage of psychosexual development, occurring between ages 1 and 3 years, whereby a child's emotional gratification is derived from bowel movements. *See also* Genital stage, Latency stage, Oral stage, Phallic stage.

Analysis of variance   A statistical measure that is used in quantitative research to examine differences or relationships between groups.

ANOVA   *See* Analysis of variance.

Antideterministic view of human nature   The view that rejects the notion that early childhood development and biological factors cause psychological problems and stresses the ability of the individual to change. This view is in opposition to the deterministic view of human nature.

APA   *See* American Psychiatric Association, American Psychological Association.

APGA   *See* American Personnel and Guidance Association.

APNA   *See* American Psychiatric Nurses Association.

Aptitude test   A type of an ability test that measures what one is capable of learning. *See* Cognitive ability test, Individual intelligence test, Multiple aptitude test, Special aptitude test.

Aquinas, Thomas   Like Augustine, during the Middle Ages, Aquinas highlighted consciousness, self-examination, and inquiry as philosophies that dealt with the human condition.

Aristotle   Has been termed the first psychologist because of his use of objectivity and reason in studying information.

Armed Services Vocational Aptitude Test Battery (ASVAB)   A type of multiple aptitude test.

Artifacts   Symbols of a culture or group that can provide multiple meanings to understanding the beliefs, values, and behaviors of that group.

Artistic   One of Holland's six personality types that describes an individual who is able to skillfully express his or her imagination.

Assimilation   The absorption of new information into an existing store of knowledge.

Assistant to specialist   A human service professional who works closely with a highly trained professional as an aide and helper in servicing clients.

Association for Counselor Education and Supervision (ACES)   Originally a division of APGA (now ACA), this organization was instrumental in originally setting standards for master's-level counseling programs.

Association for Multicultural Counseling and Development (AMCD)   A division of ACA that developed 31 multicultural counseling competencies that are considered imperative in the preparation of human service professionals.

ASVAB   *See* Armed Services Vocational Aptitude Test Battery.

Augustine   During the Middle Ages, he highlighted consciousness, self-examination, and inquiry as philosophies that dealt with the human condition.

Autonomy versus shame and doubt (ages 1–3 years)   Erikson's second stage of psychosocial development where the child begins to gain control over his or her body and explore the environment. Significant caretakers either promote or thwart autonomy during this stage.

Avocation   An activity pursued for satisfaction that does not have a monetary goal.

Bandura, Albert   Early learning theorist who examined the role of modeling or social learning as another behavioral approach.

Beck, Aaron   Cognitive therapist who stresses that our thoughts affect our feelings and behavior.

Behavior changer   A human service professional who uses intervention strategies and counseling skills to facilitate client change.

Behavioral approach   The use of classical conditioning, operant conditioning, or modeling to bring about behavior change.

Behavioral family therapy   An approach to family counseling that is based on learning and cognition.

Binet, Alfred   Developed the first individual intelligence test.

Block grant   Federal funding to states that allows the state to decide which programs to fund.

Boundaries   Barriers that mediate information flow into and out of a system.

Brief treatment   Short-term counseling that involves working on very focused problems and aims for practical change to relieve problems.

Broker   A human service professional who helps clients find and use services.

Buckley Amendment   *See* Family Educational Rights and Privacy Act.

Buspar   A psychotropic medication that is an antianxiety agent.

CAI   *See* Career Assessment Inventory.

Career   The totality of work and life roles through which the individual expresses himself or herself.

Career Assessment Inventory (CAI)   A type of interest inventory.

Career awareness   The consciousness that one has about his or her career-related decisions that can be facilitated through self-examination, particularly through examining one's values, preferences, knowledge of occupations and life roles, and interests.

Career counseling   An individual or group counseling relationship in which the focus of the helping relationship is on the career development process and the goals are to increase career awareness and to foster decision making relative to career goals.

Career Decision-Making System (CDM)   A type of interest inventory.

Career development   All the psychological, sociological, educational, physical, economic, and other factors that are at play in shaping one's career over the life span.

Career guidance   A program designed by helpers that offers information concerning any aspect of career development and facilitates career awareness for individuals. Career guidance can be provided individually or in group settings.

Career path   The sequence of positions or jobs that are available to persons within an organization or business. This path, which typically signifies potential advancement, defines an individual's sequence of jobs or occupational roles.

Caregiver   A human service professional who offers direct support, encouragement, and hope to clients.

Carkhuff, Robert   Developed a 5-point scale to measure empathy.

Case management   The overall process involved in maintaining the optimal functioning of clients. Includes (1) treatment planning (2) diagnosis, (3) monitoring medication, (4) case report writing, (5) managing client contact hours, (6) monitoring progress toward client goals, (7) making referrals, (8) follow-up, and (9) time management.

Causal-Comparative Research   A kind of quantitative research that examines intact groups instead of randomly assigning subjects to groups. Also called *Ex post facto research*.

CDM   *See* Career Decision-Making System.

Certification   Usually set by states or by national organizations, a more rigorous credentialing than registration but less rigorous than licensing.

Chaos   The first stage of developing an eclectic counseling approach in which no theory is used and the clinician's responses are based on moment-to-moment subjective judgments that can be harmful to the client.

Charity Organization Society (COS)   Arising in the United States in the 1800s, an organization of volunteers who tried to alleviate the conditions of poverty by entering the poorer districts of cities and helping the residents there.

Children of alcoholics (COAs)   Children who are at a greater risk for chemical dependency as well as other adjustment problems because of having parents that are alcoholics.

Classical conditioning   Behavior change brought about by pairing a conditioned stimulus (such as the sound of a bell) with an unconditioned stimulus (such as the sight of food) until the conditioned stimulus alone evokes a response (such as salivation).

Closed questions   Questions that delimit the kinds of responses a client can make.

Closure stage   The stage of group development in which the leader summarizes the learning that has occurred and facilitates the separation process.

Coalescent stage   The second stage of developing an eclectic approach to counseling in which the clinician becomes comfortable with one approach and begins to integrate techniques from other orientations into his or her theoretical style.

COAs   *See* Children of alcoholics.

Coding   The process ethnographic researchers use to break down large pieces of data into smaller parts that hold meaning to the research question.

Cognitive ability test   A type of aptitude test that measures general intellectual ability and is usually given in group settings in schools to assess an individual's ability to do well in school.

Cognitive approach   A counseling approach that stresses the importance of helping a client understand his or her thinking process to facilitate change.

Cognitive complexity   The ability to understand the world, and for human service professionals, clients, in complex ways. One of the eight characteristics identified for being an effective helper.

Collaborative process   The joint effort between helper and client that determines what goals would best meet the client's needs.

College counseling   A subspecialty in the counseling field.

Commitment to relativism   The third stage of William Perry's theory of adult cognitive development, where a person maintains a relativistic outlook and commits to specific values and behaviors in his or her own life. *See also* Dualism, Relativism.

Communication perspective to family therapy   An approach to family counseling that broadly follows the guidelines from general systems theory.

Community Mental Health Centers Act Passed in 1963, this act provided federal funds for the creation of comprehensive mental health centers across the country, which greatly changed the delivery of mental health services.

Community planner A human service professional who designs, implements, and organizes new programs to service client needs.

Compassion fatigue/vicarious traumatization syndrome The name given to the stress-related syndrome that affects mental health professionals as a result of working in a profession where one witnesses the saddest aspects of humanity.

Competence Being knowledgeable of the most recent professional research and being able to apply it with clients. Having a thirst for knowledge. One of the eight characteristics identified for being an effective helper.

Concrete-operational stage Jean Piaget's third stage of cognitive development (ages 7–11 years) when a child starts developing logical thinking. *See also* Formal-operational stage, Preoperational stage, Sensorimotor stage.

Conditions of worth Carl Rogers's term for how conditions and opinions of significant others lead to incongruity in an individual because of the individual's need to be loved.

Confidentiality The ethical guideline that stresses discretion when retaining information from clients.

Confrontation A counseling technique that emphasizes challenging others without being judgmental, argumentative, or aggressive.

Congruent The quality of being in sync with one's feelings and behaviors. *See also* Genuine, Transparent.

Conservation The notion that liquids and solids can be transformed in shape without changing their volume or mass.

Constructivism A cognitive view that states that one's construction of reality is based on a complex interaction of thoughts, actions, and feelings thus creating a unique meaning-making system.

Constructivist career development theorists Theorists who believe that career decision-making is related to how individuals make meaning out of the world of work.

Consultant A human service professional who seeks and offers knowledge and support to other professionals and meets with clients and community groups to discuss and solve problems.

Control theory William Glasser's recent adaptation of his Reality Therapy approach in which he examines the process of understanding the world through our unique filters. An antideterministic approach. *See* Reality therapy and Antideterministic view of human nature.

Conventional One of Holland's six personality types that describes individuals who are concrete and prefer clerical tasks.

Conventional level Lawrence Kohlberg's second level of moral development (ages 9–18 years) when a person makes a moral decision based on peer approval or disapproval (Stage 3) or on established rules of what is right or wrong (Stage 4). *See also* Preconventional level, Postconventional level.

Conversion disorder A term for the process by which emotions become transformed into physical manifestations (for example, paralysis of a limb, blindness).

Correlation coefficient Used in correlational research to show the strength of the relationship between two or more sets of scores.

Correlational research Used to explore the relationship between two variables (simple correlational studies) or to predict scores on a variable from scores obtained from other variables (predictive correlational studies).

Correlations *See* Correlational research.

COS *See* Charity Organization Society.

Council for Standards in Human Service Education (CSHSE) Founded in 1979, this organization was established to help human service educators and college administrators achieve maximum educational quality and relevance to the service delivery system in their communities.

Counseling group Similar to a therapy group but with less self-disclosure and personality reconstruction expected; a meeting of individuals whose purpose is to effect behavior change and increase self-awareness.

Counselor An individual who has a master's degree in counseling, including school counselors, mental health counselors, college counselors, and rehabilitation counselors.

Counterconditioning The conditioning of new adaptive behavior through the use of behavioral techniques.

Countertransference The process in which the helper's own issues interfere with effectively helping his or her clients.

Covert rules Unconscious or unspoken rules of behavior created by families that are partially responsible for the ways in which family members related to one another. *See also* Overt rules.

Credentialing Usually regulated by state or national legislation, a method of ensuring minimum competence in a field. Three types of credentialing are certification, licensure, and registration.

Criterion-referenced test A test where the examinee's score is compared with the accomplishment of specific goals the examinee must attain.

CSHSE *See* Council for Standards in Human Service Education.

Cultural anthropology *See* Ethnographic research.

Cultural fairness Whether or not a test measures what it is supposed to measure in a consistent manner for all subgroups for which the test is given.

Cultural mosaic A society that has many diverse values and customs.

Culture The common values, norms of behavior, symbols, language, and life patterns that people may share.

DAT *See* Differential Aptitude Test.

Data manager A human service professional who develops systems to gather facts and statistics as a means of evaluating programs.

Deceleration stage Stage 5 of Donald Super's career development theory, occurring between age 64 and time of death, where the individual starts to separate self from the job and focuses more on retirement and avocational activities. *See also* Establishment stage, Exploration stage, Growth stage, Maintenance stage.

Decision-making theory The postulation that an individual's decision-making process is crucial in making career choices.

Defense mechanism An often unconscious mental process that allows a person to make compromises to avoid anxiety and to protect the ego. *See* Denial, Projection, Rationalization, Regression, Repression.

Deinstitutionalization A social change occurring in the late 1970s whereby patients who were held against their wills and were not in danger of hurting themselves or others were released from psychiatric hospitals.

Denial A defense mechanism that refuses to admit the truth or see reality to protect the ego.

Dependent variable In true experimental research, a quantity that is measured following manipulation of the independent variable; an outcome measure.

Descriptive statistics Used in the reporting of survey research and often includes measures of variability, measures of central tendency, percentages, and frequencies.

Deterministic view of human nature The view that instincts, genetics, and early childhood development are so influential that there is little ability for the person to change. This view is in opposition to the antideterministic view of human nature.

Developmental approach to career development The concept that career development is a life-span process that involves a series of predictable stages through which people pass. Two developmental theorists are Donald Super and Eli Ginzberg. *See also* Personality approach to career development.

Developmental crisis A predictable lifespan problem with which the family must deal.

Developmental cycles Salvadore Minuchin's family systems theory term for the process of a family experiencing predictable struggles as it ages and progresses through the life stages.

Developmental readiness The state where the client is ready to advance to a higher developmental stage.

Developmental stages In the psychodynamic approach, the psychological and physical tasks an individual must accomplish in the life span.

Diagnostic and Statistical Manual-IV (DSM-IV-TR) Developed by the American Psychiatric Association, a manual that details the different types of mental illnesses and emotional problems.

Diagnostic test A type of an achievement test that assesses suspected problem areas and is usually given one-to-one by a highly trained, experienced examiner.

Dictionary of Holland Occupational Codes Written by John Holland, it lists, by Holland code, thousands of jobs.

Dictionary of Occupational Titles (DOT) Published by the federal government, a comprehensive classification system for approximately 30,000 occupations.

Differential Aptitude Test (DAT) Used in the career assessment process to determine one's aptitude in a variety of domains.

Direct questions Simple, frank, and straightforward questioning of clients.

Generally, not as effective as indirect questions.

Directive approach Aimed at guiding clients through the change process by teaching them about and steering them toward healthier ways of living. This view is in opposition to nondirective counseling.

Discover A comprehensive computer-based career awareness program.

Discrimination (as used in learning theory) The ability of a person to respond selectively to one stimulus but not respond to a similar stimulus.

Discrimination (as used in understanding diversity issues) An active behavior that negatively affects individuals of ethnic, cultural, and racial groups.

Documents Records of events that are generally housed in libraries or archival centers and include such things as letters, diaries, autobiographies, journals and magazines, films, recordings, paintings, and institutional records.

Dogmatism Not allowing others to express their points of view. Insisting on your point of view. *See also* Nondogmatic.

DOT *See* Dictionary of Occupational Titles.

DSM-IV *See* Diagnostic and Statistical Manual-IV.

Dual relationships The ethical guideline that stresses the importance of helpers avoiding dual relationships such as friendships and social relationships with clients.

Dualism The first stage in William Perry's theory of adult cognitive development, where a person views the world in terms of black or white, or right or wrong, and has little tolerance for ambiguity. *See also* Commitment to relativism, Relativism.

Dysfunctional family The term used to describe families that have relational problems. Usually, such problems are the result of unfinished business that husbands and wives bring into the marriage that affects their marriage and, in turn, the family.

EAP   *See* Employee assistance program.

Eclecticism   The selection of what appears to be the best of several methods, approaches, or styles and their integration into one counseling approach.

Education for All Handicapped Children Act   Enacted in 1975, a federal law that guarantees an education in the least restrictive environment to individuals with a disability between the ages of 3 and 21 years. This act mandates the states to fund the services.

Educational Resources Information Center (ERIC)   An electronic search that can assist when you are conducting research in educational-related literature.

Ego   According to Freudian theory, the conscious portion of the psyche that is the mediator between the person and reality, especially in the functioning of the person's perception of and adaptation to reality. *See also* Id, Superego.

Eigenwelt   As used by the existentialist, a word for an individual's uniqueness.

Einfühlung   A German word meaning "to feel within," from which the word empathy was derived.

Elavil   A psychotropic medication that is an antidepressant.

Ellis, Albert   Founder of rational emotive behavior therapy.

Empathic   One of eight characteristics of the effective human service professional that is empirically and theoretically related to effectiveness as a helper.

Empathic person   An individual who has a deep understanding of another person's point of view.

Empathy   The ability to understand another person's feelings and situation in the world. *See also* Empathic and Empathic person.

Empirical or Empirically   *See* Empiricism.

Empiricism   The practice of relying on observation and experiment to test out a hypothesis.

Employee assistance program (EAP)   A program run by business or industry that provides primary prevention and early referral for treatment.

Encounter group   A group in which expressions of feelings are encouraged, which leads to new self-awareness.

Encouragement, affirmation, and self-esteem building   Three ways of expressing positive attitudes toward clients to help them integrate a more constructive outlook toward life.

Enhanced Guide for Occupational Exploration   The Enhanced GOE offers job descriptions based on skills, abilities, physical requirements, environment, salary, and job outlook for approximately 2500 jobs.

Enterprising   One of Holland's six personality types that describes those who are persuasive and like to lead.

ERIC   *See* Educational Resources Information Center.

Erikson, Erik   Founder of the psychosocial developmental model (see specific stages).

Erogenous zones   The psychoanalytic term used to describe places on the body from which sexual satisfaction is derived as a result of the individual's psychosexual development.

Establishment stage   Stage 3 of Donald Super's career development theory, occurring between ages 24 and 44 years, where the individual stabilizes career choice and advances in the chosen field. *See also* Deceleration stage, Exploration stage, Growth stage, Maintenance stage.

Ethical guidelines   *See* Ethical standards.

Ethical Standards   Codes developed by professional associations to aid the professional in making sound ethical decisions.

Ethical Standards of Human Service Professionals   Ethical guidelines adopted by NOHSE in 1995 that reflect the unique perspective of the human service professional.

Ethnocentric worldview   The potentially harmful assumption that one's view of the world is the same as his or her client's.

Ethnographic interviews A common method used by ethnographers for collecting data.

Ethnographic research Involves the description and understanding of human cultures through immersion within the cultures. Sometimes called *Cultural anthropology.*

Ethnicity Long-term patterns of behavior that have some historical significance and may include similar religious, ancestral, language, or cultural characteristics.

Etiology The origin(s) of a disease.

Evaluator A human service professional who assesses client programs and ensures that agencies are accountable for services provided.

Existentialism The philosophical belief centering on the individual's existence in an incomprehensible universe and on the plight of the individual to assume full responsibility for his or her acts without certain knowledge of what is moral or immoral.

Experiential family therapy An approach to family counseling developed by Carl Whitaker and others.

Exploration stage Stage 2 of Donald Super's career development theory, occurring between ages 14 and 24 years, where the individual tentatively tests occupational fantasies through work, school, and leisure activities and later chooses an occupation or more professional training. *See also* Deceleration stage, Establishment stage, Growth stage, Maintenance stage.

Ex-post facto research *See* Causal-comparative research.

Extinction A principle of operant conditioning that causes behavior to cease because of a lack of reinforcement.

Family Educational Rights and Privacy Act Also known as the Buckley Amendment, this 1974 federal act grants parents the right to access their children's educational records.

Feminist therapy A gender-awareness approach that focuses on specific tasks to be achieved in the helping relationship.

Fixated When one's maturity is hindered because of unresolved issues in a developmental stage.

Formal-operational stage Jean Piaget's fourth stage of cognitive development (ages 11–16 years), when a child can think abstractly, consider more than one aspect of a problem at one time, and understand more complex meanings. *See also* Concrete-operational stage, Preoperational stage, Sensorimotor stage.

Formative evaluation *See* Process evaluation.

Freedom of Information Act Enacted in 1974, this federal law allows individuals to have access to any records maintained by a federal agency that contain personal information about the individual.

Freud, Sigmund Founder of psychoanalytic counseling.

Friendly Visitors Volunteers who worked with the poor and deprived for Charity Organization Societies. Frequently stressed moral judgment and religious values while helping these individuals.

GATB *See* General Aptitude Test Battery.

Galt, John Minson, II Tried to employ more humane methods of treating the mentally ill in the public mental hospitals of the 1800s.

Galton, Sir Francis One of the first experimental psychologists.

Gender-aware therapy Counseling methods with specific guidelines that address differences in gender. Includes feminist therapy and men's issues therapy.

General Aptitude Test Battery (GATB) Published by the U.S. Department of Labor, Employment and Training Administration, it is an aptitude test that allows an individual to examine whether occupational preferences match his or her abilities.

General systems theory The postulation that any living system (individual, family, community, institution, and so on) has regulatory mechanisms that maintain homeostasis while it interacts with other systems.

Generalization The tendency for stimuli that are similar to a conditioned stimulus to take on the power of the conditioned stimulus.

Generativity versus stagnation (middle/late adulthood) Erikson's seventh stage of psychosocial development where the healthy adult becomes concerned about the meaningfulness of his or her life through such activities as work, volunteering, parenting, and community activities.

Genital stage Sigmund Freud's fifth and final stage of psychosexual development, occurring at puberty and continuing through the life span, where sexual energy is focused on social activities and love relationships and where unresolved issues of earlier stages emerge. *See also* Anal stage, Latency stage, Oral stage, Phallic stage.

Genuine The quality of expressing one's true feelings. Being congruent with one's feelings, thoughts, and behaviors. One of the eight characteristics identified for being an effective helper. *See also* congruent, transparent.

Ginzberg, Eli Formulated an early developmental model of career development.

GIS *See* Guidance Information System.

Glasser, William Founder of reality therapy.

GOE *See* Guide for Occupational Exploration.

Graduate Record Exam A type of cognitive ability test used for admission into graduate school.

GRE *See* Graduate Record Exam.

Great Society The term given to the numerous social programs generated by President Lyndon Johnson.

Grigg v. Duke Power Company A Supreme Court decision that asserted that tests used for hiring and advancement at work must show that they can predict job performance for all groups.

Group dynamics The ways in which groups interact.

Group leadership styles The various techniques adopted by group leaders that are based on the personality of the leader and on the stage of group development.

Group membership behavior The behaviors taken on by group members that are a function of the personality of the member and the stage of group development. Behaviors often mimic those in one's "real" life.

Growth stage Stage 1 of Donald Super's career development theory, occurring between birth and age 14 years, where the individual becomes aware of interests and abilities related to the world of work and begins to compare his or her abilities with those of peers. *See also* Deceleration stage, Establishment stage, Exploration stage, Maintenance stage.

Guidance Information System (GIS) A comprehensive computer-based career awareness program.

Guide for Occupational Exploration (GOE) A sourcebook to examine interests as they relate to potential jobs.

Haldol A psychotropic medication that is an antipsychotic.

Head Start Program A federally funded program, started in the 1970s, that provides an intellectually stimulating and nurturing environment to disadvantaged preschool children.

Health maintenance organization (HMO) A managed health care system that offers subscribers a pool of designated providers from which they can choose.

Heuristic The process of gathering information that can be used in an investigation. Something that is researchable.

Hierarchy In systems, how the system defines who is the rule maker and who is in charge.

Hierarchy of needs In Abraham Maslow's hierarchical theory, the postulation that lower-order needs must be fulfilled before higher-order needs; the order is (1) physiological needs,

(2) safety needs, (3) love and belonging, (4) self-esteem, and (5) self-actualization.

Historical research Relies on the systematic collection of information through a literature review to describe and analyze conditions and events from the past in an effort to answer a research question.

Hippocrates One of the first individuals in recorded history to reflect on the human condition.

HMO *See* Health maintenance organization.

Holland code A code used in describing one's personality type that can be matched to specific jobs.

Homeostasis The tendency for a system to maintain equilibrium.

Hull House A settlement house established by Jane Addams in Chicago in 1899.

Humanistic approach Developed by Carl Rogers and others, this approach tends to be more nondirective, facilitative, and present-centered; as when compared with the more directive and past-focus approach of psychoanalysis. *See also* Psychoanalysis.

Humanistic counseling and education Founded by Carl Rogers, Abraham Maslow, and others, this philosophy of counseling and education advocates that individuals are born with positive qualities that would be expressed in a nurturing environment. If such an environment was not present in early childhood, such qualities could be developed later in life in a nurturing environment. *See also* Actualizing tendency.

Human service professional/worker A person who has an associate's or bachelor's degree in human services or a closely related field.

Hypothesis An assumption or proposition that is derived from prior research and allows us to examine phenomena. *See also* Research question.

Id According to Freudian theory, the unconscious portion of the psyche that is the source of instinctual drives and needs. *See also* Ego, Superego.

IDEA *See* Individuals with Disabilities Education Act.

Identified patient In a family, the individual who is blamed for a behavior problem when actually the family "owns" the problem.

Identity versus role confusion (adolescence) Erikson's fifth stage of psychosocial development where adolescents begin to identify the temperament, values, interests, and abilities they hold. Self-understanding can lead to a strong sense of identity whereas lack of self-understanding can lead to role confusion.

Imperial stage Stage 2 of Robert Kegan's constructive model of development, where a person can begin to control impulses and where needs, interests, and wishes become primary. *See also* Incorporative stage, Impulsive stage, Institutional stage, Interindividual stage, Interpersonal stage.

Impulsive stage Stage 1 of Robert Kegan's constructive model of development, where a person has limited control over his or her actions and acts spontaneously to have needs met. *See also* Incorporative stage, Imperial stage, Institutional stage, Interindividual stage, Interpersonal stage.

Incongruity As pertains to conditions of worth, the state of being inconsistent within oneself; that is, ignoring true beliefs and values and accepting significant others' beliefs and values to be accepted.

Incorporative stage Stage 0 of Robert Kegan's constructive model of development, where a person is self-absorbed and has no sense of being separate from the outside world. *See also* Imperial stage, Impulsive stage, Institutional stage, Interindividual stage, Interpersonal stage.

Independent variable In true experimental research, the variable that is being manipulated to examine its effect on some outcome measure. *See also* Dependent variable.

Indirect questions Questions that border on being an empathic response and do not challenge the client directly.

Individual intelligence test A type of aptitude test that measures general intellectual ability and is usually given one-to-one by a highly trained, experienced examiner; often given to identify individuals with learning disabilities or individuals who are gifted.

Individuals with Disabilities Education Act (IDEA) A federal law that has ensured the rights of individuals with disabilities to receive educational services within the least restrictive environment.

Inductive analysis Used in qualitative data collection to determine the patterns and categories that emerge from data.

Industry versus inferiority (ages 6–12 years) Erikson's fourth stage of psychosocial development where the child begins to examine what he or she does well. High self-worth or feelings of inferiority can be formed in this stage.

Informal test An assessment measure that varies in the way it is administered; the results may not necessarily be compared with those of a norm group.

Information flow The manner in which information flows into and out of systems. Affected by boundaries, hierarchies, and system rules.

Information giving The communication of factual knowledge.

Informed consent Notifying clients of and getting clients' agreement on some of the basic issues related to the helping relationship before the interview.

InfoTrac An electronic search to assist when one is conducting research in educational-related literature.

Initial stage The beginning stage of group development.

Initiative versus guilt (ages 3–5 years) Erikson's third stage of development where the child explores the environment and gains an increased sense of independence. Caretakers either encourage or thwart exploration.

Institutional racism When an agency or organization purposely, or out of ignorance, supports policies or behaviors that are racist.

Institutional stage Stage 4 of Robert Kegan's constructive model of development, where a person has separated his or her values from others' and has a strong sense of personal autonomy and self-reliance. *See also* Incorporative stage, Imperial stage, Impulsive stage, Interindividual stage, Interpersonal stage.

Integrative approach An eclectic technique in which a counselor borrows from varying viewpoints in developing his or her own method of counseling.

Integrity versus despair (later life) Erikson's last stage of psychosocial development where the older person examines whether or not he or she has successfully mastered the preceding developmental tasks. Such mastery will lead to a sense of integrity whereas lack of mastery will lead to despair.

Interest inventory A type of personality test that measures an individual's likes, dislikes, and orientation to occupational choices. Often this test compares an individual's interests or personal characteristics to people in varying occupations to gain a sense of which occupations best fit that person.

Interindividual stage Stage 5 of Robert Kegan's constructive model of development, where a person maintains a separate sense of self while accepting feedback from others in order to grow and change. *See also* Incorporative stage, Imperial stage, Impulsive stage, Institutional stage, Interpersonal stage.

Internality Being internally oriented.

Internalize To incorporate feelings or values within the self.

Internally oriented A characteristic of the effective human service professional that focuses on relying on one's own inner sense in making decisions.

Interpersonal stage Stage 3 in Robert Kegan's constructive model of development, where a person cannot separate his or her own sense of being from family, friends, or community groups. *See also* Incorporative stage, Imperial stage, Impulsive stage, Institutional stage, Interindividual stage.

Intimacy versus isolation (early adulthood/adulthood)   Erikson's sixth stage of psychosocial development where, if the young adult has achieved a sense of self, he or she is ready to develop intimate relationships. Lack of self-understanding leads to isolation.

Introjection   Unconsciously adopting significant others' beliefs and values.

Introspective   *See* Introspective person.

Introspective person   An individual who is open to his or her deeper feelings and is willing to be self-critical and receive feedback from others.

Investigative   One of Holland's six personality types, which describes individuals as introverted and interested in problem solving.

Iowa Test of Basic Skills (ITBS)   A type of survey battery achievement test.

ITBS   *See* Iowa Test of Basic Skills.

Ivey, Allen   Developed a model to help professionals use their knowledge of life span development in the helping relationship.

Job   Positions within a work environment that are similar in nature.

Jung, Carl   Founder of the Jungian analytical approach.

Kegan, Robert   An adult developmental theorist.

Kitchener, Karen   Examined the role of moral principles in the making of ethical decisions.

Kohlberg, Lawrence   Examined moral development through the life span.

Kohut, Heinz   Adopted a psychodynamic approach to counseling that highlights the way people attach and separate from important others in their lives.

Kuhn, T. S.   Developed the concept of the paradigm shift.

Laing, R. D.   Viewed abnormal behavior as a normal response to a stressful situation.

Latency stage   Sigmund Freud's fourth stage of psychosexual development, occurring between ages 5 years through puberty, where the child replaces sexual feelings with socialization. *See also* Anal stage, Genital stage, Oral stage, Phallic stage.

LCSW   *See* Licensed clinical social worker.

Leisure   Time taken from required effort to pursue self-chosen activities that express one's abilities and interests.

Lewin, Kurt   Developed the National Training Laboratory (NTL) to examine group dynamics or the ways in which groups tend to interact.

Licensed clinical social worker (LCSW)   An individual who has a master's degree in social work and has met specific state requirements to obtain licensure.

Licensed professional counselor (LPC)   An individual who has a master's degree in counseling and has met specific state requirements to obtain licensure.

Licensure   This most rigorous form of credentialing is generally set by the state and requires a minimum educational level, usually a state or national exam, and additional documentation of expertise such as evidence of posteducation supervision. *See also* Certification, Registration, Credentialing.

Life-span development theories   Models of understanding the development of the person that stress that individuals continue to grow throughout their lives.

Listening skills   A counseling technique that stresses being able to hear the client and enable the establishment of a trusting, open relationship.

Logical analysis   The process used in qualitative research to understand the information collected. It involves reviewing the data, synthesizing results, and drawing conclusions and generalizations

Loose boundary   As pertains to general systems theory, a framework that allows information to flow too easily into and out of the system, thus causing difficulty in the system's sense of identity. *See also* Rigid boundary, Semipermeable boundary.

LPC   *See* Licensed professional counselor.

Maintenance stage   Stage 4 of Donald Super's career development theory, occurring between ages 44 and 64 years, where the individual confirms career choice and hopes to avoid stagnation. *See also* Deceleration stage, Establishment stage, Exploration stage, Growth stage.

Major depression   A mood disorder characterized by feelings of sadness, diminished interest in pleasure, a significant increase or decrease in appetite, diminished ability to concentrate, feelings of worthlessness, or suicidal thoughts.

Managed health care   Includes HMOs, PPOs, and EAPs, which are designed to help contain health care costs.

Maslow, Abraham   Founder of humanistic counseling.

Maslow's hierarchy   A humanistic approach that stresses a hierarchy of needs and has greatly affected the human service and mental health fields. *See* Hierarchy of needs.

May, Rollo   A leader in the humanistic approach to counseling.

McKinney Act   Enacted in 1987, this act provides to the poor and homeless funds for job training, literacy programs, child care, and transportation and subsidizes counseling.

McPheeters, Harold   Received a grant for the funding of some of the first mental health programs at community colleges and, thus, is considered by some to be the founder of the human services field.

Mead, Margaret   Made ethnographic research popular through her studies of aboriginal youth in Samoa.

Mean   A statistical property, the average of all test scores of the group. *See also* Measures of central tendency, Median, Mode.

Measures of central tendency   Those statistical concepts that provide information about the middle range of scores. *See also* Mean, Median, Mode.

Measures of variability   Those statistical concepts that provide information on how much scores vary. *See also* Range, Standard deviation.

Median   A statistical property, the middle test score the point where 50% of examinees score above and 50% score below the group. *See also* Mean, Measures of central tendency, Mode.

Medical model   The view, often held by adherents of the deterministic view of human nature and contrasted to the wellness approach, that mental illness is most likely caused by genetic/biological factors and therefore can be diagnosed and treated as an illness.

Meichenbaum, Donald   A cognitive therapist who believes that it is not only the behavior of the individual that becomes reinforced, but the ways in which the individual thinks.

Melting pot   The misnomer that various values and customs of different cultures become integrated and subsumed into the larger culture.

Men's issues therapy   A gender-aware approach that focuses on specific tasks to be achieved in the helping relationship relating to men.

Mental health counseling   A subspecialty in the counseling profession.

Mental Health Study Act   Passed in 1955, this act was a broadly based effort to study the diagnosis and treatment of mental illness.

Mesmer, Franz   A contemporary of Freud's who influenced him to practice hypnosis. The name from which the word *mesmerized* was derived.

Metatheory stage   The fourth stage of developing an eclectic approach to counseling in which the counselor develops a full appreciation of many theories and ties together commonalities among them into a single integrative approach.

Milgram, Stanley   Conducted controversial deceptive research that was one factor that eventually led to restraints on the ways research could be conducted.

Miller v. California   The 1973 Supreme Court case that declared that local municipalities have the right to set their own standards concerning what is considered obscene.

Minnesota Multiphasic Personality Inventory-II (MMPI-II)   An objective test that measures psychopathology.

Minority   Any group of people who are being singled out because of their cultural or physical characteristics and who are being systematically oppressed by those individuals who are in a position of power.

Minuchin, Salvadore   Developed the structural approach to family counseling and highlighted the importance of understanding situational crises and developmental milestones when working with families.

Mitwelt   As used by the existentialist, a word that describes the common experiences held in groups and cultures.

MMPI-II   *See* Minnesota Multiphasic Personality Inventory-II.

Mobilizer   A human service professional who organizes client and community support to provide needed services.

Mode   A statistical property, the most frequent test score of the group. *See also* Mean, Measures of central tendency, Median.

Modeling   The acquisition of behavior patterns through the viewing of models in social situations.

Moral dilemma   A problem of a moral nature that has no clear-cut answer.

MSW   Masters in social work.

Multicultural counseling competencies   Thirty-one skills determined to be essential in the training of mental health professionals that were developed by the Association for Multicultural Counseling and Development (AMCD).

Multigenerational family therapy   An approach to family counseling that

follows general systems theory guidelines.

Multiple aptitude test   A type of aptitude test that measures a broad range of abilities and how those abilities might be associated with occupational choice.

Multisystem approach   An approach that addresses a wide range of needed social services. Used in setting where clients need many services such as in prisons.

Myers Briggs Type Indicator   An objective type personality test used to measure common personality qualities.

NASW   *See* National Association of Social Workers.

National Association of Social Workers (NASW)   The professional association for social workers.

National Certified Counselor (NCC)   Certification as a counselor that requires a master's degree and additional training and supervision.

National Defense Education Act (NDEA)   Passed in 1958 as a direct response to the Soviet Union's launching of Sputnik, the act provided funds for the expansion of counseling programs in schools in order to identify gifted students.

National Institute of Mental Health (NIMH)   Created by the U.S. Congress in the late 1940s, this agency was the federal government's first real effort in confronting mental health issues and resulted in systematic research and training in the mental health field.

National Organization for Human Service Education (NOHSE)   Founded in 1975, this professional association provides a link between human service organizations and practitioners, promotes the improved education of human service professionals, advocates the development of human service organizations, and supports creative approaches toward meeting human service needs.

National Training Laboratory (NTL)   Founded in the 1940s by Kurt Lewin and other prominent theorists, this institution examines group dynamics and trains individuals to understand the special interactions that occur in groups.

National Vocational Guidance Association (NVGA) Founded in 1913 as a professional association for vocational guidance counselors, it is considered to be the forerunner of ACA.

NCC *See* National Certified Counselor.

NDEA *See* National Defense Education Act.

Negative reinforcement The removal of a stimulus that yields an increase in behavior.

Networking The process of becoming involved in numerous professionally related activities in an effort to become more knowledgeable about the field and possibly develop job and graduate school opportunities.

NIMH *See* National Institute of Mental Health.

NOHSE *See* National Organization for Human Service Education.

Nondirective approach Aimed at trusting the client's ability to develop the strategies for change in the helping process. This view is in opposition to directive counseling.

Nondogmatic A characteristic of the effective human service professional that stresses the importance of allowing others to express their points of view and the lack of the need to change others to one's own point of view.

Nondogmatic people Individuals who allow others to express their points of view, do not need to change others to their own viewpoint, and are open to criticism and change.

Nonverbal behavior Behavior exhibited through posture, tone of voice, eye contact, personal space, and touching.

Norm group A group to which one compares oneself. Often used in testing. A peer group.

Norm-referenced test Assessment instruments in which examinees' scores can be compared to their peer or norm group.

NTL *See* National Training Laboratory.

NVGA *See* National Vocational Guidance Association.

Objective personality test Usually given in multiple choice or true/false format, this type of personality test usually compares an individual's traits with those of a norm group.

Observation In qualitative research, this is an examination of a situation that uses descriptive information gathering.

Occupation A group of similar jobs within a workplace that can connote the kinds of work a person is pursuing. The jobs are identifiable and exist independently from the person.

***Occupational Outlook Handbook* (OOH)** Published by the federal government, a sourcebook on approximately 300 occupations that includes future outlook, nature of the work, type of training needed, and wage/employment conditions.

Offering alternatives A response that suggests to the client that there may be a number of ways to tackle the problem and suggests a variety of alternatives from which the client can choose.

O★NET Developed by the U. S. Department of Labor (2002), this on-line resource is intended to eventually replace the DOT. O★NET offers comprehensive information on job skills and job requirements.

OOH *See* Occupational Outlook Handbook.

Open questions Questions that allow for a wide variety of responses.

Open-mindedness Being nonjudgmental and allowing others to have their points of view; being willing to change your viewpoint. One of the eight characteristics identified for being an effective helper.

Operant conditioning The shaping of behavior, which is brought about through the use of positive reinforcement and/or negative reinforcement.

Operationalize To take an abstract construct (for example, empathy) and develop a means to define, measure, and quantify it.

Oral histories   In qualitative research, an interview with an individual who has participated in the event or observed the event in question.

Oral stage   Sigmund Freud's first stage of psychosexual development, occurring between birth and age 1 years, whereby a child's emotional gratification is derived from intake of food, by sucking, and later by biting. *See also* Anal stage, Genital stage, Latency stage, Phallic stage.

Outcome evaluation   The assessment of a program after it is completed. Also called *summative evaluation*.

Outreach worker   A human service professional who might go into communities to work with clients.

Overt rules   Clearly defined rules made by families that affect how members in the family related. *See also* Covert rules.

Paradigm shift   The concept that knowledge builds on itself, that new discoveries are based on past knowledge, and that when current knowledge no longer explains the way things work, a new view of understanding the world is in order.

Parsons, Frank   Founder of vocational guidance and trait-and-factor approach to career guidance.

Participant observation   Research where information is gathered by the researcher who joins and interacts with a group.

Pause time   The amount of silence between statements made during an interview; may vary according to differing cultures.

Pavlov, Ivan   A behavioral researcher who discovered classical conditioning.

Perry, William   An adult development theorist who's emphasis is on the learning process and cognitive development of college students. *See also* Dualism, Commitment, and Relativism.

Personal growth group   A special kind of support group that offers support to group members while encouraging expression of feeling and exploration of individual growth.

Personality approach to career development   The concept that career choice is greatly affected by personality development. Two personality theorists are Ann Roe and John Holland. *See also* Developmental approach to career development.

Personality assessment   Tests that measure the affective realm and include objective tests, projective tests, and interest inventories.

Person-centered approach   Developed by Carl Rogers and part of the humanistic approach to counseling, this is a way to facilitate change through the counseling relationship, whereby empathy, unconditional positive regard, and genuineness are necessary and sufficient personality characteristics to effect growth.

Phallic stage   Sigmund Freud's third stage of psychosexual development, occurring between ages 3 and 5 years, when the child becomes aware of his or her and the opposite sex's genitals and receives pleasure from self-stimulation. *See also* Anal stage, Genital stage, Latency stage, Oral stage.

Phenomenology   The philosophical study of the development of human consciousness and self-awareness.

Piaget, Jean   A cognitive developmental theorist who examined child development.

PL94–142   *See* Public Law 94–142.

Plato   An early Greek philosopher who considered problems of the human condition to have physical, moral, and spiritual origins.

Poor Laws   Established by the English government in 1601, this was one of the first attempts at legislating aid for the poor. In many ways, the American system of social welfare was modeled after the Poor laws.

Portfolio   Materials such as a résumé, transcripts, and reports put together in an application package for potential employers, graduate schools, and others.

Positive regard   A trait humanists consider necessary for creating a nurturing environment.

Positive reinforcement   The presentation of a stimulus that yields an increase in behavior.

Postconventional level   Lawrence Kohlberg's third level of moral development (age 14 years and older) when a person makes a moral decision based on acceptance of a social contract that is related to democratically recognized universal truths (Stage 5), or individual conscience based on universal principles and moral values that are not necessarily held by others (Stage 6). *See also* Conventional level, Preconventional level.

Power differentials   The control, authority, or influence over others.

Power dynamics   The force of individuals, institutions, or society that places, on some individuals, undue demands that cause stressful behaviors that many people call abnormal.

Practicality   The usefulness of a test, considering such factors as cost, length, ease of administration, and ease of interpretation.

Preconventional level   Lawrence Kohlberg's first level of moral development (ages 2–9) when a person makes a moral decision based on perceived power others hold and the desire to avoid punishment (Stage 1), or the egocentric desire to satisfy one's own need to gain personal rewards. *See also* Conventional level, Postconventional level.

Predictive correlational studies   Used to predict scores on a variable from scores obtained from other variables.

Pregroup stage   The stage of group development in which the group leader screens potential group members before forming the group.

Prejudice   As pertains to stereotyping and racism, negative opinions and attitudes held about members of ethnic or cultural groups.

Preoperational stage   Jean Piaget's second stage of cognitive development (ages 2–7 years) when a child develops language ability and can maintain mental images. A child in this stage responds intuitively rather than acting in a manner that might seem to be logically correct. *See also* Concrete-operational stage, Formal-operational stage, Sensorimotor stage.

Primary prevention   Concentrating on the prevention of emotional problems and promoting a wellness outlook.

Primary sources   Using original records, as opposed to secondary sources, in collecting data for historical research.

Privileged communication   As determined by the state, the legal right of a professional (lawyer, priest, physician, or licensed therapist) to not reveal information about a client.

Probability level   The statistical level set to determine significance between groups and whether or not the results could be found by chance alone.

Problem solving   The use of counseling skills to aid a client in working through issues.

Process evaluation   The assessment of a program during its implementation to gain feedback about its effectiveness and to allow for change in the program as needed.

Program accreditation   As set by the Council for Standards in Human Service Education, program accreditation acknowledges that human service programs have met minimal standards in the training of human service professionals.

Program evaluation   Assessing a program to determine if it has achieved its goals and objectives and has worth and value.

Professional disclosure statement   A written statement, given to the client, describing such issues as the limits of confidentiality, the length of the interview, the helper's credentials, the limits of the relationship, the helper's theoretical orientation, legal concerns, fees for service, and agency rules that might affect the client.

Projection   A defense mechanism, the viewing of one's own unacceptable qualities (ideas, emotions, attitudes) as belonging to others to protect the ego.

Projective test   A type of personality test where the individual gives an unstructured response to a stimulus. These responses are then interpreted by an experienced clinician to uncover personality characteristics. Examples are the Rorschach Inkblot test and sentence completion test.

Prozac   A psychotropic medication that is an antidepressant.

Psyche   The conscious and unconscious emotions, thoughts, and sensations of an individual.

Psychiatric nurse   A nurse who has specialized training as a mental health professional.

Psychiatrist   A physician who generally has completed a residency in psychiatry that is, has completed extensive training in some kind of mental health setting.

PsychINFO   An electronic search used to review psychology-related literature.

Psychoanalysis   Developed by Sigmund Freud, a method of analyzing psychological problems, based on early childhood experiences and instinctual aggressive and sexual drives, where the client talks freely about himself or herself especially about childhood experiences. *See also* Psychosexual stages of development, Structures of personality.

Psychobiology   The study of the mind/body interactions that influence the development and functioning of the personality.

Psychodynamic approach   The belief that drives (instinctual like sex and aggression, social, attachment/separation), which are at least somewhat unconscious, motivate behavior.

Psychodynamic family therapy   An approach to family counseling based on psychodynamic theory and practiced by A.C. Robin Skynner and others.

Psychoeducational groups   Groups that are focused on educating participants to prevent future problems.

Psychologist   Generally, a person who has a doctoral degree in psychology, has completed an internship at a mental health facility, and has passed specific state requirements to obtain licensure as a psychologist.

Psychological adjustment   Being willing to look at oneself in a therapeutic context and work on one's issues. Living a lifestyle that leads towards psychological healthy living. One of the eight characteristics identified as being related to counselor effectiveness.

Psychopathology   Unusual or abnormal mental health problems.

Psychosexual stages of development   As posited by Sigmund Freud, the five stages of individual development: oral stage, anal stage, phallic stage, latency stage, and genital stage. *See also* Psychoanalysis.

Psychosocial development   Erik Erikson's model of human development, based on the antideterministic view of human nature and opposed to Freud's deterministic view of human nature, positing that both psychological and social forces are major motivators in individual development throughout the life span.

Psychotherapist   Although generally not licensed by states, on a practical level, a person who has an advanced degree in psychology, social work, or counseling and who works in a mental health setting or in private practice, providing individual, marital, or group counseling.

Psychotropic medications   Medications that affect psychological functioning. (*See* Buspar, Elavil, Haldol, Prozac, Tranxene, Thorazine, Valium, Zoloft)

Public Law 94–142 (PL 94–142)   The Education for All Handicapped Children Act which ensures the right to an education within the least restrictive environment for individuals between the ages of 3 and 21 who have a disability. Recently updated with the Individuals with Disabilities Education Act (IDEA).

Punishment   Applying an aversive stimulus following a behavior in an effort to decrease a specific behavior. An ineffective method of changing behavior as it can lead to undesirable side effects (e.g., counteraggression).

Qualitative research   Field research that relies on the researcher's observations and descriptions of phenomena and his or her interpretation of the phenomena within a social context.

Quantitative research   Research that relies on controlled research designs and can be applied in a laboratory setting or in the field.

Questions   A counseling skill that should be used carefully if it is to be effective. *See* Closed and Open questions.

Race   Traditionally, a division of people who share common genetic and biological characteristics.

Racism   The irrational dislike or hate held about or directed at people of a particular race.

Range   A statistical property, the spread of test scores from highest to lowest for the group. *See also* Measures of variability, Standard deviation.

Rationalization   A defense mechanism attributing one's actions and thoughts to apparent, but not real, creditable motives to protect the ego.

Readiness test   A type of an achievement test that measures an individual's readiness to advance to the next educational level.

Real self   One's genuine, true self.

Realistic   One of Holland's six personality types that describes individuals who are practical and have good physical skills.

Reality therapy   Developed by William Glasser, a proponent of the antideterministic view of human nature, a treatment that helps the individual cope with the stress of living through the use of behavior-change strategies.

Registration   The least vigorous type of credentialing. *See also* Certification, Licensure, and Credentialing.

Regression   A defense mechanism of reverting to an earlier stage of development with less demanding ways of responding to anxiety.

Rehabilitation Act   Enacted in 1973, this law ensured access to vocational rehabilitation for adults, based on three conditions: a severe physical or mental disability, a disability that interferes with obtaining or maintaining a job, and employment that is feasible.

Rehabilitation counseling   A subspecialty in the counseling field.

Reinforcement contingencies   Those stimuli in the environment that shape (reinforce) one's behavior.

Relationship building   Finding a mechanism that allows one to build effective relationships with clients. Relationships are formed in many different ways depending on the personality of the helper. One of the eight characteristics identified as being related to counselor effectiveness.

Relativism   The second stage in William Perry's theory of adult cognitive development, where a person begins to think abstractly, allows for differing opinions, and understands there are many ways to view the world. *See also* Dualism, Commitment to relativism.

Reliability   The consistency of test scores; a measure of the accuracy of a test.

Relics   Any of a variety of objects that can provide evidence about the past event in question.

Repression   A defense mechanism the result of thrusting painful memories usually early childhood experiences into the unconscious.

Research design   After developing a hypothesis or research question and doing a review of the literature, the approach one takes to study and evaluate a particular question. *See also* Quantitative and Qualitative research.

Research question   Based on prior research and theory, a question that is developed to examine a particular problem. *See also* Hypothesis.

Review of the literature   A thorough examination of major research done in a particular area, found in books, articles, and computerized abstracts.

Richmond, Mary Developed one of the first social work training programs.

Rigid boundary As pertains to general systems theory, a framework that does not allow information to flow easily into and out of the system, thus causing difficulty in a change process. *See also* Loose boundary, Semipermeable boundary.

Roe's psychodynamic approach A career developmental theory that bases career choice on the type of early parenting received and classifies individuals in one of eight orientations toward the world of work.

Rogers, Carl Founder of Person-Centered Counseling.

Role-playing A way of rehearsing new behaviors.

Rorshach Test A projective test where an inkblot is shown to a client and interpretations are made about the individual's personality.

Rules In systems theory, how the system defines itself as a result of boundaries, information flow, and homeostasis. Rules can be overt or covert. *See* Overt rules and Covert rules.

Rush, Benjamin Known for his progressive and humanistic treatment of the mentally ill in the first "modern" mental institutions.

SAT *See* Scholastic Aptitude Test.

Satir, Virginia A social worker who was instrumental in popularizing a systemic approach to counseling. Developed the communication approach to family counseling.

Scapegoat An individual within a system who is unconsciously given the blame for problems in the system.

Schedules of reinforcement The numerous ways in which a stimulus can be arranged to reinforce behavior that is based on elapsed time and frequency of responses.

Schemata The organized, mental ways of perceiving and responding to complex situations or stimulants.

Schizophrenia A psychotic disorder characterized by misrepresentation of and retreat from reality, delusions, hallucinations, and withdrawn, bizarre, or regressive behavior; popularly and erroneously called split personality.

Scholastic Aptitude Test (SAT) A type of cognitive ability test used for admission into college.

School counseling A subspecialty in the counseling field.

SDS *See* Self-directed search.

Secondary prevention Focuses on the control of nonsevere mental health problems.

Secondary sources Documents or verbal information obtained from sources that did not actually experience the event which researchers use in collecting data for historical studies.

Self-actualized person Abraham Maslow's term for a person who is in touch with himself or herself, can hear feedback from others, is nondogmatic, has a strong internal locus of control, and is empathic and introspective.

Self-disclosure The act in which the helper reveals to the client personal information about himself or herself in order to show more effective ways of coping.

Self-Directed Search (SDS) A type of interest inventory.

Self-efficacy theory The postulation that an individual's belief system greatly affects the types of choices he or she makes.

Self-esteem How a person values and feels about oneself.

Self-help groups Sometimes called support groups, their purpose is to educate, affirm, and enhance the existing strengths of the group members.

Selye, Hans Stated that stress is a healthy response to a changing situation, but can become unhealthy if not properly dealt with by the individual.

Semipermeable boundary As pertains to general systems theory, a framework that allows information to enter the system and be processed and incorporated. *See also* Loose boundary, Rigid boundary.

Sensorimotor stage   Jean Piaget's first stage of cognitive development (ages birth to 2 years) when the child responds to only physical and sensory experiences. *See also* Concrete-operational stage, Formal-operational stage, Preoperational stage.

Sentence completion   A projective test where an individual is asked to complete the end of a sentence and interpretations are made about the individual's personality.

Settlement movement   Arising in the United States in the 1800s, the attempt by social activists, while living with the poor, to change communities through community action and political activities.

Shamans   Individuals who have special status because of their healing and sometimes mystical powers.

Sheehy, Gail   An adult developmental theorist.

SIGI-Plus   *See* System of Interactive Guidance and Information-Plus.

Silence   A skill used to help a client reflect on what he or she has been saying; it allows the helper to process the session and formulate his or her next response.

Simon, Sid   A founding figure of the values clarification movement.

Simple correlational studies   A type of correlational research that explores the relationship between two variables.

Situational crisis   An unexpected problem, with which the family must deal, that is condition-specific.

Situational theory   The postulation that often the career choices we make are out of our control and are related more to conditions in society.

Skills standards   Twelve competencies identified in a national project as being important to the work of the human services professional.

Skinner, B. F.   The well-known behaviorist who believed that one's personality is developed through reinforcement contingencies. Developed operant conditioning theory.

Social   One of Holland's six personality types that describes individuals who are verbally skilled, like social situations, and care for others.

Social casework   Having its roots in charity organization societies, the process by which the needs of a client are examined and a treatment plan is designed to facilitate client growth.

Social class   The grouping of people according to such things as wealth, ancestry, rank, and status.

Social learning   The learning gained from watching the behavior of others and then acting out those behaviors.

Social worker   Generally, a person who has a master's degree in social work.

Southern Region Education Board (SREB)   SREB identified 13 roles and functions necessary for a qualified human service professional relative to human service education.

Special aptitude test   A type of aptitude test that measures a specific ability (for example, hand-eye coordination) and is often used for job placement and acceptance into specialty schools.

Spontaneous recovery   After treatment for behavior change, the recurrence of former, unwanted behaviors.

SREB   *See* Southern Region Education Board.

Stages of group development   The typical stages that a group progesses through in the group process, including the pregroup stage, initial stage, transition stage, work stage, and closure stage.

Stages of psychosocial development   As developed by Erik Erikson, eight stages of life-span development that affect the formation of the personality of a human being.

Standard deviation   A statistical property, the amount, on average, that test scores vary from the mean. *See also* Measures of variability, Range.

Standardized test   An assessment instrument that is administered in the same way every time it is given; the test results may be compared with those of a norm group. An example is the Scholastic Aptitude Test (SAT).

Stanford Achievement Test A type of survey battery achievement test.

Stanford–Binet This individual intelligence test is based on the original Binet scale and is one of the more popular tests of intelligence in use today.

Stereotypes Rigidly held beliefs about a group of people that falsely assumes that most or all members of the group have certain behaviors or beliefs that tend to be unique to that group.

Strategic family therapy An approach to family counseling developed by Jay Haley that focuses on strategies for change.

Stress The normal physiological and psychological response to changing situations. In moderation, it is a healthy response; however, too much stress can cause psychological and physical problems.

Strong Vocational Interest Inventory An interest inventory.

Structural family therapy An approach to family counseling developed by Salvadore Minuchin that focuses on the structure and hierarchy of the family.

Structure of the interview The general process of an interview, which involves four stages: opening, information-gathering, goal setting, and closure.

Structures of personality The id, ego, and superego. *See also* Psychoanalysis.

Subception Carl Rogers's term for the professional's ability to perceive feelings and deeper meanings beyond what the individual experiences.

Subcultures Groups of people whose behaviors and values may differ from the larger culture.

Subject/object theory The basis for Robert Kegan's constructive model of development, the conjecture that individuals pass through specific developmental stages in constructing their unique way of making meaning of the world.

Summative evaluation Sometimes called *outcome evaluation,* it involves the assessment of a total training program after it is finished in an effort to show its effectiveness.

Super's developmental self-concept theory A five-stage career development theory that is founded in the belief that we make career choices based on how we view our self through the life span.

Super, Donald Formulated an early developmental model of career development that is still in use today.

Superego According to Freudian theory, the partly conscious portion of the psyche that internalizes parental and societal rules and serves as the rewarder or punisher through a system of moral attitudes, conscience, and a sense of guilt. *See also* Ego, Id.

Supervisee The individual whose work is being overseen by another in a supervisory relationship.

Supervision The process of having one's work overseen by a superior who assesses and evaluates the supervisee's performance to (1) help the supervisee become a better human service professional and (2) facilitate client growth.

Support group A meeting of individuals whose purpose is to educate and affirm group members; an example is Alcoholics Anonymous.

Survey battery test A type of an achievement test that measures general knowledge and is usually given in large-group settings in schools.

Survey research Research where specific information is gathered from a target population, using a questionnaire.

System of Interactive Guidance and Information-Plus (SIGI-Plus) A comprehensive computer-based career awareness program.

Szaz, Thomas Believes that abnormal behavior is a function of power dynamics in relationships. A system proponent of the understanding of maladaptive behavior.

Tabula rasa   From the Latin meaning "smoothed or erased tablet," the mind in its blank, or empty state before receiving outside impressions.

Tarasoff case   The landmark case that set a precedent for the responsibility that mental health professionals have regarding confidentiality and acting to prevent a client from harming self or others.

Teacher/educator A human service professional who tutors, mentors, and models new behavior for clients.

Tertiary prevention   Concentrates on the control of serious mental health problems.

Theoretical integration stage   The third stage of developing an eclectic approach to counseling in which the clinician has thoroughly learned one theory and is comfortable integrating one or more other theories into his or her approach.

Theory   A comprehensive system of doing counseling that enables the helper to understand his or her clients, apply techniques, predict change, and evaluate results.

Therapy group   A meeting of individuals whose purpose is to effect behavior change and increase self-awareness; similar to a counseling group but with more self-disclosure and personality reconstruction expected.

Thorazine   A psychotropic medication that is an antipsychotic.

Token economy   A technique to bring about positive behavior changes. The client is given a token for each success, and at the end of a specified time, the tokens are turned in for a higher-level reinforcer (for example, money).

Trait-and-factor approach   As developed by Frank Parsons, a systematic approach to vocational guidance that involves knowing oneself, knowing job characteristics, and making a match between the two through "true reasoning."

Transferable skills   Skills from one job or activity that are similar enough to allow transferability to skills in another job and activity.

Transference   The redirection of both negative and positive feelings and desires, especially those unconsciously retained from childhood, toward a helper.

Transition stage   The third stage of group development in which goals and rules are understood by group members, some anxiety and resistance still exists, and an effort is made to assist members in focusing on themselves and moving toward the working stage.

Transparent   The quality of embodying genuineness and congruence. *See also* genuine, congruent.

Tranxene   A psychotropic medication that is an antianxiety agent.

Treatment planning   The accurate assessment of client needs leading toward the formation of client goals.

Triad model   A training model that provides a safe environment for the counselor so that he or she can learn to better understand culturally different clients. The team members are the client; the counselor; the anticounselor, who highlights the differences in values and expectations between the counselor and client; and a procounselor, who highlights the similarities.

True experimental research   Research where one manipulates the independent variable(s) and randomly assigns subjects to particular groups, to measure the effect of the outcome. *See* Dependent variable, Independent variable.

Trust versus mistrust (ages birth–1 year)   Erikson's first stage of psychosocial development where the infant develops a sense of trust or mistrust based on the type of caretaking received.

T-tests   A statistical measure that is used in quantitative research to examine differences between groups.

Umwelt   As used by the existentialist, a term for individuals' shared universal experiences.

Unconditional positive regard   Carl Rogers's term for the characteristic of the helper to unconditionally accept the helpee, with "no strings attached."

Unconscious   The drives that we are unaware of that motivate our behavior.

Unconscious factors   A concept that much of our behavior is caused by factors beyond our everyday awareness.

Unfinished business   Unresolved problems and experiences brought from an earlier life stage that affect interpersonal relationships.

Validity   The ability of a test to measure what it is supposed to measure.

Valium   A psychotropic medication that is an antianxiety agent.

Values clarification   An approach that helps a person understand and accept his or her own perspectives and worldview while encouraging openness to view the world in other ways.

Variable   Any characteristics or quality that can be measured.

View of Human Nature   The manner in which an individual makes sense out of the world. In counseling theory, the way that an individual applies his or her meaning of the world to the counseling relationship.

Wellness approach   The view, supported by adherents of the antideterministic view of human nature and contrasted to the medical model, that espouses the ability of the individual to change.

Wheel of Wellness   A model used to assess one's level of health in the areas of spirituality, work and leisure, friendship, love, and self-direction.

"Why" questions   A type of question sometimes used in the helping relationship. "Why" questions, however, are generally not recommended because they tend to make clients feel defensive.

Work   Effort expended in pursuit of a job, occupation, or avocation to produce or accomplish something.

Work stage   The fourth stage of group development in which trust and group cohesion emerge and change and growth occur.

Wundt, William   One of the first experimental psychologists.

Zoloft   A psychotropic medication that is an antidepressant.

References

ACA (American Counseling Association). (1995). *Code of ethics and standards of practice* (Rev. ed.). Alexandria, VA: Author.

ACA (American Counseling Association) (1999). *Ethical standards for Internet on-line counseling.* Retrieved, December 6, 2002, from the World Wide Web: http://www.counseling.org/resources/internet.htm

ACA (American Counseling Association). (2002). *Mission and vision statements.* Retrieved November 21, 2002, from the World Wide Web: http://www.counseling.org/about/mission.htm

ACES (Association for Counselor Education and Supervision) (1995). Ethical guidelines for counseling supervisors. *Counselor Education and Supervision,* 34, 270–276.

ACT Discover Center (1998). *Discover, colleges and adults.* Hunt Valley, MD: Author.

Addams, J. (1911). *Twenty years at Hull House.* New York: Macmillan.

ADL (Anti-Defamation League) (1992). *Anti-defamation league survey on anti-Semitism and prejudice in America.* New York: Author.

Adler, A. (1964). *Social interest: A challenge to mankind.* New York: Capricorn.

Adler, A. (1994). *Understanding human nature.* Boston: Oneworld Publications.

Albert, K. A., & Luzzo, D. A. (1999). The role of perceived barriers in career development: A social cognitive perspective. *Journal of Counseling & Development,* 77(4), 431–36.

Allen, J. P., & Turner, E. J. (1988). *We the people: An atlas of America's ethnic diversity.* New York: Macmillan.

Alinsky, S. (1970). *The professional radical: Conversations with Saul Alinsky.* New York: Harper & Row.

Alinsky, S. (1971). *Rules for radicals.* New York: Random House.

Altekruse, M. K., & Wittmer, J. (1991). Accreditation in counselor education. In F. O. Bradley (Ed.), *Credentialing in counseling* (pp. 81–85). Alexandria, VA:

Association for Counselor Education and Supervision.

Americans with Disabilities Act. (1992, July). Americans with Disabilities Act. *The Resource,* p. 1. Norfolk, VA: Old Dominion University Office of Personnel Services.

AMHCA (American Mental Health Counselors Association) (2000). *Code of ethics of the American Mental Health Counselors Association.* Retrieved, June 1, 2002, from the World Wide Web: www.amhca.org/ethics.html

Anastasi, A. (1992). What counselors should know about the use and interpretation of psychological tests. *Journal of Counseling and Development,* 70, 610–615.

Anastasi, A., & Urbina, S. (1997). *Psychological testing* (7th ed.). Englewood Cliffs, NJ: Prentice-Hall.

Andrews, H. B. (1995). *Group design and leadership: Strategies for creating successful common theme groups.* Boston: Allyn & Bacon.

Ansell, C. (1984). Ethical practices workbook. In *Preparatory course for the national and state licensing examinations in psychology* (Vol. IV). Los Angeles: Association for Advanced Training in the Behavioral Sciences.

APA (American Psychiatric Association). (2000). *Diagnostic and statistical manual of mental disorders* (4th ed., text revision). Washington, DC: Author.

APA (American Psychological Association) (1954). *Technical recommendations for psychological tests and diagnostic techniques.* Washington, DC: Author.

APA (American Psychological Association) (2002). *Ethics code of psychologists.* Retrieved November 22, 2002, from the World Wide Web: http://apa.org/ethics

APNA (American Psychiatric Nurses Association). (2002). *Mental health care: A consumers guide.* Retrieved March 8, 2002, from the World Wide Web: www.apna.org/guide.htm

Appignanesi, R., & Oscar, Z. (1999). *Introducing Freud.* Duxford, England: Icon Books.

Arches, J. (1997). Burnout as a public issue. *Human Service Education,* 16(1), 37–45.

ASGW (Association for Specialists in Group Work) (2000). *Professional standards for the training of group workers.* Retrieved June 1, 2002 from the World Wide Web: http://asgw.educ.kent.edu.

Associations Unlimited (2002a). *National Association of Social Workers.* Retrieved March 8, 2002, from the World Wide Web: Available online through most libraries.

Associations Unlimited (2002b). *American Psychological Association.* Retrieved March 8, 2002, from the World Wide Web: Available online through most libraries.

Associations Unlimited (2002c). *American Psychiatric Association.* Retrieved March 8, 2002, from the World Wide Web: Available online through most libraries.

Associations Unlimited (2002d). *American Psychiatric Nurses Association.* Retrieved March 8, 2002, from the World Wide Web: Available online through most libraries.

Assouline, M., & Meir, E. I. (1987). Meta-analysis of the relationship between congruence and well-being measures. *Journal of Vocational Behavior,* 31, 319–332.

Atkinson, D. R. (1985). A meta-review of research on cross-cultural counseling and psychotherapy. *Journal of Multicultural Counseling and Development,* 13, 138–153.

Atkinson, D. R., Morten, G., & Sue, D. W. (1998). *Counseling American minorities: A cross-cultural perspective* (5th ed.). Dubuque, IA: McGraw-Hill.

Atkinson, D. R., Poston, W. C., Furlong, M. J., & Mercado, P. (1989). Ethnic group preferences for counselor characteristics. *Journal of Counseling Psychology,* 36(1), 68–72.

Axelson, J. A. (1999). *Counseling and development in a multicultural society* (3rd ed.). Pacific Grove, CA: Brooks/Cole.

Axelson, L. J., & Dail, P. W. (1988). The changing character of homelessness in the United States. *Family Relations,* 37, 463–469.

Baker, S. B., & Shaw, M. C. (1987). *Improving counseling through primary prevention.* Columbus, OH: Merrill.

Baltimore, M. L., Hickson, J., George, J. D., & Crutchfield, L. B. (1996). Portfolio assessment: A model for counselor education. *Counselor Education and Supervision, 36,* 113–121.

Bandura, A. (1997). *Self-efficacy: The exercise of control.* New York: Freeman.

Bandura, A., Ross, D., & Ross, S. A. (1963). Imitation of film-mediated aggressive models. *Journal of Abnormal and Social Psychology, 67,* 3–11.

Barker, P. (1998). *Basic family therapy* (4th ed.). New York: Oxford University Press.

Baruth, L. G., & Huber, C. H. (1984). *An introduction to marital theory and therapy.* Prospect Heights, IL: Waveland Press.

Baruth, L. G., & Manning, L. M. (1998). *Multicultural counseling and psychotherapy: A lifespan perspective* (2nd ed.). Paramus, NJ: Prentice-Hall.

Barz, M. L. (2001). Assessing suicide hotline volunteers' empathy and motivations. *Dissertation Abstracts International: Section B: the Sciences & Engineering, 62*(3-B), 1563, US: Univ Microfilms International No. AAI3009882

Baxter, N. J., Toch, M. U., & Perry, P. A. (1997). *Opportunities in counseling and development careers* (rev. ed.). Lincolnwood, IL: VGM Career Horizons.

Beck, A. T. (1976). *Cognitive therapy and emotional disorders.* New York: International Universities Press.

Beck, A. T., & Weishaar, M. E. (2000). Cognitive therapy. In R. J. Corsini & D. Wedding (Eds.), *Current psychotherapies* (6th ed.) (pp. 229–261). Itasca, IL: Peacock.

Benack, S. (1988). Relativistic thought: A cognitive basis for empathy in counseling. *Counselor Education and Supervision, 27*(3), 216–232.

Benjamin, A. (1987). *The helping interview with case illustrations* (4th ed.). Boston: Houghton Mifflin.

Bennett, B. D., Bryant, B., VandenBos, G. R., & Greenwood, A. (1995). *Professional liability and risk management.* Washington, DC: American Psychological Association.

Benson, H., & Klipper, M. S. (2000). *The relaxation response.* New York: Morrow Avon.

Bernard, J. M., & Goodyear, R. K. (1998). *Fundamentals of clinical supervision.* Boston: Allyn & Bacon.

Bertalanffy, L. von. (1934). *Modern theories of development: An introduction to theoretical biology.* London: Oxford University Press.

Bertalanffy, L. von. (1968). *General systems theory.* New York: Braziller.

Best, J. W., & Kahn, J. V. (1997). *Research in education* (8th ed.) Englewood Cliffs, NJ: Prentice-Hall.

Biegeleisen, J. I. (1991). *Job resumes: How to write them, how to present them, preparing for interviews.* New York: Berkley.

Binswanger, L. (1962). *Existential analysis and psychotherapy.* New York: Dutton.

Binswanger, L. (1963). *Being-in-the-world. Selected papers.* New York: Basic Books.

Black, C. (1979). Children of alcoholics. *Alcohol Health and Research World,* Fall, 23–27.

Blasi, G. L. (1990). Social policy and social science research on homelessness. *Journal of Social Issues, 46*(4), 207–219.

Bloom, J. (1997). *Credentialing Professional Counselors for the 21st Century* (Report No. ISBN-1–56109–070–0). Greensboro, NC: ERIC Clearinghouse on Counseling and Counseling and Student Services. (ERIC Document Reproduction Service No. Ed 399–498).

Bolles, R. N. (2002). *What color is your parachute?: A practical manual for job-hunters and career changers* (2002 ed.). Berkeley, CA: Ten Speed Press.

Borders, L. D. (1994). *The good supervisor* (Report No. EDO-CG-94–18). Greensboro, NC: ERIC Clearinghouse on Counseling and Student Services. (ERIC Document Reproduction Service No. ED 372–350)

Borders, L. D., & Larrabee, M. J. (1993). A research perspective for the Journal of Counseling and Development. *Journal of Counseling and Development, 72,* 5–6.

Bowen, M. (1976). Theory in the practice of psychotherapy. In P. J. Guerin (Ed.),

Family therapy: Theory and practice (pp. 42–90). New York: Gardner Press.

Bowen, M. (1978). *Family therapy in clinical practice.* New York: Jason Aronson.

Bradley, F. O. (Ed.) (1991). *Credentialing in counseling.* Alexandria, VA: Association for Counselor Education and Supervision.

Bradley, L. J., & Gould, L. J. (1994). *Supervisee resistance* (Report No. EDO-CG-94-12). Greensboro, NC: ERIC Clearinghouse on Counseling and Student Services. (ERIC Document Reproduction Service No. ED 372-344)

Brammer, L. M., & MacDonald, G. (1999). *The helping relationship* (7th ed.). Boston: Allyn & Bacon.

Brammer, L. M., Shostrom, E. L., & Abrego, P. L. (1989). *Therapeutic psychology: Fundamentals of counseling and psychotherapy* (5th ed.) Englewood, Cliffs: NJ: Prentice-Hall.

Britton, P. J. (2000). Staying on the roller coaster with clients: Implications of the new HIV/AIDS medical treatments for counseling. *Journal of Mental Health Counseling, 22*(1), 85–94.

Britton, P. J., Rak, C. F., Cimini, K. T., & Shepherd, J. B. (1999). HIV/AIDS education for counselors: Efficacy of training. *Counselor Education and Supervision, 39,* 53–65.

Brown, D. (2003). *Career information, career counseling, and career development* (8th ed.). Boston MA: Allyn & Bacon.

Brown, N. (1992). *Teaching group therapy: Process and practice.* New York: Praeger.

Brown, N. (1998). *Psychoeducational group counseling.* Bristol, PA: Taylor & Francis.

Browning, C., Reynolds, A. L., & Dworkin, S. H. (1995). Affirmative psychotherapy for lesbian women. In D. R. Atkinson, Atkinson & G. Hackett (Eds.). *Counseling diverse populations* (pp. 289–306). Madison, WI: Brown & Benchmark.

Budman, S. H., & Gurman, A. S. (1988). *Theory and practice of brief therapy.* New York: Guilford Press.

Burger, W. R., & Youkeles, M. (2000). *Human services in contemporary America.* Pacific Grove, CA: Brooks/Cole.

Burgess, R. G. (1995). *In the field: An introduction to field research.* New York: Routledge.

Buscaglia, L. (1972). *Love.* Thorofare, NJ: Slack.

Byrne, R. H. (1995). *Becoming a master counselor: Introduction to the profession.* Pacific Grove, CA: Brooks/Cole.

Cameron, S. C., & Wycoff, S. M. (1998). The destructive nature of the term race: Growing beyond a false paradigm. *Journal of Counseling and Development, 76*(3), 277–285.

Capuzzi, D., & Gross, D. R. (Eds.) (2002). *Introduction to group counseling* (3rd ed.). Denver, CO: Love Publishing.

Carkhuff, R. R. (1969). *Helping and human relations* (Vol. 2). New York: Holt, Rinehart & Winston.

Carkhuff, R. (2000). *The art of helping* (8th ed.). Amherst, MA: Human Resource Development Press.

Carlson, J., & Sperry, L. (Eds.) (2000). *Brief therapy with individuals and couples.* Phoenix, AZ: Zeig, Tucker, and Theisen.

Carroll, J. (1996). Managed care and service delivery: An interview with Dr. Shelly Kleine. *Human Service Education, 16*(1), 3–9.

Casey, J. A. (1999). Computer assisted simulation for counselor training of basic skills. *Journal of technology in counseling, 1*(1), 1–7.

Cass, V. C. (1979). Homosexual identity formation: A theoretical model. *Journal of Homosexuality, 4,* 219–235.

Cayleff, S. E. (1986). Ethical issues in counseling, gender, race, and culturally distinct groups. *Journal of Counseling and Development, 64*(5), 345–347.

Centers for Disease Control (2002). *Division of HIV/AIDS prevention.* Retrieved May 23, 2002, from the World Wide Web: www.cdc.gov/nchstp/od/news/At-a-Glance.pdf

Chambers, C. A. (1963). *Seedtime of reform: American social service and social action, 1918–1933.* Minneapolis: University of Minnesota Press.

Claiborn, C. D. (1991). The Buros tradition and the counseling profession. *Journal of*

Counseling and Development, 69,
456–457.

Close, G. (2001). Community development.
In T. McClam & M. Woodside (Eds.),
Human service challenges in the 21st century
(pp. 243–252). Birmingham, AL: Ebsco
Media.

Clubok, M. (1984). Four-year human
services programs: How they differ from
social work. *Journal of the National
Organization of Human Service Educators,*
6, 1–6.

Clubok, M. (1987). Human services: An
"aspiring" profession in search of a
professional identity. In R. Kornick
(Ed.), *Curriculum development in human
services education.* Council for Standards
in Human Service Education,
Monograph Series, Issue 5.

Clubok, M. (1990). Development of
professional organizations for human
service educators and workers. In S.
Fullerton & D. Osher (Eds.)., *History of
the human services movement* (pp. 71–83).
Council for Standards in Human
Service Education, Monograph Series,
No. 7.

Clubok, M. (1997). Baccalaureate-level
human services and social work:
Similarities and differences. *Human
Service Education,* 17(1), 7–18.

Clubok, M. (2001). The aging of America. In
T. McClam & M. Woodside (Eds.),
Human service challenges in the 21st century
(pp. 339–346). Birmingham, AL: Ebsco
Media.

Cobia, D. C., Carney, J. S., & Shannon, D. M.
(2000). In G. McAuliffe, K. Eriksen, &
Associates. *Preparing counselors and
therapists: Creating constructivist and
developmental programs* (pp. 135–147).
Virginia Beach, VA: Donning Company.

Cogan, D. B. (1989). A theoretical
perspective on the supervision of field
work students. In C. Tower (Ed.), *Field
work in human service education* (pp.
40–52). Knoxville, TN: Council for
Standards in Human Service Education.

Cogan, D. B., & O'Connell, G. R. (1982).
Models of supervision: A five-year
review of the literature. *Journal of the
National Organization of Human Service
Educators,* 4, 12–17.

Cohen, E. D. (1990). Confidentiality,
counseling, and clients who have AIDS:
Ethical foundations of a model rule.
Journal of Counseling and Development,
68(3), 282–286.

Cole, S. (1975). *The sociological method.*
Chicago: Rand McNally.

Collison, B. B., & Garfield, N. J. (Eds.).
(1996). *Careers in counseling and human
services* (2nd ed.). Washington, DC:
Taylor & Francis.

Committee on Government Operations
(1997). *A citizen's guide on using the
Freedom of Information Act and the Privacy
Act of 1974 to request government records*
(4th report). House Report 102–146.
Washington, DC: Government Printing
Office.

Community Support Skills Standards
(2002). *The community support skill
standards: creating pathways to careers in
human services: framing competencies for
direct service workers.* Retrieved June 1,
2002, from the World Wide Web:
www.nohse.com/newskil.html

Compton's Encyclopedia (1996, December 14).
Religion [Online]. Available: America
Online

Consulting Psychologists Press (1994). *The
Strong Interest Inventory.* Stanford, CA:
Author.

Conwill, W. (2001). Millennial mandates for
mental health. in T. McClam and
M. Woodside (Eds.), *Human service
challenges in the 21st century*
(pp. 175–192). Birmingham, AL: Ebsco
Media.

Corey, G. (2000). *Theory and practice of group
counseling* (5th ed.). Pacific Grove, CA:
Brooks/Cole.

Corey, G. (2001). *Theory and practice of
counseling and psychotherapy* (6th ed.).
Pacific Grove, CA: Brooks/Cole.

Corey, M. S., & Corey, G. (2002). *Groups,
process & practice* (6th ed.). Pacific Grove,
CA: Brooks/Cole.

Corey, G., Corey, M., & Callanan, P. (2003).
Issues and ethics in the helping professions
(6th ed.). Pacific Grove, CA:
Brooks/Cole.

Cormier, W. H., & Cormier, L. S. (1998). *Interviewing strategies for helpers* (4th ed.). Pacific Grove, CA: Brooks/Cole.

Cottone, R. R. (2001). A social constructivism model of ethical decision making in counseling. *Journal of counseling and development, 79*(1), 39–45.C

Cottone, R. R., & Claus, R. E. (2000). Ethical decision-making models: A review of the literature. *Journal of Counseling and Development, 78,* 275–283.

Cottone, R. R., & Tarvydas, V. M. (1998). *Ethical and professional issues in counseling.* Upper Saddle River, NH: Merrill.

Couch, R. D. (1995). Four steps for conducting a pregroup screening interview. *Journal for Specialists in Group Work, 20*(1), 18–25.

CSHSE (2002a). *Standards goals and objectives.* Retrieved December 7, 2002, from the World Wide Web: http://www.cshse.org/goals.html#top

CSHSE (2002b). *Overview of standards.* Retrieved December 7, 2002, from the World Wide Web: http://www.cshse.org/overview.html

CSHSE (2002c). *Summary of standards.* Retrieved December 7, 2002, from the World Wide Web: http://www.cshse.org/standards.html

Dahir, C. A. Sheldon, C. B., & Valiga, M. J. (1998). *Vision into action: Implementing the national standards.* Alexandria: American School Counselor Association.

D'Andrea, M. (1996, November 19). *Multicultural counseling.* Presentation at Old Dominion University, Norfolk, VA.

D'Andrea, M., & Daniels, J. (1991). Exploring the different levels of multicultural counseling training in counselor education. *Journal of Counseling and Development, 70*(1), 78–85.

D'Andrea, M., & Daniels, J. (1992, September). *The structure of racism: A developmental framework.* Paper presented at the Association for Counselor Education and Supervision National Conference, San Antonio, TX.

D'Andrea, M., & Daniels, J. (1999). Exploring the psychology of white racism through naturalistic inquiry. *Journal of Counseling and Development, 77*(1), 93–101.

Davidson, B. (1992). What can be the relevance of the psychiatric nurse to the life of a person who is mentally ill? *Journal of Clinical Nursing, 1*(4), 199–205.

Davis, F. J. (1978). *Minority-dominant relations: A sociological analysis.* Arlington Heights, IL: AHM.

Davison, G. C., & Neale, J. M. (2001). *Abnormal psychology* (8th ed.). New York: John Wiley.

DeAngelis, T. (1996). Psychoanalysis adapts to the 1990s. *APA Monitor, 27*(9), 1, 43.

Deutsch, C. J. (1984). Self-reported sources of stress among psychotherapists. *Professional Psychology: Research & Practice, 15*(6), 833–845.

Diambra, J. F. (2000). Human services: A bona fide profession in the 21st century. *Human Service Education, 20,* 3–9.

Diambra, J. F. (2001). Human services: The past as prelude. In T. McClam & M. Woodside (Eds.), *Human service challenges in the 21st century* (pp. xvii–xxii). Birmingham, AL: Ebsco Media.

DiGiovanni, J. (2001). About the Council for Standards in Human Service Education. In T. McClam & M. Woodside (Eds.), *Human service challenges in the 21st century* (pp. ix–xii). Birmingham, AL: Ebsco Media.

Dinkmeyer, D. C., Dinkmeyer, D. C., Jr., & Sperry, L. (1987). *Adlerian counseling and psychotherapy* (2nd ed.). Columbus, OH: Merrill.

Dipietro, K. A., & Nelson, J. T. (2001). Technology and human services: Advancements in a partnership for the new millenium. In T. McClam & M. Woodside (Eds.), *Human service challenges in the 21st century* (pp. 347–358). Birmingham, AL: Ebsco Media.

Donaho, M. W., & Meyer, J. L. (1990). *How to get the job you want: A guide to resumes, interviews, and job-hunting strategy.* Englewood Cliffs, NJ: Prentice-Hall.

Donaldson v. O'Connor, 422 U.S. 563 (U.S. Supreme Ct., 1975).

Donley, R. J., Horan, J. J., & DeShong, R. L. (1990). The effect of several self-disclosure permutations on counseling process and outcome. *Journal of Counseling and Development, 67,* 408–412.

Donlon, P. T., Schaffer, C. B., Ericksen, S. E., Pepitone-Arreola-Rockwell, F., & Schaffer, L. C. (1983). *A manual of psychotropic drugs: A mental health resource.* Bowie, MD: Robert J. Brady.

Doster, J. A., & Nesbitt, J. G. (1979). Psychotherapy and self-disclosure. In J. Chelune & Associates (Eds.), *Self-disclosure: Origins, patterns, and implications of openness in interpersonal relationships* (pp. 177–242). San Francisco: Jossey-Bass.

Downing, N. E., & Roush, K. L. (1985). From passive acceptance to active commitment: A model of feminist identity development for women. *Counseling Psychologist,* 13(4), 695–709.

Doyle, R. E. (1998). *Essential skills and strategies in the helping process* (2nd ed.). Pacific Grove, CA: Brooks/Cole.

Drum, D. J. (1992). A review of Leo Goldman's article "Qualitative assessment: An approach for counselors." *Journal of Counseling & Development,* 70(5), 622–623.

Drummond, R. J. (1996). *Appraisal procedures for counselors and helping professionals.* Columbus, OH: Merrill.

Durkin, H. E. (1972). Analytic group therapy and general systems theory. In C. J. Sager & H. S. Kaplan (Eds.) *Progress in group and family therapy* (pp. 9–17). New York: Brunner/Mazel.

Dykeman, W. (1997). Poverty: What are we to make of its gnawing existence in our midst? *Human Service Education,* 17(1), 3–5.

Dyne, W. A. (1990). (Ed.). *Encyclopedia of Homosexuality: Volume 1.* New York: Garland.

Educational Testing Services (1998–1999). *SIGI-Plus.* Princeton, NJ: Author.

Egan, G. (2002). *The skilled helper: A Problem-Management and Opportunity-Development Approach to Helping* (7th ed.). Pacific Grove, CA: Brooks/Cole.

Eidson-Claxton, S., & Bridges, L. (2001). Organ transplantation: Issues impacting human service professions. In T. McClam & M. Woodside (Eds.), *Human service challenges in the 21st century* (pp. 133–146). Birmingham, AL: Ebsco Media.

Ellis, A. (1996). *How to stubbornly refuse to make yourself miserable about anything yes anything!* Secaucus, NJ: Carol.

Ellis, A., & Harper, R. A. (1997). *A guide to rational living* (3rd ed.). No. Hollywood, CA: Wilshire.

Ellwood, R. S. (1993). *Introducing religion from inside and outside* (3rd ed.). Englewood Cliffs, NJ: Prentice-Hall.

Encyclopedia of Black America (1981). New York: McGraw-Hill.

Erikson, E. H. (1968). *Identity: Youth and crisis.* New York: Norton.

Erikson, E. H. (1998). *The life cycle completed.* New York: Norton.

Essandoh, P. K. (1996). Multicultural counseling as the "fourth force": A call to arms. *Counseling Psychologist, 24,* 126–138.

Ethical standards of human . . . (1996). Ethical standards of human service professionals. *Human Service Education,* 16(1), pp. 11–17.

Evans, D. R., Hearn, M. T., Uhlemann, M. R., & Ivey, A. E. (1998). *Essential interviewing* (5th ed.). Pacific Grove, CA: Brooks/Cole.

Faith, M. S., Wong, F. Y., & Carpenter, K. M. (1995). Group sensitivity training: Update, meta-analysis, and recommendations. *Journal of Counseling Psychology, 42,* 390–399.

Fava, G. A., & Sonino, N. (2000). Psychosmatic medicine: Emerging trends and perspectives. *Psychotherapy and Psychosomatic,* 69(4), 184–187.

FBI (Federal Bureau of Investigation) (1999). *Uniform crime reports: Hate crime statistics.* Retrieved June 1, 2001, from the World Wide Web: http://www.fbi.gov/ucr/99hate.pdf

Federal Register. (1977). *Regulation Implementing Education for All Handicapped Children Act of 1975* (PL94–142), 42(163), 42474–42518.

Field, S. (2000). *100 best careers for the 21st century* (2nd ed.). New York: IDG Books.

Fitzgerald, L. F., & Nutt, R. (1995). The division 17 Principles concerning the counseling/psychotherapy of women: Rationale and implementation. In D. R. Atkinson & G. Hackett (Eds.), *Counseling diverse populations* (pp. 229–261). Madison, WI: Brown & Benchmark.

Flavell, J. H. (1963). *The developmental psychology of Jean Piaget.* New York: Van Nostrand.

Forrest, D. V., & Stone, L. A. (1991). Counselor certification. In F. O. Bradley (Ed.), *Credentialing in counseling* (pp. 23–52). Alexandria, VA: Association for Counselor Education and Supervision.

Foster, S., & Gurman, A. S. (1985). Family therapies. In S. J. Lynn & J. P. Garske (Eds.), *Contemporary psychotherapies: Models and methods* (pp. 377–418). Columbus, OH: Merrill.

Fowler, J. (1995). *Stages of faith: The psychology of human development and the quest for meaning.* New York: Harper & Row. (Original work published in 1981).

Frankl, V. E. (1984). *Man's search for meaning: An introduction to logotherapy.* New York: Simon & Schuster.

French, M. (1993, April). *How to get the job you want: Using a portfolio.* Symposium conducted at the annual spring conference of the Southern Organization for Human Services Education, Port Richey, FL.

Freud, S. (1947). *The ego and the id.* London: Hogarth Press.

Fullerton, S. (1990a). A historical perspective of the baccalaureate-level human service professional. *Human Service Education, 10*(1), 53–62.

Fullerton. S. (1990b). Development of baccalaureate-level professional education in human services. In S. Fullerton & D. Osher (Eds.), *History of the human services movement* (pp. 57–70).

Council for Standards in Human Service Education, Monograph Series, Issue No. 7.

Gabbard. G. O. (1995). What are boundaries in psychotherapy? *The Menninger Letter, 3*(4), 1–2.

Gable, R. A., & Hendrickson, J. M. (Eds.). (1990). *Assessing students with special needs: A sourcebook for analyzing and correcting errors in academics.* New York: Longman.

Gall, J. P., Gall, M. D., & Borg, W. R., & (1999). *Educational research* (4th ed.). Boston: Allyn & Bacon.

Garcia, M. H., Wright, J. W., & Corey, G. (1991). A multicultural perspective in an undergraduate human services program. *Journal of Counseling and Development, 70*(1), 86–90.

Garfield, S. L. (1989). *The practice of brief psychotherapy.* New York: Pergamon Press.

Garner, G. O. (2001). *Careers in social and rehabilitation services* (2nd ed.). Lincolnwood, IL: VGM Career Horizons.

Garretson, D. J. (1993). Psychological misdiagnosis of African Americans. *Journal of Multicultural Counseling and Development, 21,* 119–126.

Gay, L. R., & Airasian, P. (2003). *Educational research: Competencies for analysis and application* (7th ed.). Upper Saddle River, NJ: Merrill.

Gazda, G. M. (1989). *Group counseling: A developmental approach* (4th ed.). Boston: Allyn & Bacon.

Gelso, C. J. (1992). Realities and emerging myths about brief therapy. *Counseling Psychologist, 20*(3), 464–471.

Gerrig, R, & Zimbardo, P. G., &. (2002). *Psychology and life* (16th ed.). Boston: Allyn & Bacon.

Gesell, A., & Ilg, F. L. (1943). *Infant and child in the culture of today.* New York: Harper.

Gibson, R. L., & Mitchell, M. (1995). *Introduction to counseling and guidance* (4th ed.). New York: Macmillan.

Gilligan, C. (1982). *In a different voice: Psychological theory and women's development.* Cambridge, MA: Harvard University Press.

Gilliland, B. E., James, R. K., & Bowman, J. T. (1994). Response to the Lazarus and Beutler article "On Technical Eclecticism." *Journal of Counseling and Development,* 72, 554–555.

Gingerich, W. J., & Eisengart, S. (2000). Solution focused brief therapy: A review of outcome research. *Family Process,* 39(4), 477–498.

Ginzberg, E. (1972). Toward a theory of occupational choice: A restatement. *Vocational Guidance Quarterly,* 20(3), 169–176.

Gladding, S. (1997). *Community and agency counseling.* Upper Saddle River, NJ: Prentice Hall.

Gladding, S. (2000). *Counseling: A comprehensive profession* (5th ed.). Upper Saddle River, NJ: Merrill.

Gladding, S. T. (2003). *Group work: A counseling specialty* (4th ed.). Uppersaddle River, NJ: Merrill.

Gladstein, G. (1983). Understanding empathy: Integrating counseling, developmental, and social psychology perspectives. *Journal of Counseling Psychology,* 30, 467–482.

Glasser, W. (1961). *Mental health or mental illness?* New York: Harper & Row.

Glasser, W. (1965). *Reality therapy: A new approach to psychiatry.* New York: Harper & Row.

Glasser, W. (1999). *Control theory: A new psychology of personal freedom.* New York: HarperPerennial.

Glasser, W. (2000). *Reality therapy in action.* New York: HarperCollins.

Goldman, L. (1992). Qualitative assessment: An approach for counselors. *Journal of Counseling and Development,* 70(5), 616–621.

Glosoff, H. L., Herlihy, B., & Spense, B. E. (2000). Privilege communication in the counselor-client relationship. *Journal of Counseling and Development,* 78(4), 454–462.

Goldstein, A. P., & Higginbotham, H. N. (1991). Relationship-enhancement methods. In F. H. Kanfer & A. P.

Goldstein (Eds.), *Helping people change* (4th ed., pp. 20–69). Needham Heights, MA: Allyn & Bacon.

Gompertz, K. (1960). The relation of empathy to effective communication. *Journalism Quarterly,* 37, 535–546.

Gonzales, M., Castillo-Canez, I., Tarke, H., Soriano, F., Garcia, P., Velasquez, R. J. (1997). Promoting the culturally sensitive diagnosis of Mexican Americans: Some personal insights. *Journal of Multicultural Counseling & Development,* 25(2), 156–161.

Good, B. J. (1997). Studying mental illness in context: Local, global, or universal. *Ethos,* 25(2), 230–248.

Good, G. E., Gilbert, L. A., & Scher, M. (1995). Gender aware therapy: A synthesis of feminist therapy and knowledge about gender. In D. R. Atkinson & G. Hackett (Eds.), *Counseling diverse populations* (pp. 262–272). Madison, WI: Brown & Benchmark.

Gottfredson, G. D., Holland, J. L., & Ogawa, D. K. (1996). *Dictionary of Holland occupational codes* (3rd ed.). Odessa, FL: Psychological Assessment Resources.

Granello, P. F. (2000). *Historical context: The relationship of computer technologies and counseling* (Report No. EDO-CG-00–10). Greensboro, NC: ERIC Counseling and Student Services Clearinghouse. (ERIC Document Reproduction Service No. ED-99-CO-0014).

Greenberg, L. S. (1994). What is "real" in the relationship? Comment on Gelso and Carter (1994). *Journal of Counseling Psychology,* 41(3), 307–309.

Greene, D. S. (1995). Human services and the liberal arts: An integration. *Human Service Education,* 15(1), 27–34.

Greenhaus, J. H. (1987) *Career Management.* New York: Dryden Press.

Griggs v. Duke Power Company, 401 U.S. 424 (1971).

Grunebaum, H. (1983). A study of therapists' choice of a therapist. *American Journal of Psychiatry,* 140, 1336–1339.

Guterman, J. T., & Kirk, M. A. (1999). Mental health counselors and the

Internet. *Journal of Mental Health Counseling,* 21, 309–325.

Guy, J. D., & Liaboe, G. P. (1986). Personal therapy for the experienced psychotherapist: A discussion of its usefulness and utilization. *Clinical Psychologist,* 39(1), 20–23.

Gysbers, N. C., Heppner, M. J., Johnson, J. A. (2003). *Career counseling: Process, Issues, and Techniques* (2nd ed.). Boston: Allyn & Bacon.

Hackney, H. L., & Cormier, L. S. (2001). *The professional counselor: A process guide to helping* (4th ed.). Needham Heights, MA: Allyn & Bacon.

Hagen, J. W. (2001). Restorative justice: Victim-offender mediation. In T. McClam & M. Woodside (Eds.), *Human service challenges in the 21st century* (pp. 41–57). Birmingham, AL: Ebsco Media.

Haley, J. (1973). *Uncommon therapy.* New York: Norton.

Haley, J. (1976). *Problem-solving therapy.* San Francisco: Jossey-Bass.

Halley, A. A., Kopp, J., & Austin, M. J. (1998). *Delivering human services: A learning approach to practice (4th ed.).* New York: Longman.

Haney, H., & Leibsohn, J. (1999). *Basic counseling responses: A multimedia learning system for the helping professional.* Pacific Grove, CA: Brooks/Cole.

Hanna, F. J., Bemak, F., & Chun, R. (1999). Toward a new paradigm for multicultural counseling. *Journal of Counseling and Development,* 77, 125–134.

Hanna, F. J., & Shank, G. (1995). The specter of metaphysics in counseling research and practice: The qualitative challenge. *Journal of Counseling and Development,* 74, 53–59.

Hannon, J. W., Ritchie, M. R., & Rye, D. A. (1992, September). *Class: The missing dimension in multicultural counseling and counselor education.* Presentation made at the national conference of the Association for Counselor Education and Supervision, San Antonio, TX.

Hansen, J. C., Stevic, R. R., & Warner, R. W. (1978). *Counseling: Theory and process.* Boston: Allyn & Bacon.

Harrington, T. F. (1995). *Assessment of abilities* (Report No. EDO-CG-95–12). Greensboro, NC: ERIC Clearinghouse on Counseling and Student Services. (ERIC Document Reproduction Service No. ED 389–960.)

Harrington, T., & O'Shea, A. (2000). *Career decision making system.* Circle Pines, MN: American Guidance Service.

Harris-Bowlsbey, J., Spivack, J. D., & Lisansky, R. S. (1991). *Take hold of your future (Leader's Manual)* (2nd ed.). Iowa City, IA: American College Testing Program.

Hashimim, J. (1991). Counseling older adults. In P. K. H. Kim (Ed.), *Serving the elderly: Skills for practice* (pp. 33–51). New York: McGraw-Hill.

Heppner, P. P., Kivlighan, D. M., & Wampold, B. E. (1992). *Research design in counseling.* Pacific Grove, CA: Brooks/Cole.

Herr, E. L., & Cramer, S. H. (1996). *Career guidance and counseling through the life span: Systematic approaches* (5th ed.). New York: HarperCollins.

Hicks-Coolick, A. & Millsap, T. (2001). Meeting the needs of incarcerated parents and their children: Challenges in the 21st century. In T. McClam & M. Woodside (Eds.), *Human service challenges in the 21st century* (pp. 19–28). Birmingham, AL: Ebsco Media.

Higgs, J. A. (1992). Dealing with resistance: Strategies for effective group. *Journal for Specialists in Group Work,* 17(2), 67–73.

Highlen, P. S., & Hill, C. E. (1984). Factors affecting client change in individual counseling. In S. D. Brown & R. W. Lent (Eds.), *Handbook of counseling psychology* (pp. 334–396). New York: Wiley.

Hohenshil, R. H. (1993). Assessment and diagnosis in the *Journal of Counseling and Development,* 72, 7.

Hohenshil, T. H. (2000). High tech counseling. *Journal of Counseling and Development,* 78, 365–368.

Holcom-McCoy, C. C., & Myers, J. E. (1999). Multicultural competence and counselor training: A national survey. *Journal of Counseling and Development,* 77, 294–302.

Holland, J. L. (1994). *The self-directed search* (Rev. ed.). Odessa, FL: Psychological Assessment Resources.

Hollis, J. W., & Dodson, T. A. (2000). *Counselor preparation 1999–2001: Programs, faculty, trends* (10th ed.). Philadelphia: Taylor & Francis.

Horst, E. A. (1995). Reexamining gender issues in Erikson's stages of identity and intimacy. *Journal of Counseling and Development, 73,* 271–278.

Hothersall, D. H. (1995). *The history of psychology* (3rd ed.). New York: McGraw-Hill.

Howard, G. S., Nance, D. W., & Myers, P. (1986). Adaptive counseling and therapy: An integrative, eclectic model. *Counseling Psychologist, 14,* 342–363.

Hughey, K. F. (2001). Comprehensive guidance and counseling programs [Special issue]. *Professional School Counseling,* 4(4).

Hutchins, D. E., & Cole, C. G. (1997). *Helping relationships and strategies* (3rd ed.). Pacific Grove, CA: Brooks/Cole.

Ihle, G. M., Sodowsky, G. R., & Kwan, K. (1996). Worldviews of women: Comparisons between White American clients, White American counselors, and Chinese international students. *Journal of Counseling and Development, 74,* 300–306.

Ivey, A. (1993). Developmental strategies for helpers: *Individual, family, and network interventions.* North Amherst, MA: Microtraining Associates.

Ivey, A., & Gluckstein, N. (1974). *Basic attending skills: An introduction to microcounseling and helping.* N. Amherst, MA: Microtraining Associates.

Ivey, A., & Ivey, M. (1999). *Intentional interviewing and counseling: Facilitating client development in a multicultural society* (4th ed.). Pacific Grove, CA: Brooks/Cole.

Jagger, L., Neukrug, E., & McAuliffe, G. (1992). Congruence between personality traits and chosen occupation as a predictor of job satisfaction for people with disabilities. *Rehabilitation Counseling Bulletin,* 36(1), 53–60.

Jayakar, P. (1986). *Krishnamurti: A biography.* New York: Harper & Row.

Jensen, J. P., Bergin, A. E., & Greaves, D. W. (1990). The meaning of eclecticism: New survey and analysis of components. *Professional Psychology: Research and Practice, 21,* 124–130.

Jetter, J. (2001, April 20). Global issues dog S. Africa on AIDS: Way is cleared for cheaper drugs, but market-medicine conflict remains. *Washington Post Foreign Service,* p. A01.

Johansson, C. B. (1996). *Career assessment inventory: Enhanced version.* Minnetonka, MN: National Computer Systems.

Jones, L. K. (1994). Frank Parsons' contribution to career counseling. *Journal of Career Development,* 20(4), 287–294.

Jourard, S. M. (1971). *The transparent self: Self disclosure and well-being* (2nd ed.). Princeton, NJ: Van Nostrand Reinhold.

Jung, C. G. (1968). *Analytical psychology: Its theory and practice: The Tavistock lectures.* New York: Pantheon Books. (Original work published 1935)

Jung, C. G. (1975). Freud and Jung: Contrasts. In R. F. C. Hull (Trans.), *Critiques of Psychoanalysis.* (Extracted from The Collected Works of C. G. Jung (Vols. 4 and 18) by W. McGuire, Ed., 1961, Princeton, NJ: Princeton University Press. (Original work published 1929)

Kahill, S. (1988a). Symptoms of professional burnout: A review of the empirical evidence. *Canadian Psychology,* 29(3), 284–297.

Kahill, S. (1988b). Interventions for burnout in the helping professions: A review of the empirical evidence. *Canadian Journal of Counselling,* 22(3), 162–169.

Kahn, M. (1997). *Between therapist and client: The new relationship* (rev. ed.). New York: W. H. Freeman.

Kain, C. D. (Ed.). (1989). *No longer immune: A counselor's guide to AIDS.* Alexandria, VA: American Association for Counseling and Development.

Kalat, J. W. (2001). *Biological psychology* (7th ed.). Pacific Grove, CA: Brooks Cole.

Kaplan, M., & Cuciti, P. L. (Eds.). (1986). *The Great Society and its legacy: Twenty years of U.S. social policy.* Durham, NC: Duke University Press.

Kegan, R. (1982). *The evolving self.* Cambridge, MA: Harvard University Press.

Kegan, R. (1994). *In over our heads.* Cambridge, MA: Harvard University Press.

Kelly, K. R., & Hall, A. S. (Eds.). (1992). Mental health counseling for men [Special Issue]. *Journal of Mental Health Counseling, 19*(2).

King, M. A. (2001). A call for services: Closing a chasm in criminal justice. In T. McClam & M. Woodside (Eds.), *Human service challenges in the 21st century* (pp. 5–17). Birmingham, AL: Ebsco Media.

King, P. M. (1978). William Perry's theory of intellectual and ethical development. In L. Knefelkamp, C. Widick, & C. L. Parker (Eds.). *Applying new developmental findings* (pp. 34–51). San Francisco: Jossey-Bass.

Kitchener, K. S. (1984). Intuition, critical evaluation and ethical principles: The foundation for ethical decisions in counseling psychology. *Counseling Psychologist, 12*(3), 43–45.

Kleinke, C. L. (1994). *Common principles of psychotherapy.* Pacific Grove, CA: Brooks/Cole.

Kohlberg, L. (1969). *Stages in the development of moral thought and action.* New York: Holt, Rinehart & Winston.

Kohut, H. (1984). *How does analysis cure?* Chicago: University of Chicago Press.

Koss, M. P. & Butcher, J. N. (1986). Research on brief psychotherapy. In S. L. Garfield & A. E. Bergin (Eds.), *Handbook of psychotherapy and behavior change* (3rd ed., pp. 627–670). New York: Wiley.

Kottler, J. A. (1994). *Advanced group leadership.* Pacific Grove, CA: Brooks/Cole.

Krathwohl, D. R. (1998). *Methods of educational and social science research: An integrated approach* (2nd ed.). New York: Longman.

Krogman, W. M. (1945). The concept of race. In R. Linston (Ed.), *The science of man in world crisis* (pp. 38–62). New York: Columbia University Press.

Kubler-Ross, E. (1997). *On death and dying.* New York: Simon & Schuster.

Kuhn, T. S. (1962). *The structure of scientific revolutions.* Chicago: University of Chicago Press.

Laing, R. D. (1967). *The politics of experience.* New York: Ballantine Books.

Lamar, J. (1992). The problem with you people. *Esquire, 117,* 90–91, 94.

Lambert, M. J., & Bergin, A. E. (1983). Therapist characteristics and their contribution to psychotherapy outcome. In C. E. Walker (Ed.), *Handbook of psychotherapy and behavior change* (pp. 205–241). Homewood, IL: Dow Jones-Irwin.

Lambert, M. J., Ogles, B. M., & Masters, K. S. (1992). Choosing outcome assessment devices: An organizational and conceptual scheme. *Journal of Counseling and Development, 70,* 527–534.

Lanci, J. R. (1997). *A new temple for Corinth: Rhetorical and archaeological approaches to Pauline imagery.* New York: Peter Lang.

Lanci, J. R. (1999). *Texts, rocks, and talk: Reclaiming biblical Christianity.* Collegeville, MN: Michael Glazier/Liturgical Press.

Landis, D., & Bhagat, R. S. (Eds.). (1996). *Handbook of intercultural training* (2nd ed.). Thousand Oaks, CA: Sage Publications.

Langer, E. (2000). Mindful learning. *Current Directions in Psychological Science, 9*(6), 220–223.

Lazarus, A. A., & Beutler, L. E. (1993). On technical eclecticism. *Journal of Counseling and Development, 71*(4), 381–385.

Leary, M. R. (2001). *Introduction to behavioral research methods* (3rd ed.). Boston: Allyn & Bacon.

Lee, V. E., Brooks-Gunn, J., Schnur, E., & Liaw, F. (1990). Are Head Start effects sustained? A longitudinal follow-up comparison of disadvantaged children attending Head Start, no preschool, and other preschool programs. *Child Development, 61,* 495–507.

Lee, W. M. L., & Mixson, R. J. (1995). Asian and Caucasian client perceptions of the effectiveness of counseling. *Journal of Multicultural Counseling and Development, 23*, 48–56.

Levinson, D. (1986). *The seasons of a man's life.* New York: Ballantine.

Linzer, N. (1990). Ethics and human service practice. *Human Service Education, 10*(1), 15–22.

Lipps, T. (1935). Empathy, inner-imitation of sense feelings. In M. Rader (Ed.), *A modern book of esthetics* (pp. 291–304). New York: Holt.

Locke, D. (1992). Counseling beyond U.S. borders. *American Counselor, 1*(2), 13–17.

Loewenberg, F., & Dolgoff, R. (1996). *Ethical decisions for social work practice* (5th ed.). Itasca, IL: Peacock.

Lombana, J. H. (1989). Counseling persons with disabilities: Summary and projections. *Journal of Counseling and Development, 68*(2), 177–179.

Lonergan, E. C. (1994). Using theories of group therapy. In H. S. Bernard & K. R. MacKenzie, *Basics of Group Psychotherapy* (pp. 191–216) New York: Guilford Press.

Loulan, J. (1987). *Lesbian passion: Loving ourselves and each other.* San Francisco: Spinsters/Aunt Lute.

Lovell, C. (1999). Empathic-cognitive development in students of counseling. *Journal of Adult Development, 6*(4), 195–203.

Lucas, J. (2001). Strategies for increasing agency multiculturalism. In T. McClam & M. Woodside (Eds.), *Human service challenges in the 21st century* (pp. 299–311). Birmingham, AL: Ebsco Media.

Lum, D. (2000). *Social work practice and people of color: A process-stage approach* (4th ed.). Pacific Grove, CA: Brooks/Cole.

Mabe, A. R., & Rollin, S. A. (1986). The role of a code of ethical standards in counseling. *Journal of Counseling and Development, 64*(5), 294–297.

Macht, J. (1990). A historical perspective. In S. Fullerton & D. Osher (Eds.), *History of the human services movement* (pp. 9–22). Council for Standards in Human Service Education, Monograph Series, No. 7.

Macionis, J. J. (2001). *Sociology* (8th ed.). Englewood Cliffs, NJ: Prentice-Hall.

Magolda, M. B., & Porterfield, W. D. (1988). *Assessing intellectual development: The link between theory and practice.* Alexandria, VA: American College Personnel Association.

Mahalik, J. R. (1990). Systematic eclectic models. *Counseling Psychologist, 18*(4), 655–679.

Mahoney, M. J. (1991). *Human change processes: The scientific foundation of psychotherapy.* New York: Basic Books.

Mahoney, M. J. (Ed.). (1995). *Cognitive and constructive psychotherapies: Theory, research, and practice.* New York: Springer.

Mandel, B. R., & Schram, B. (1985). *An introduction to human services: Policy and practice.* Needhan Heights, MA: Allyn & Bacon.

Maslow, A. H. (1954). *Motivation and personality.* New York: Harper & Row.

Maslow, A. (1968). *Toward a psychology of being* (2nd ed.). Princeton, NJ: Van Nostrand.

Maslow, A. (1970). *Motivation and personality* (Rev. ed.). New York: Harper & Row.

Maze, M., & Mayall, D. (Eds.) (1995). *Enhanced guide for occupational exploration.* Indianapolis, IN: JIST Publishing.

McAuliffe, G. (1992). Assessing and changing career decision making self-efficacy expectations. *Journal of Career Development, 19*, 25–36.

McAuliffe, G. (1993). Constructive development and career transition. Implications for counseling. *Journal of Counseling and Development, 72*, 29–36.

McAuliffe, G. (1999). Toward a constructivist and developmental identity for the counseling profession: The context-phase-stage-style assessment model. *Journal of Counseling & Development 77*(3), 267–280.

McAuliffe, G., & Eriksen, K. (Eds.) (2000). *Preparing counselors and therapists: Creating constructivist and developmental programs.* Virginia Beach, VA: Donning Company.

McBride, B. C., & Martin, G. E. (1990). A framework for eclecticism: The importance of theory to mental health counseling. *Journal of Mental Health Counseling, 12*(4), 495–505.

McClam, T. (1997a). Human service education: Back to the future. *Human Service Education, 17*(1), 29–35.

McClam, T. (1997b). Baccalaureate-level human services and social work: Similarities and differences. *Human Service Education, 17*(1), 29–36.

McClam, T. (1999). Let's talk credentialing: An interview with Mary DiGiovanni. *Human Service Education, 19*, 3–10.

McClam, T., & Woodside, M. R. (1989). A conversation with Dr. Harold McPheeters. *Human Service Education, 9*(1), 1–9.

McClam, T., & Woodside, M. R. (2001). *Human service challenges in the 21st century.* Birmingham, AL: Ebsco Media.

McDaniels, C., & Watts, G. A. (1994). Frank Parsons: Light, information, inspiration, cooperation [Special issue]. *Journal of Career Development, 20*(4).

McGrath, P. R. (1991–1992). *Human service education: Stage of the discipline—a survey of faculty members of the National Organization of Human Service Education.* Unpublished doctoral dissertation. National-Louis University, Evanston, IL.

McKenzie, K. (1999). Moving the misdiagnosis debate forward. *International Review of Psychiatry, 11*(2–3), 153–161.

McMillan, J. H., & Schumacher, S. (2001). *Research in education* (5th ed.). New York: Harper Collins.

McMillen, D. P. (2001). The future of human services: Models of service delivery. In T. McClam & M. Woodside (Eds.), *Human service challenges in the 21st century* (pp. 229–242). Birmingham, AL: Ebsco Media.

McNamara, K., & Rickard, K. M. (1989). Feminist identity development: Implications for feminist therapy with women. *Journal of Counseling and Development, 68*, 184–189.

McPheeters, H. (1990). Developing the human services generalist concept. In S. Fullerton & D. Osher (Eds.), *History of the human services movement* (pp. 31–40). Council for Standards in Human Service Education, Monograph Series, No. 7.

Mead, M. (1961). *Coming of age in Samoa: A psychological study of primitive youth for Western civilization.* New York: Morrow.

Medical Economics Staff (2001). *HMO/PPO directory, 2001.* Montvale, NJ: Author.

Mehrens, W. A. (1992). Leadership to researchers and practitioners. *Journal of Counseling and Development, 70*(3), 439–440.

Meichenbaum, D. (1977). *Cognitive behavior modification: An integrative approach.* New York: Basic Books.

Midgette, T. E., & Meggert, S. S. (1991). Multicultural counseling instruction: A challenge for faculties in the 21st century. *Journal of Counseling and Development, 70*(1), 136–141.

Milgram, S. (1965). Some conditions of obedience and disobedience to authority. *Human Relations, 18*, 56–76.

Milgram, S. (1974). *Obedience to authority.* New York: Harper & Row.

Miller v. California, 413 U.S. 15, (1973).

Miller, N. (2001). Children of the incarcerated. In T. McClam & M. Woodside (Eds.), *Human service challenges in the 21st century* (pp. 29–40). Birmingham, AL: Ebsco Media.

Minuchin, S. (1974). *Families and family therapy.* Cambridge, MA: Harvard University Press.

Minuchin, S. (1981). *Family therapy techniques.* Cambridge, MA: Harvard University Press.

Moore, D., & Haverkamp, B. E. (1989). Measured increases in male emotional expressiveness following a structured group intervention. *Journal of Counseling and Development, 67*, 513–517.

Morrow, K. A., & Deidan, C. T. (1992). Bias in the Counseling Process: How to Recognize and Avoid It. *Journal of Counseling and Development, 70*(5), 571–77.

Morse, P. S., & Ivey, A. E. (1996). *Face to face: Communication and conflict resolution in the schools.* Thousand Oaks, CA: Corwin Press.

Mulkey, S. W. (2001). Medical influence on human service outcomes. In T. McClam & M. Woodside (Eds.), *Human service challenges in the 21st century* (pp. 105–114). Birmingham, AL: Ebsco Media.

Mussen, P. H., Conger, J. J., & Kagan, J. (1969). *Child development and personality.* New York: Harper & Row.

Myers, J. E., & Schwiebert, V. (1996). *Competencies for gerontological counseling.* Alexandria, VA: American Counseling Association.

Myers, J. E., Sweeney, T. J., & Witmer, J. M. (2000). The wheel of wellness counseling for wellness: A holistic model for treatment planning. *Journal of Counseling and Development, 78,* 251–266.

Napier, A., & Whitaker, C. (1978). *The family crucible.* New York: Harper & Row.

National Institute of Mental Health (1995). *Decade of the brain* (3rd ed.). [Brochure]. Rockville, MD: Author.

NASW (National Association of Social Workers) (1999). Code of ethics. Retrieved June 1, 2001, from the World Wide Web: www.naswdc.org/code.htm

Neukrug, E. (1980). *The effects of supervisory style and type of praise upon counselor trainees' level of empathy and perception of supervisor.* Unpublished doctoral dissertation, University of Cincinnati, Cincinnati, OH.

Neukrug, E. (1987). The brief training of paraprofessional counselors in empathic responding. *New Hampshire Journal for Counseling and Development,* 15(1), 15–19.

Neukrug, E. (1991). Computer-assisted live supervision in counselor skills training. *Counselor Education and Supervision,* 31(2), 132–138.

Neukrug, E. (1996). A developmental approach to the teaching of ethical decision making. *Human Service Education,* 16(1), 19–36.

Neukrug, E. (2001). Medical breakthroughs: Genetic research and genetic counseling, psychotropic medications, and the mind-body connection. In T. McClam & M. Woodside (Eds.), *Human service challenges in the 21st century* (pp. 115–132). Birmingham, AL: Ebsco Media.

Neukrug, E. (2002). *Skills and techniques for human service professionals.* Pacific Grove, CA: Brooks/Cole.

Neukrug, E. (2003a). *The world of the counselor* (2nd ed.). Pacific Grove, CA: Brooks/Cole.

Neukrug, E. (2003b). *Experiencing the world of the counselor: A workbook for counselor educators and students* (2nd ed.). Pacific Grove, CA: Brooks Cole.

Neukrug, E. S., Barr, C. G., Hoffman, L. R., & Kaplan, L. S. (1993). Developmental counseling and guidance: A model for use in your schools. *School Counselor, 5,* 356–362.

Neukrug, E., Lovell, C., & Parker, R. (1996). Employing ethical codes and decision-making models: A developmental process. *Counseling and Values, 40,* 98–106.

Neukrug, E., & McAuliffe, G. (1993). Cognitive development and human service education. *Human Service Education,* 13(1), 13–26.

Neukrug, E., Milliken, T., & Shoemaker, J. (2001). Counseling seeking behavior of NOHSE practitioners, educators, and trainees. *Human Service Education, 21,* 45–48.

Neukrug, E., & Milliken, T., & Walden, S. (2001). Ethical practices of credentialed counselors: An updated survey of state licensing boards. *Counselor Education and Supervision,* 41(1), 57–70.

Neukrug, E., & Williams, G. (1993, October). Counseling counselors: A survey of values. *Counseling and Values,* 38, 51–62.

Nichols, M. P., & Schwartz, R. C. (2001). *Family therapy: Concepts and methods* (5th ed.). Boston: Allyn & Bacon.

Nigg, J. T., & Goldsmith, H. H. (1994). Genetics of personality disorders:

Perspectives from personality and psychopathology research. *Psychological Bulletin,* 115, 346–380.

Niles, S. G., & Harris-Bowlsbey, J. (2002). *Career development interventions in the 21st century.* Upper Saddle River, NJ: Prentice Hall.

NIMH (National Institute of Mental Health) (1998, August 15). *Mental illness in America* [On-line]. Available: www.nimh.nih.gov/research/amer.htm

Nooe, R. M. (2001). Mental illness and homelessness. In T. McClam & M. Woodside (Eds.), *Human service challenges in the 21st century* (pp. 205–214). Birmingham, AL: Ebsco Media.

NOHSE (National Organization of Human Service Education). (2002). *NOHSE.* Retrieved March 8, 2002, from the World Wide Web: www.nohse.org

Norcross, J. C. (Ed.). (1986). *Handbook of eclectic psychotherapy.* New York: Brunner/Mazel.

Norcross, J. C., Prochaska, J. O., & Gallagher, K. M. (1989). Clinical psychologists in the 1980s. Theory, research, and practice. *Clinical Psychologist,* 42, 45–53.

Norcross, J. C., Strausser, D. J., & Faltus, F. J. (1988). The therapist's therapist. *American Journal of Psychotherapy,* 42(1), 53–66.

Nova. (2000). *Cracking the code of life.* Burlington, VT: Public Broadcasting, Nova.

Nye, R. D. (1996). *Three psychologies: Perspectives from Freud, Skinner, and Rogers* (5th ed.). Pacific Grove, CA: Brooks/Cole.

Nye, R. D. (2000). *Three psychologies: Perspectives from Freud, Skinner, and Rogers* (6th ed.). Pacific Grove, CA: Brooks/Cole.

Occupational Outlook Handbook (2002–2003a). *Occupational Outlook Handbook, 2002–2003 edition.* Retrieved June 1, 2001, from the World Wide Web: http://www.bls.gov/oco

Occupational Outlook Handbook. (2002–2003b). *Occupational Outlook Handbook, 2002–2003 edition.* Retrieved June 1, 2001, from the World Wide Web: www.bls.gov/oco. (Note: type in "social

and human service assistant" in "search by occupation.")

Osher, D. (1990). More than needs and service: The antecedent and concurrent social conditions that influeneced the human services movement. In S. Fullerton & D. Osher (Eds.), *History of the human services movement* (pp. 23–30). Council for Standards in Human Service Education, Monograph Series, Issue No. 7.

Osherson, S. (1986). *Finding our fathers.* New York: Faucett Columbine.

Parsons, F. (1909). *Choosing a vocation.* Boston: Houghton Mifflin.

Parsons, F. (1989). *Choosing a vocation.* Garrett Park, MD: Garrett Park. (Original work published 1909)

Peavy, R. V. (1994). A constructivist perspective for counseling. *Education and Vocational Guidance Bulletin,* 55, 31.

Peck, M. S. (1998). *People of the lie.* New York: Simon & Schuster.

Pedersen, P. B. (1981). Triad counseling. In R. Corsini (Ed.), *Handbook of innovative psychotherapies.* (pp. 840–854). New York: Wiley.

Pedersen, P. (1983). Intercultural training of mental-health providers. In D. Landis & R. W. Brislin (Eds.), *Intercultural training: Vol. 2. Issues in training* (pp. 325–352). Elmsford, NY: Pergamon Press.

Pedersen, P. B. (1987). Intercultural criteria for mental-health training. In P. Pedersen (Ed.), *Handbook of cross-cultural counseling and therapy* (pp. 315–321). New York: Praeger.

Pedersen, P. B., Draguns, J. G., Lonner, J., & Trimble, J. E. (1996). *Counseling across cultures* (4th ed.). Thousand Oaks, CA: Sage Publications.

Pedersen, P. B. (2000). *A handbook for developing multicultural awareness* (3rd ed.). Alexandria, VA: American Counseling Association.

Pennebaker, J. W., Colder, M., & Sharp, L. K. (1990). Accelerating the coping process. *Journal of Personality and Social Psychology,* 58, 528–537.

Pennebaker, J. W., & Susman, J. R. (1988). Disclosure of traumas and psychosomatic processes. *Social Science and Medicine,* 26, 327–332.

Petrie, R. D. (1984). Competence and curriculum. *Journal of the National Organization of Human Service Educators,* 6, 8–13.

Petrie, D. (1987). Life cycle simulation: Human growth and development course design and method. *Human Service Education,* 8(1), 21–25.

Phelps, R. E., Taylor, J. D., & Gerard, P. A. (2001). Cultural mistrust, ethnic identity, racial identity, and self-esteem among ethnically diverse black university students. *Journal of Counseling and Development,* 79, 209–216.

Piaget, J. (1954). *The construction of reality in the child.* New York: Basic Books.

Plaud, J. J., & Eifert, G. H. (1998). *From behavior theory to behavior therapy.* Boston: Allyn & Bacon.

Pollak, J., Levy, S., & Breitholtz, T. (1999). Screening for medical and neuro-developmental disorders for the professional counselor. *Journal of Counseling and Development,* 77, 350–356.

Pope, M. (1995). The "salad bowl" is big enough for us all: An argument for the inclusion of lesbians and gay men in any definition of multiculturalism. *Journal of Counseling and Development,* 73, 301–303.

Poston, W. S. C., Craine, M., & Atkinson, D. R. (1991). Counselor dissimilarity, confrontation, client cultural mistrust, and willingness to self-disclose. *Journal of Multicultural Counseling and Development,* 19, 65–73.

Pottick, K. J. (1988). Jane Addams revisited: Practice theory and social economics. *Social Work with Groups,* 11, 11–26.

Pressly, P. K., & Heesacker, M. (2001). The physical environment and counseling: A review of theory and research. *Journal of Counseling and Development* 79, 148–160.

Pritts, T. A., Wang, Q., Sun, X., Moon, M. R., Fischer, D. R., Fischer, J. E., Wong, H. R., & Hasselgren, P. O. (2000). Induction of the stress response in vivo decreases nuclear factor-kappa B activity in jejunal mucosa of endotoxemic mice. *Archives of Surgery,* 135(7), 860–866.

Prochaska, J. O., & Norcross, J. C. (1983). Contemporary psychotherapists: A national survey of characteristics, practices, orientations, and attitudes. *Psychotherapy: Theory, Research and Practice,* 20(2), 161–173.

Quintana, S. M., & Bernal, M. E. (1995). Ethnic minority training in counseling psychology: Comparison with clinical psychology and proposed standards. *Counseling Psychologist,* 23(1), 102–121.

Raths, L. E., Harmin, M., & Simon, S. B. (1966). *Values and teaching.* Columbus, OH: Merrill.

Remley, T. P. (1991). An argument for credentialing. In F. O. Bradley (Ed.), *Credentialing in counseling* (pp. 81–85). Alexandria, VA: Association for Counselor Education and Supervision.

Reynolds, J. F., Mair, D. C., & Fischer, P. C. (1995). *Writing and reading mental health records: Issues and analysis* (2nd ed.). Mahwah, NJ: Erlbaum Associates.

Rice, F. P. (2001). *Human development: A life-span approach* (4th ed.). Upper Saddle River, NJ: Prentice Hall.

Riverside Publishing Company (1997). *Guidance information systems.* Itasca, IL: Author.

Robertiello, R. C., & Schoenewolf, G. (1992). *101 Common therapeutic blunders: Countertransference and counterresistance in psychotherapy.* Northvale, NJ: Jason Aronson.

Roe, A. (1956). *The psychology of occupations.* New York: Wiley.

Roe, A., & Siegelman, M. (1964). *The origin of interests.* APGA Inquiry Studies No. 1. Washington, DC: American Personnel and Guidance Association.

Rogers, C. R. (1942). *Counseling and psychotherapy.* Boston: Houghton Mifflin.

Rogers, C. R. (1951). *Client-centered therapy.* Boston: Houghton Mifflin.

Rogers, C. R. (1957). The necessary and sufficient conditions of therapeutic personality change. *Journal of Consulting Psychology,* 21(2), 95–103.

Rogers, C. R. (1959). A theory of therapy, personality and interpersonal relationships as developed in the client-centered framework. In S. Koch (Ed.), *Psychology: A study of science: Vol. 3. Formulations of the person and the social context* (pp. 184–256). New York: McGraw-Hill.

Rogers, C. R. (1961). Ellen West and loneliness. In H. Kirschenbaum & V. L. Henderson (Eds.), *The Carl Rogers reader* (pp. 157–167). Boston: Houghton Mifflin.

Rogers, C. R. (1970). *Carl Rogers on encounter groups.* New York: Harper & Row.

Rogers, C. R. (1980). *A way of being.* Boston: Houghton Mifflin.

Rogers, C. R. (1986). Reflection of feelings. *Person-Centered Review,* 1(4), 375–377.

Romano, G. (1992). Description of D. Locke's "Counseling beyond U.S. borders." *American Counselor,* 1(2), 13–17.

Rose, P. I. (1964). *They and we: Racial and ethnic relations in the United States.* New York: Random House.

Rossi, P. H. (1990). The old homeless and the new homelessness in historical perspective. *American Psychologist,* 45(8), 954–959.

Rowe, W., Murphy, H. B., & De Csipkes, R. A. (1975). The relationship of counseling characteristics and counseling effectiveness. *Review of Educational Research,* 45, 231–246.

Russell-Miller, M. (2001). Social service trends and the implications for staffing needs within the social service subsystem: Provision of services to the elderly. In T. McClam & M. Woodside (Eds.), *Human service challenges in the 21st century* (pp. 253–262). Birmingham, AL: Ebsco Media.

Sadow, D., Ryder, M., Stein, J., & Geller, M. (1987). Supervision of mental health students in the context of an educational milieu. *Human Service Education,* 8(2), 29–36.

Safran, J. D., & Muran, J. C. (2000). *Negotiating the therapeutic alliance: A relational treatment guide.* New York: Guilford.

Samovar, L. A., & Porter, R. E. (Eds.). (2001), *Intercultural communication: A reader* (9th ed.) Belmont, CA: Wadsworth.

Sampson, J. P., Kolodinsky, R. W., & Greeno, B. P. (1997). Counseling on the information highway: Future possibilities and potential problems. *Journal of Counseling and Development,* 75, 203–212.

Sanders, J. R. (1994). *The program evaluation standards: How to assess evaluations of educational programs* (2nd ed.). Thousand Oaks, CA: Sage Publications.

Sandhu, D. S. (1997). Psychocultural profiles of Asian and Pacific Islander Americans: Implications for counseling and psychotherapy. *Journal of Multicultural Counseling & Development,* 25(1), 7–22.

Satir, V. (1967). *Conjoint family therapy.* Palo Alto, CA: Science and Behavior Books.

Satir, V. (1972a). *Peoplemaking.* Palo Alto, CA: Science and Behavior Books.

Satir, V. (1972b). Family systems and approaches to family therapy. In G. D. Erickson, and T. P. Hogan (Eds.), *Family therapy: An introduction to theory and technique* (2nd ed., pp. 211–225). Pacific Grove, CA: Brooks/Cole. (original work published 1967).

Savage, D. (1992, November 10). Court lets firms cut health care. *Los Angeles Times,* Section A, pp. 1, 18–19.

Savickas, M. L., & Walsh, W. B. (Eds.). (1996). *Handbook of career counseling theory and practice.* Palo Alto, CA: Cavies-Black.

Schatzberg, A. F., & Nemeroff, C. B. (1998). *Textbook of psychopharmacology* (2nd ed.). Washington, DC: American Psychiatric Press.

Scher, M. (1979). On counseling men. *Personnel and Guidance Journal,* 57, 252–254.

Scher, M. (1981). Men in hiding. *Personnel and Guidance Journal,* 60, 199–202.

Schlossberg, N. K. (1995). *Counseling adults in transition* (2nd ed.). New York: Springer.

Schmidt, J. J. (1999). Two decades of CACREP and what do we know? *Counselor Education and Supervision, 39*(1), 34–45.

Schram, B., & Mandel, B. R. (1996). *An introduction to human services: Policy and practice* (3rd ed.). Needham Heights, MA: Allyn & Bacon.

Schulz, C. (1993, June 12). *Peanuts cartoon.* New York: United Media.

Schweinhart, L. J., (2001). *Recent evidence on preschool programs* (Report No. ED-99-CO-0020). ERIC Clearinghouse on Elementary and Early Childhood Education, Champaign, IL. (ERIC Document Reproduction Service No. Ed 458–056)

Scissons, E. D. (1993). *Counseling for results.* Pacific Grove, CA: Brooks/Cole.

Sears, S. (1982). A definition of career guidance terms: A national vocational guidance association perspective. *Vocational Guidance Quarterly, 31*(2), 137–143.

Seem, S. R., & Johnson, E. (1998). Gender bias among counseling trainees: A study of case conceptualization. *Counselor Education and Supervision, 37,* 257–268.

Selye, H. (1956). *The stress of life.* New York: McGraw-Hill.

Selye, H. (1974). *Stress without distress.* New York: Lippincott.

Sexton, T. (1993). A review of the counseling outcome research. In G. R. Walz & J. C. Bleuer (Eds.), *Counselor efficacy: Assessing and using counseling outcomes research* (Report No. ISBN-1–56109–056–5). Ann Arbor, MI: ERIC Clearinghouse on Counseling and Personnel Services. (ERIC Document Reproduction Service No. Ed 362–821)

Sexton, T., & Whiston, S. C. (1991). A review of the empirical basis for counseling: Implications for practice and training. *Counselor Education and Supervision, 30,* 330–354.

Sexton, T., & Whiston, S. C. (1994). The status of the counseling relationship: An empirical review, theoretical implications, and research directions. *Counseling Psychologist, 22,* 6–78.

Shaffer, J. B. P., & Galinsky, M. D. (1974). *Models of group therapy and sensitivity training.* Englewood Cliffs, NJ: Prentice-Hall.

Shannon, J. W., & Woods, W. J. (1995). Affirmative psychotherapy for gay men. In D. R. Atkinson & G. Hackett (Eds.), *Counseling diverse populations* (pp. 307–324). Madison, WI: Brown & Benchmark

Sheehy, G. (1976). *Passages: Predictable crises of adult life.* New York: Bantam Books.

Shostrom, E. (1974). *Manual for the Personal Orientation Inventory: An inventory for the measurement of self-actualization.* San Diego, CA: Educational and Industrial Testing Service.

Simon, P. (1969). *The boxer.* New York: Paul Simon Music.

Simon, S. B., Howe, L. W., & Kirschenbaum, H. W. (1995). *Values clarification: A practical, action-directed workbook* (Rev. ed.). New York: Warner Books.

Singer, B. L., & Deschamps, D. (1994). *Gay and lesbian stats: A pocket guide to facts and figures.* New York: New Press.

Skillings, J. H., & Dobbins, J. E. (1991). Racism as a disease: Etiology and treatment implications. *Journal of Counseling and Development, 70*(1), 206–215.

Skinner, B. F. (1953). *Science and human behavior.* New York: Macmillan.

Skinner, B. F. (1960). Pigeons in a pelican. *American Psychologist, 15,* 28–37.

Skinner, B. F. (1971). *Beyond freedom and dignity.* New York: Knopf.

Skynner, A. C. (1976). *Systems of marital and family psychotherapy.* New York: Brunner/Mazel.

Skynner, A. C. R. (1981). An open-systems, group-analytic approach to family therapy. In A. S. Gurman & D. P. Kniskern (Eds.), *Handbook of family therapy* (pp. 39–84). New York: Brunner/Mazel.

Slater, J. R., & Spetalnick, D. (2001). Compassion fatigue: A personal perspective. In T. McClam & M. Woodside (Eds.), *Human service challenges in the 21st century* (pp. 215–224). Birmingham, AL: Ebsco Media.

Sodowsky, G. R., & Taffe, R. C. (1991). Counselor trainees' analysis of multicultural counseling videotapes. *Journal of Multicultural Counseling and Development, 19,* 115–129.

Sokal, M. M. (1992). Origins and early years of the American Psychological Association, 1890–1906. *American Psychologist, 47*(2), 111–122.

Solomon, A. (1992). Clinical diagnosis among diverse populations: A multicultural perspective. *Families in Society: The Journal of Contemporary Human Services, 73*(6), 371–377.

Sommer, B., & Sommer, R. (2002). *A practical guide to behavioral research: Tools and techniques* (5th ed.). New York: Oxford University Press.

Special Committee on Aging, U.S. Senate. (1997). *Developments in aging, 1997.* Washington, DC: Government Printing Office.

Speight, S. L., Myers, J., Cox, C. I., & Highlen, P. S. (1991). A redefinition of multicultural counseling. *Journal of Counseling and Development, 70*(1), 29–36.

Spiegler, M. D. (1998). *Contemporary behavior therapy* (3rd ed.). Pacific Grove, CA: Brooks/Cole.

Spokane, A. R. (1985). A review of research on person-environment congruence in Holland's theory of careers. *Journal of Vocational Behavior, 26,* 306–343.

Sprinthall, R. C., & Sprinthall, N. A. (1998). *Educational psychology: A developmental approach* (7th ed.). Boston: McGraw-Hill.

SREB (Southern Regional Educational Board) (1969). *Roles and functions for different levels of mental health workers.* Atlanta, GA: Author.

Steenbarger, B. N. (1992). Toward science-practice integration in brief counseling and therapy. *Counseling Psychologist, 20*(3), 403–450.

Steinem, G. (1992). *Revolution from within: A book on self-esteem.* Boston: Little, Brown.

Stokes, D., Rowe, D., Romero, D., Gonzales, M., Adams, M., & Lyons, S. (1987).

Establishing a university multicultural peer counseling program: A brief description. *Human Service Education, 8,* 26–29.

Strong, S. R. (1991). Theory-driven science and naive empiricism in counseling psychology. *Journal of Counseling Psychology, 38*(2), 204–210.

Sue, D. (1978). Counseling across cultures. *Personnel and Guidance Journal, 56,* 451.

Sue, D. W. (1992). The challenge of multiculturalism: The road less traveled. *American Counselor, 1*(1), 6–15.

Sue, D. W., Arredondo, P., & McDavis, R. J. (1992). Multicultural counseling competencies and standards: A call to the profession. *Journal of Multicultural Counseling and Development, 20,* 64–88.

Sue, D. W., Bernier, J. E., Durran, A., Feinberg, L., Pedersen, P., Smith, E. J., & Vasquez-Nuttall, E. (1982). Professional forum: Position paper: Cross-cultural counseling competencies. *Counseling Psychologist, 10*(2), 45–52.

Sue, D. W., & Sue, D. (1999). *Counseling the culturally different: Theory and practice* (3rd ed.). New York: John Wiley.

Sullivan, W., Wolk, J., & Hartmann, D. (1992). Case management in alcohol and drug treatment: Improving client outcome. *Families in Society: The Journal of Contemporary Human Services, 73,* 195–204.

Super, D. E. (1976). *Career education and the meaning of work.* Monographs on Career Education. Washington, DC: Office of Career Education, U.S. Office of Education.

Super, D. E. (1990). A life-span, life-space approach to career development. In D. Brown, L. Brooks, & Associates, *Career choice and development: Applying contemporary theories to practice.* San Francisco: Jossey-Bass.

Super, D. E., Savickas, M. L., & Super, C. M. (1996). The life-span, life-space approach to careers. In D. Brown, L. Brooks, & Associates (Eds.), *Career choice and development* (3rd ed.) (pp. 121–178). San Francisco, CA: Jossey-Bass.

Sweeney, T. J. (1991). Counselor credentialing: Purpose and origin. In

O. F. Bradley (ed.), *Credentialing in counseling* (pp. 81–85). Alexandria, VA: American Counseling Association.

Sweeney, T. J. (1992). CACREP: Precursors, promises, and prospects. *Journal of Counseling and Development, 70,* 667–672.

Sweitzer, H. F., & McKinney, W. L. (1991). A survey of human service graduates: Implications for curriculum planning. *Human Service Education,* 11(1), 3–16.

Swenson, L. C. (1997). *Psychology and law for the helping professions* (2nd ed.). Pacific Grove, CA: Brooks/Cole.

Szaz, T. (1961). *The myth of mental illness.* New York: Hoeber.

Szaz, T. (Speaker) (1990). A conversation with an officially dominated schizophrenic patient (Cassette Recording No. PC289-W9AD). Phoenix, AZ: Milton H. Erickson Foundation.

Tafoya, T. (1996, June). *New heights in human services: Multiculturalism.* Keynote address at National Organization of Human Services Annual Conference, St. Louis, MO.

Tarasoff et al. v. Regents of University of California, 529 P.2d 553 (Calif. 1974), vacated, reheard en banc, and affirmed 551 P.2d 334 (1976).

Taylor, M., Bradley, V., & Warren, R. (Eds.). (1996). *The community support skill standards: Tools for managing change and achieving outcomes: Skill standards for direct service workers in the human services.* Cambridge, MA: Human Services Research Institute.

Thomas, R. M. (1990). *Counseling and life-span development.* New York: Sage Publications.

Thompson, J. J. (1973). *Beyond words: Nonverbal communication in the classroom.* New York: Citation Press.

Thompson, R. (1996). *Counseling techniques: Improving relationships with others, ourselves, our families and our environment.* Washington, DC: Accelerated Development.

Thorndike, R. M., Cunningham, G. K., Thorndike, R. L., & Hagen, E. P. (1997).

Measurement and evaluation in psychology and education (6th ed.). Uppersaddle, NJ: Merrill.

Tiedeman, D. V., & O'Hara, R. P. (1963). *Career development: Choice and adjustment.* New York: College Entrance Examination Board.

Tiedeman, D. V., & Miller-Tiedeman, A. (1984). Career decision making: An individualistic perspective. In D. Brown & L. Brooks (Eds.), *Career choice and development: Applying contemporary theories to practice* (Chap. 10). San Francisco: Jossey-Bass.

Tillitski, C. J. (1990). A meta-analysis of estimated effect sizes for group versus individual versus control treatments. *International Journal of Group Psychotherapy,* 40(2), 215–224.

Toseland, R. W., & Siporin, M. (1986). When to recommend group treatment: A review of the clinical and research literature. *International Journal of Group Psychotherapy,* 36, 171–201.

Trotzer, J. P. (1989). *The counselor and the group* (2nd ed.). Muncie, IN: Accelerated Development.

Tuckman, B. W., & Jensen, M. A. C. (1977). Stages of small-group development revisited. *Group and Organizational Studies,* 2, 419–427.

UNAIDS. (2002). *AIDS epidemic update.* Retrieved December 5, 2002, from the World Wide Web: http://www.unaids .org/worldaidsday/2002/press/update/ epiupdate2002_en.doc

U.S. Census Bureau (2000a). *Resident population estimates of the United States by age and sex: April 1, 1990 to July 1, 1999, with short-term projection to November 1, 2000.* Retrieved June 1, 2001, from the World Wide Web: http://www.census .gov/population/estimates/nation/ intfile2–1.txt

U.S. Census Bureau (2000b). *Historical poverty tables.* Table 2. Poverty status of people by family relationship, race, and Hispanic origin: 1959 to 1999. Retrieved June 1, 2001, from the World Wide Web: www.census.gov/hhes/ poverty/histpov/hstpov2.html

U.S. Census Bureau (2000c). *Projections of the total resident population by 5-year age groups, and sex with special age categories: middle series, 2025 to 2045.* Retrieved June 1, 2001, from the World Wide Web: www.census.gov/population/projections/nation/summary/np-t3-f.txt

U.S. Census Bureau (2000d). *Historical poverty tables.* Table 2. Poverty status of people by family relationship, race, and Hispanic origin: 1959 to 1999. Retrieved June 1, 2001, from the World Wide Web: www.census.gov/hhes/poverty/histpov/hstpov2.html

U.S. Census Bureau (2000e). *Historical poverty tables.* Table 14. Distribution of the poor by race and Hispanic origin:1966 to 1999 Retrieved June 1, 2001, from the World Wide Web: www.census.gov/hhes/poverty/histpov/hstpov14.html

U.S. Census Bureau (2001a). Table 1. Prevalence of disability by age, sex, race, and Hispanic origin: 1997. Retrieved June 1, 2001, from the World Wide Web: www.census.gov/hhes/www/disable/sipp/disab97/ds97t1.html

U.S. Census Bureau (2001b). *Resident population estimates of the United States by sex, race, and Hispanic origin: April 1, 1990 to July 1, 1999, with short-term projection to November 1, 2000.* Retrieved June 1, 2001, from the World Wide Web: http://www.census.gov/population/estimates/nation/intfile3–1.txt

U.S. Census Bureau (2001c). *Projections of the resident population by race, Hispanic origin, and nativity: middle series, 2050 to 2070.* Retrieved June 1, 2001, from the World Wide Web: www.census.gov/population/projections/nation/summary/np-t5–g.txt

U.S. Census Bureau (2001d). *Immigrants, fiscal year 1998.* Retrieved June 1, 2001, from the World Wide Web: http://www.ins.usdoj.gov/graphics/aboutins/statistics/imm98.pdf

U.S. Census Bureau (2001e). *Prevalence of disability by age, sex, race, and Hispanic origin:* 1997. Table 1. Retrieved June 1, 2001, from the World Wide Web: www.census.gov/hhes/www/disable/sipp/disab97/ds97t1.html

U. S. Census Bureau. (2002). *USA statistics in brief: Population and vital statistics. Retrieved* December 8, 2002, from the World Wide Web: http://www.census.gov/statab/www/poppart.html

U.S. Administration on Aging (1999).

U.S. Department of Commerce (1991). *Statistical abstracts of the United States* (111th ed.). Washington, DC: Bureau of Census. Government Printing Office.

U.S. Department of Health and Human Services. (2000). *Health and human services fact sheet: Substance abuse.* Retrieved June 1, 2001, from the World Wide Web: http://www.hhs.gov/news/press/2000pres/00fsmtf.html

U.S. Department of Health and Human Services (2001). *Health and human services fact sheet: Substance abuse.* Retrieved June 1, 2001, from the World Wide Web: drinkers,http://www.hhs.gov/news/press/2000pres/00fsmtf.html

U.S. Department of Justice (1992). *Americans with Disabilities Act requirements fact sheet.* Washington, DC: Civil Rights Division, Coordination and Review Section.

U.S. Department of Justice (2001). Correction statistics. Retrieved June 1, 2001, from the World Wide Web: http://www.ojp.usdoj.gov/bjs/pub/pdf/cj-3.pdf

U.S. Department of Labor (1992).

U.S. Department of Labor (1998–1999). *Occupational outlook handbook.* Retrieved November 21, 2002, from the World Wide Web: http://www.umsl.edu/services/govdocs/ooh9899/38.htm#training.

U.S. Department of Labor (1999). *Dictionary of occupational titles* (4th ed.). Indianapolis, IN: JIST Publishing.

U.S. Department of Labor (2002). *O*NET at a glance.* Retrieved June 1, 2002 from the World Wide Web: www.doleta.gov/programs/onet/glance.asp.

U.S. Department of Labor, Bureau of Labor Statistics (1998–99). *Occupational outlook handbook.* Washington, DC: Government Printing Office.

Usher, C. H. (1989). Recognizing cultural bias in counseling theory and practice: The case of Rogers. *Journal of Counseling and Development,* 17(2), 62–71.

Vander Kolk, C. J. (1990). *Introduction to group counseling and psychotherapy.* Prospect Heights, IL: Waveland Press.

Voydanoff, P. (2001) Conceptualizing community in the context of work and family. *Community, Work & Family,* 4(2), 133–156.

VanZandt, C. E. (1990). Professionalism: A matter of personal initiative. *Journal of Counseling and Development,* 68(3), 243–245.

Vroman, C. S., & Bloom, J. W. (1991). A summary of counselor credentialing legislation. In F. Bradley (Ed.), *Credentialing in counseling* (pp. 86–102). Alexandria, VA: Association for Counselor Education and Supervision.

Wallen, J. (1993). *Addiction in human development: Developmental perspectives on addiction and recovery.* New York: Haworth Press.

Wallerstein, J. S., & Blakeslee, S. (1989). *Second chances: Men, women, and children a decade after divorce.* New York: Ticknor & Fields.

Wallerstein, J. S., & Blakeslee, S. (1996). *Second chances: Men, women, and children a decade after divorce.* Boston: Houghton Miflin.

Walsh, W. B., & Betz, N. E. (1995). *Tests and assessment* (3rd ed.). Englewood Cliffs, NJ: Prentice-Hall.

Ward, D. E. (1982). A model for the more effective use of theory in group work. *Journal for Specialists in Group Work,* 7, 224–230.

Warnath, C. F. (1975). Vocational theories: Direction to nowhere. *Personnel and Guidance Journal,* 53, 422–428.

Webster. (2002). *Miriam-Webster Collegiate Dictionary.* Retrieved May 1, 2002, from the World Wide Web: www.m-w.com.

Wertheimer, M. (1978). *A brief history of psychology.* New York: Holt, Rinehart & Winston.

Westwood, M. J., & Ishiyama, F. I. (1990). The communication process as a critical intervention for client change in cross-cultural counseling. *Journal of Multicultural Counseling and Development,* 18, 163–171.

Wheeler, S. (1991). Personal therapy: An essential aspect of counsellor training, or a distraction from focusing on the client? *Journal for the Advancement of Counselling,* 14, 193–202.

Whitaker, C. (1976). The hindrance of theory in clinical work. In P. J. Guerin (Ed.), *Family therapy* (pp. 154–164). New York: Gardner Press.

Whitfield, W., McGrath, P., & Coleman, V. (1992, October). *Increasing multicul-tural sensitivity and awareness.* Symposium presented at the annual conference of the National Organization for Human Service Education, Alexandria, VA.

Whitson, S. C., & Coker, J. K. (2000). Reconstructing clinical training: Implications from research. *Counselor Education and Supervision,* 39, 228–253.

Widick, C. (1975). The Perry scheme: A foundation for developmental practice. *Counseling Psychologist,* 6(4), 35–38.

Williams, R. C., & Myer, R. A. (1992). The men's movement: An adjunct to traditional counseling approaches. *Journal of Mental Health Counseling,* 14, 393–404.

Wilson, F. R. (1995). Internet information sources for counselors. *Counselor Education and Supervision,* 34(4), 369–387.

Wilson, L. L., & Stith, L. L. (1991). Culturally sensitive therapy with black clients. *Journal of Multicultural Counseling and Development,* 19, 32–43. (Original work published 1991)

Wise, R., Charner, I., & Randour, M. A. (1978). A conceptual framework for career awareness in career decision-making. In J. Whiteley & A. Resnikoff (Eds.), *Career counseling* (pp. 216–231). Pacific Grove, CA: Brooks/Cole.

Woititz, J. G. (1991). *Adult children of alcoholics* (Expanded edition). Boston: G. K. Hall & Co.

Wolpe, J. (1969). *The practice of behavior therapy.* New York: Pergamon Press.

Woodside, M., & McClam, T. (1998a). *An introduction to human services* (3rd ed.). Pacific Grove, CA: Brooks/Cole.

Woodside, M., & McClam, T. (1998b). *Generalist case management: A method of human service delivery.* Pacific Grove, CA: Brooks/Cole.

World Health Organization (2001). *AIDS epidemic update: December 2000.* Retrieved June 1, 2001, from the World Wide Web: http://www.unaids.org/wac/2000/wad00/files/WAD_epidemic_report.htm

Wylie, M. S. (1995, September/October). The new visionaries. *Family Therapy Networker,* 20–29, 32–35.

X, Malcom, & Haley, A. (1992). *The autobiography of Malcolm X.* New York: Ballantine.

Yalom, I. D. (1995). *The theory and practice of group psychotherapy* (4th ed.). New York: Basic Books.

Yeaton, W. H. (1994). The development and assessment of valid measures of service delivery to enhance inference in outcome-based research: Measuring attendance at self-help group meetings. *Journal of Consulting and Clinical Psychology, 62,* 686–694.

Yutrzenka, B. A. (1995). Making a case for training in ethnic and cultural diversity in increasing treatment efficacy. *Journal of Consulting and Clinical Psychology,* 63(2), 197–206.

Zunker, V. G. (2002). *Career counseling: Applied concepts for life planning.* Pacific Grove, CA: Brooks Cole.

Zwelling, S. S. (1990). *Quest for a cure: The public hospital in Williamsburg, Virginia, 1773–1885.* Williamsburg, VA: Colonial Williamsburg Foundation.

Credits

Chapter 9

261: Source: Edwin L. Herr and Stanley L. Cramer, *Career Guidance and Counseling Through the Life Span: Systematic Approaches*, 5/e. Published by Allyn and Bacon, Boston, MA. Copyright © 1996 by Pearson Education. Reprinted by permission of the publisher.

Chapter 10

297: Source: Reprinted from *The Wheel of Wellness* (p. 10), by J. M. Witmer, T. J. Sweeney, and J. E. Myers, 1998, Greensboro, NC: Authors. Copyright 1998 by Witmer et al. Reprinted with permission of American Counseling Association and the authors. No further reproduction authorized without written permission of the American Counseling Association. 317: Source: Reprinted by permission of Lynn McKinney, President of National Organization for Human Service Education. 325, 327: Source: Council for Standards in Human Service Education (CSHSE). 331: Source: Reprinted with permission from the *Diagnostic and Statistical Manual of Mental Disorders*, Fourth Edition, Text Revision. Copyright 2000 American Psychiatric Association.

PHOTO CREDITS

Chapter 1

16: Carl Rogers Memorial Library. 19: UPI-Bettmann/CORBIS.

Chapter 2

33: National Library of Medicine. 39: Bettmann/CORBIS. 44: Dr. Harold McPheeters.

Chapter 3

68: Bettmann/CORBIS. 71: B. F. Skinner Foundation.

Chapter 4

103: Bettye Lane.

Chapter 5

131: Kristina Williams-Neukrug. 135: Harvard Graduate School of Education. 143: Ed Neukrug.

Chapter 6

162: Avanta Network, 310 Third Avenue NE, Issaquah, WA 98027. 171: Joel Becker.

Chapter 7

196: Cheryl Evans. 199: Joel Becker. 216: © Mike Spinelli/Courtesy of NEA Today.

Chapter 8

233: Bettmann/CORBIS.

Chapter 9

264: Ed Kamper Photography/Charles M. Super. 271: Diana Mara Henry.

Chapter 10

284: bottom, AP/Wide World Photos; top, Ed Kashi/CORBIS. 286: © Michael Siluk. 288: Jewish Community Center of Tidewater, Norfolk, VA. 291: Courtesy Lisa Lyons.

Index